Diagnostic and
Operative Hysteroscopy

System requirement:
- **Windows XP or above**
- **Power DVD player (Software)**
- **Windows media player 11.0 version or above (Software)**

Accompanying DVD ROM is playable only in Computer and not in DVD player.

Kindly wait for few seconds for DVD to autorun. If it does not autorun then please do the following:
- Click on my computer
- Click the **CD/DVD drive** and after opening the drive, kindly double click the file **Jaypee**

DVD CONTENTS

Diagnostic and Operative Hysteroscopy

SECOND EDITION

Editors

Tirso Pérez-Medina PhD
Professor
Senior Gynecologist
Universidad Autonoma De Madrid
Puerta de Hierro University Hospital
Madrid, Spain

Enrique Cayuela Font PhD
Chairman
Department of Obstetrics and Gynecology
L´ Hospitalet de Llobregat
General Hospital
Barcelona, Spain

Forewords

Jose Manuel Bajo-Arenas
Victor Gomel

JAYPEE BROTHERS MEDICAL PUBLISHERS (P) LTD
New Delhi • Panama City • London

Jaypee Brothers Medical Publishers (P) Ltd

Headquarter

Jaypee Brothers Medical Publishers (P) Ltd
4838/24, Ansari Road, Daryaganj
New Delhi 110 002, India
Phone: +91-11-43574357
Fax: +91-11-43574314
Email: jaypee@jaypeebrothers.com

Overseas Offices

JP Medical Ltd
83 Victoria Street, London
SW1H 0HW (UK)
Phone: +44-2031708910
Fax: +02-03-0086180
Email: info@jpmedpub.com

Jaypee-Highlights Medical Publishers Inc.
City of Knowledge, Bld. 237, Clayton
Panama City, Panama
Phone: 507-317-0160
Fax: +50-73-010499
Email: cservice@jphmedical.com

Website: www.jaypeebrothers.com
Website: www.jaypeedigital.com

Publisher: Jitendar P Vij
Publishing Director: Tarun Duneja
Cover Design: Seema Dogra, Sumit Kumar

Diagnostic and Operative Hysteroscopy

First Edition: 2007

Second Edition: **2012**

ISBN 978-93-80704-69-2

Printed at Replika Press Pvt. Ltd.

Dedicated to

Nuria, Tirso, Natalia and Nurita
Only with their patience can this book see the light

CONTRIBUTORS

Maria Alejo Sánchez
Department of Pathology
Vic General Hospital
Barcelona, Spain

Carmen Alvarez
Attending Gynecologist
12 De Octubre University Hospital
Madrid, Spain

Nuria De Argila Fernandez-Durán
Qualified in Infirmary
Master in Infirmary Sciences

Pilar Arranz-Garcia
Qualified in Infirmary
Professor of Medical-Surgical Infirmary (Predegree)
and Sanitary Technology (Postdegree)
Madrid, Spain

Josefina Autonell Reixach
Department of Pathology
Vic General Hospital
Barcelona, Spain

Enrique Cayuela Font
Chairman
Department of Obstetrics and Gynecology
L'Hospitalet General Hospital
Barcelona, Spain

Ramón Cos Plans
Senior Gynecologist
Parc Tauli Hospital, Sabadell
Barcelona, Spain

Joan Carles Ferreres Piñas
Department of Pathology
Hospital Universitari Vall D'hebron
Barcelona, Spain

Concepción Garcia-Zarza
Qualified in Infirmary
Outpatient Surgery Unit
Santa Cristina University Hospital
Madrid, Spain

Josep Grau Galtes
Staff Physician
Senior Gynecologist
Obstetrics and Gynecology Department
Vic General Hospital
Barcelona, Spain

Cristina Gonzalez Macho
Attending Gynecologist
12 De Octubre University Hospital
Madrid, Spain

Carmen Guillen Gamez
Attending Gynecologist
12 De Octubre University Hospital
Madrid, Spain

Miguel Angel Huertas
Head
Department of Obstetrics and Gynecology
Getafe University Hospital
Madrid, Spain

Federico Heredia Prim
Senior Gynecologist
Parc Tauli Hospital
Sabadell, Barcelona, Spain

Enrique Iglesias Goy
Professor
Senior Gynecologist
Universidad Autonoma De Madrid
Puerta de Hierro University Hospital
Madrid, Spain

Jesus S Jimenez
Associate Professor
Senior Gynecologist
Universidad Complutense De Madrid
12 De Octubre University Hospital
Madrid, Spain

Gregorio Lopez Gonzalez
Attending Gynecologist
12 De Octubre University Hospital
Madrid, Spain

Sonia Moros
Senior Gynecologist
Vic General Hospital, Barcelona, Spain

Tirso Pérez-Medina
Professor
Senior Gynecologist
Universidad Autonoma De Madrid
Puerta de Hierro University Hospital
Madrid, Spain

Juncal Pineros Manzano
Senior Gynecologist
Department of Obstetrics and Gynecology
L'Hospitalet General Hospital
Barcelona, Spain

Alberto Puig Menem
Associate Professor, Senior Gynecologist Department
of Obstetrics and Gynecology
L'Hospitalet General Hospital
Barcelona, Spain

Jennifer Rayward
Specialist in Reproduction, Procrea T
Madrid, Spain

Purificación Regueiró Espin
Senior Gynecologist
Department of Obstetrics and Gynecology
L'Hospitalet General Hospital
Hospitalet, Barcelona, Spain

Mar Rios Vallejo
Attending Gynecologist
Puerta de Hierro University Hospital
Madrid, Spain

Francisco Salazar Arquero
Attending Gynecologist
Infanta Leonor Hospital
Madrid, Spain

Teresa Tijero
Staff Anesthesiologist
Santa Cristina University Hospital
Madrid, Spain

Rafael F Valle
Professor Emeritus
Department of Obstetrics and Gynecology
Northwestern University Medical School
Chicago, Illinois, USA

Marta De Vicente
Staff Anesthesiologist
Santa Cristina University Hospital
Madrid, Spain

FOREWORD

It is often said that the few people who have the privilege of experiencing memorable professors while training are not later blessed with good pupils during their practice. Fortunately, destiny has been generous with me and has given me both. It is an honor for me to write this introductory note for two magnificent coworkers and pioneers in the field of hysteroscopy, who, in this book, share their knowledge and extensive experience in this fast-growing and extensive field.

Without forgetting any of the solid, theoretical principles, the book is full of practical advice and much wisdom acquired from the many hours these authors have spent operating.

The iconography in the book is outstanding and the images seize the know-how of the technique of the authors. Due to their great experience, they have personally contributed to the improvement of hysteroscopy equipment by sharing their ideas with the industry. Through some of their ideas, improvement of the optics involved in image capturing was achieved.

Thanks to their belief in this method, their enthusiasm and their teachings, they have helped spread the technique. At present, hysteroscopy is performed by many specialists that had in them their educational teachers.

While writing the foreword of *Diagnostic and Operative Hysteroscopy*, I cannot help but remember the days when I was head of Obstetrics and Gynecology at the old Red Cross Hospital, Madrid, Spain. I will coin a phase from King Phillip II, a XVII century Spanish King, to describe hysteroscopy in those days, when he spoke of the "Invincible Armada" he said it was a heroic act "fighting against the elements". This was certainly true of hysteroscopy at its beginnings in our hospital system. The optics and the instruments were very basic and what was worse, there was constant opposition from the "old school" who thought that hysteroscopy was little more than a passing craze. Thanks to perseverance, and lots of hard work hysteroscopy has consolidated into an indispensable technique in gynecology and at present, the hospitals of both authors are reference centers for the practice and teaching of the technique in Spain.

I believe that the book will help give the readers, students, physicians and specialists a comprehensive overview of the present focus of diagnostic and surgical hysteroscopy and it is my hope that the readers will enjoy this book as much as I have.

Jose Manuel Bajo-Arenas
President of the Spanish Society of Gynaecology and Obstetrics
Chief of the Department of Obstetrics and Gynaecology
Autónoma University of Madrid
Santa Cristina University Hospital
Madrid, Spain

FOREWORD

The wish to look into the human body is as old as human history. The Talmud describes an instrument that was used to view the cervix. More than 2000 years old specula, with elegant decorative engravings, were recovered from the ashes of Pompeii.

In 1805, Bozzini described a technique of examining the interior of the urethra. He reflected the light from a candle with a mirror directing the rays along a metal tube. His ingenuity was rewarded by the medical faculty of Vienna by censoring him for "undue curiosity". Desormeaux, almost 60 years later, fared rather better. He designed a functioning cystoscope; the *Academie Imperiale de Medicine de Paris* rewarded him with a share of the *Argenteuil* prize. In 1869, in Ireland, Pantaleoni used this scope to view the uterine cavity of a 60-year-old woman complaining of vaginal bleeding and was able to identify polyps within her uterus. Nitze improved the instrument; in 1879, he replaced the cumbersome external, alcohol and resin fuelled lamp with an incandescent platinum filament sited on the distal tip of the cystoscope.

Strides in medicine frequently follow technical improvements and innovations. These two disciplines are synergistic and stimulate each other. Endoscopy in general, greatly benefited from early technical innovations that included the development of the incandescent light bulb by Edison (1880); introduction of the "cold light" concept, a method of transmitting intense light by means of a quartz rod, by Fourestier, Gladu and Vulmière in France in 1952; and the same year, the application of fiberoptics to endoscopy by Hopkins and Kapani in England.

Although hysteroscopy preceded gynecologic laparoscopy, its utilization and acceptance lagged behind that of laparoscopy until the introduction of effective uterine distention media, which permitted proper visualization of the cavity.

In 1970, Lindemann introduced a system using pressurized carbon dioxide to distend the uterus, while the same year Edström and Fernström used high molecular dextran for the same purpose. Despite these improvements, application of the technique, which at the time was purely diagnostic, remained limited. This was due to significant improvements in non-invasive imaging techniques such as ultrasonography, and the use of a vaginal transducer for the assessment of the pelvic organs. At the time, hysteroscopy was described as "a technique looking for an indication".

Yet the impact of hysteroscopy in our specialty has been radical. This came about when hysteroscopy started to be used as a new mode of surgical access into the uterus. This revolutionized and greatly simplified many procedures that previously required a laparotomy and a hysterotomy to access the uterine cavity: Lysis of severe uterine synechiae, metroplasty for septate uterus, excision of symptomatic intrauterine fibroids. These, after all, are common conditions; hysteroscopy has simplified these procedures and significantly reduced their morbidity. Direct access to the uterus led to the introduction of interventions such as endometrial excision and endometrial ablation that offer a less invasive, yet effective alternative to hysterectomy in the treatment of abnormal (dysfunctional) uterine bleeding refractory to medical treatment. It permitted the introduction of a simple technique of permanent tubal sterilization.

All of this was made possible by further technical improvements and innovations. Improvement in lens systems resulted in the production of endoscopes of significantly smaller caliber and better optics. This evolution permitted hysteroscopy to be performed without anesthesia, which eventually led to the introduction of "office hysteroscopy".

The introduction of the lightweight mini video cameras and high resolution television monitors permitted the surgeon and others assisting at the procedure to view the operative field in one or more television monitors and work in concert as a team. These developments, together with the production of new and better equipment and instruments, allowed these intrauterine procedures to be performed more easily, more quickly and with greater safety.

The advent of operative hysteroscopy has changed medical practice in the treatment of certain conditions. Bleeding from submucous fibroids and dysfunctional uterine bleeding refractory to medical treatment frequently led to a hysterectomy in the past. Today many of these cases may be successfully treated by hysteroscopic excision of the fibroids and endometrial ablation respectively, techniques that are much less invasive yet fairly effective. In medicine, as in life, nothing remains static. Hysteroscopic endometrial ablation is already being replaced by several new simpler endometrial ablation techniques such as "global ablation" or (better) nonhysteroscopic ablation, these techniques appear to yield outcomes similar to those resulting from hysteroscopic endometrial resection or roller ball ablation. Quoting Arthur Schopenhauer "change alone is eternal, perpetual, immortal".

The book is comprehensive, to the extent of including chapters on the *Anatomy, Histology, Physiology and Pathology of the Endocervix and Uterine Cavity* (Chapter 1), on *Maintenance of Hysteroscopy Equipment* (Chapter 2), on *Imaging of the Uterus* (Chapter 4) and on *Transcervical Embryoscopy* (Chapter 16). The book is well written. It has a distinguished Spanish authorship, and includes a chapter by a well-known non-Spanish author: Rafael F Valle, a pioneer in operative hysteroscopy. The book is practical and well-illustrated. I am certain that it will prove to be a valuable text for residents in gynecology and practicing gynecologists.

Victor Gomel
Professor
Department of Obstetrics and Gynecology
Faculty of Medicine, University of British Columbia
Vancouver BC, Canada

PREFACE TO THE SECOND EDITION

The aim of this book is to critically review different aspects of hysteroscopy with recognized experts from the United States and Europe. The main objective is to provide a balanced view of current clinical opinion and to review the rapidly expanding world of hysteroscopy.

Since the pioneer clinical work performed in the late seventies and up until a few years ago when hysteroscopy found its own in the field of gynecology, the use of this technique has broadly expanded. We have been performing diagnostic hysteroscopy since the late eighties and surgical hysteroscopy since the early nineties. Today it has become the standard of reference for both diagnostic and therapeutic purposes for most pathology located in the uterine cavity. New fields of application of this technique are constantly being created.

This book begins with an extensive review of the anatomy, histology, physiology, and pathology of the endocervix and uterine cavity. Then the role of the OR nurse and personnel is outlined, setting out disinfection and sterilization guidelines of the different elements of the hysteroscopy.

Evaluation of the uterine cavity is necessary when abnormal uterine hemorrhage occurs or when the fertility is being studied. Since the endometrium evolves constantly and cyclically under the influence of the sex hormones, its structure and thickness also change. When dishomogenic growth appears, it is mandatory to thoroughly assess those problems especially those that predispose the patient to malignant transformation of the lesion.

As with what happened with gynecological laparoscopy a few years ago, hysteroscopy is no longer conceived of uniquely as a diagnostic procedure. The access to microsurgical instruments that can be inserted by accessory sheaths and the development of liquid continuous flow has transformed ambulatory hysteroscopy into a diagnostic and an operating procedure. A small number of selected intrauterine operations and in most cases without the need of anesthesia can be performed at the same time as diagnosis, following the "see and treat" principle. Thus, hysteroscopy may now be included in the concept of ambulatory surgery.

Hysteroscopy offers direct vision of the uterine cavity and the possibility to perform directed biopsies of suspicious areas. There are special hysteroscopes that evaluate lesions to different degrees and some even reach the nucleus-cytoplasm level. Other benign alterations like endometrial polyps or submucous fibromyomas can also produce pathological conditions that require treatment. Chapter 4 is devoted to different image methods that can be used as screening tests (TVUS, HSSG) or as an aid to define diagnosis (HSG, MRI).

The use of hysteroscopy in reproductive problems is studied in Chapter 5. Different indications for these problems are described, both diagnostic and operative, in infertility and repeated pregnancy loss patients.

Other chapters include specific pathologies in this field as uterine septa or intrauterine adhesions. There are several genital tract malformations in which hysteroscopy is an effective method of diagnosis and treatment when infertility is evaluated. In the field of reproduction, synechiolysis or septolysis are well-known applications. Salpingoscopy, tubal cannulation, or hysteroscopic sterilization are examples of how this technique is continuously growing. The transcervical embryoscopy is also studied.

Chapters 6 and 7 offer an extensive revision for the hysteroscopic diagnosis and management of endometrial hyperplasia and endometrial adenocarcinoma, given the different presentations that these pathologies can show. Bear in mind that hysteroscopy was initially developed to diagnose the endometrial cancer to avoid blind techniques that have been overcome nowadays.

When surgery is recommended, understanding the principles of electricity is essential. The specific anesthesia required for each technique is also outlined in another specific chapter.

For endometrial resection or ablation, this book is limited to hysteroscopic techniques and not to other techniques. There has been worldwide interest in a simple surgical alternative to abdominal, laparoscopic, or vaginal hysterectomy. High technology is involved in endometrial ablation by hysteroscopy and because the use of video cameras is needed, surgeons must master these surgical skills. Ablation should be considered in women whose only alternative would be hysterectomy due to heavy bleeding which causes anemia and limits social activity. If patients are carefully selected, an annual recurrence rate of only 5 or 8% in the first four years is reported. This is an acceptable rate especially when ablation is performed in perimenopausal women. It is important to note that endometrial ablation is a proven, safe technique that allows the resolution of the problem in 3 out of 4 patients. It is important to acquire the know-how and to offer this solution to patients.

Long-term complication rates are not available as yet. The experience of individual surgeons is relatively small, but it is hoped that national surveys will soon be published to provide a database from which the potential complications can be calculated. Although it is a safe technique, hysteroscopy is not problem-free, so it will be important for its future to be able to assess with precision the possible incidents that may occur and be prepared to resolve them.

National and international laparoscopic and hysteroscopic societies have been founded by enthusiastic practitioners. These physicians organize meetings and training courses. The future of hysteroscopy is brilliant and many new frontiers will be able to be explored with creative, skilled and well-trained physicians— this is a task in which all of us must participate.

Tirso Pérez-Medina
Enrique Cayuela Font

CONTENTS

1

Anatomy of the Uterus

María Alejo Sánchez
Joan Carles Ferreres Piñas
Josefina Autonell Reixach

GROSS ANATOMY

The mature, non gravid uterus is pear-shaped, weighing 40-80 g and about 8-9 cm in length, 4-5 cm in width and 2-3 cm in thickness. These measurements vary considerably as a function of age, phase of the menstrual cycle and parity. The uterus is a hollow, muscular organ and divided into three parts: the cervix, corpus, and fundus. Part of the corpus which connects the origin of the two fallopian tubes is called the fundus. The cornua are the two lateral regions of the fundus associated with the intramural portion of the fallopian tubes. The uterine cavity is triangular, the length is approximately 6.0 cm and the lumen communicates with the lumina of the fallopian tubes at the two cornua and with the endocervical canal at the internal os. The mucosa of the corpus (endometrium) is smooth, orange-tanned and varies in thickness, depending on the phase of the menstrual cycle and ranges between 1-8 mm, frequently is thickest in the fundus. The narrowed region between the cervix and body is called the isthmus or lower uterine segment and corresponds to the level of the internal os of the cervix or the opening between the cervical canal and the uterine cavity, and the transition is gradual without anatomic demarcation. The isthmus measures about 1 cm in length and is very narrow in the nulliparous woman. The mucosa is smooth compared to highly folded endocervix. The cervix is cylindrical in shape and measures 3-4 cm in height and 2 cm in diameter. The terminus of the cervix is round and has a circular or transverse opening, the external os. There are two lips, the anterior, which is shorter and thicker, and the posterior, which is longer and thinner. The mucosa is whitish pink and deeply clefted to form the plicae palmatae. Retention cysts are frequently visible within the canal.

The walls of the uterus (myometrium) are heavily muscled and measure about 2 cm thick. The myometrium consists of an outer longitudinal muscle layer, an inner circular submucosal muscle layer, and an interposed thick middle layer, richly populated by vessels.

The uterine arteries, which arise from the internal iliac arteries, are the main blood supply to the uterus.

The veins drain the uterovaginal venous plexus at the base of the broad ligament. The uterine veins ultimately open into the internal iliac veins. Uterine lymphatics drain from a subserosal uterine plexus into the pelvic and periaortic lymph nodes; a few lymphatics from the fundus accompany the round ligament of the uterus and drain into the superficial inguinal nodes.

The myometrium has a rich autonomic innervation that appears to be predominantly, if not exclusively, sympathetic.

Histology

The mucosa of the uterus (endometrium) is made up of glands and stroma. The surface is covered by a single layer of low columnar cells. It is divided into a deeply basal layer and a superficial functional layer. The basal layer is composed of tubular glands, occasionally branching, lined by simple to pseudostratified epithelium in dark, compact stroma. The epithelium shows no evidence of secretory or mitotic activity in either glands or stroma, but constitutes the "reserve cell layer" of the endo-metrium. The junction of the basalis and myo-metrium is irregular, may give the false impression that endometrial tissue is pathologically isolated within the myometrium. The functional layer is composed of the superficial compact layer and the deeper spongy layer. This distinction is only noticeable in the late secretory phase.

The myometrium is composed of smooth muscle cells. These cells are spindled, with blunt-ended fusiform nuclei. Scattered normal mitotic figures may be encountered, mainly during the secretory phase of the endometrial cycle.

ENDOMYOMETRIAL SPECIMENS

The endometrium is a composite tissue that requires architectural integrity. If any of these components are lacking or if the relation among them is disrupted, the validity of a histological diagnosis is compromised. Problems therefore arise in the interpretation of endometrial tissue, if the specimen is very scanty, broken or traumatized during its collection. Another very important question is the information given to the pathologist. The indications for endometrial biopsy are abnormal uterine bleeding, endometrial evaluation in infertile patients, and assessment of endometrial response to hormonal treatment. The knowledge of an adequate clinical history is mandatory for the pathologist (age, menstrual/ menopausal status, pattern and amount of bleeding, hormonal treatment or contraceptive use) as well as the indication for endometrial study.

Very important is the knowledge of the hysteroscopic appearance of the lesions and the presumptive diagnosis. The specimen should be fixed after removal to avoid autolytic artefacts that may hamper an accurate histopathologic diagnosis.

As less tissue is obtained, greater is the difficulty of interpretation of samples and less is the degree of reassurance that there is no pathology present in the uterine cavity. In hysteroscopic specimens, it is frequent to see usual artefacts like dissociation and telescoping artefacts. The first of them consists of disruption of the stroma and alteration of the relation among glands that lie closer together than normal. This false crowding may give a back-to-back appearance and lead to diagnosis of atypical hyperplasia or carcinoma. Telescoping artefact consists of gland-within-gland images, because of intussusception. Both artefacts are the trauma effect on the endometrium, at the time of sampling.

A particular problem in the interpretation of hysteroscopic specimens is when the lesion is not present in the sample. It is frequent when the lesion is not placed in the endometrium, but in the subjacent stroma or in the myometrium. Also in postmenopausal state, it is frequent to obtain only small pieces of surface and glandular epithelium with a little quantity of stroma. Usually, the glandular component is markedly artefacted.

The endometrium responds to endogenous hormonal levels in women in the reproductive age. These, estrogens and progesterone, induce cycle changes (proliferative, secretory and menstrual phases). Any situation that disturbs the hormonal status leads morphological changes in the endometrium, moving it away from normal appearance.

Dysfunctional endometrium is a range of morphological changes as a result of inadequate hormonal levels or inadequate endometrial response to hormones. Exogenous hormonal agents (oral contraceptives, hormone replacement therapy and hormonal agents used in the prevention of breast cancer as tamoxifen or raloxifene) induce a broad spectrum of morphological changes in endometrium. For the accurate interpretation of endometrial biopsy, it is necessary to know the kind of treatment that the patient receives.

By hysteroscopic examination, the majority of lesions that affect the endometrial cavity or the submucosal myometrium can be detected (TABLE 1.1). Nevertheless, some endometrial pathology may go unnoticed if the examination is done without biopsy sampling (TABLE 1.2).

Table 1.1: Physiological and pathological findings in endometrial cavity detected by hysteroscopical examination

Physiological endometrium
- Cycling endometrium
- Exaggerated secretory pattern and late proliferative phase (polypoid appearance)
- Cystic atrophy

Pathological intracavitary findings
- Epithelial endometrial lesions
  - Endometrial metaplasias (squamous, osseous...)
  - Endometrial polyps
  - Atypical polypoid adenomyoma
  - Endometrial hyperplasia
  - Endometrial carcinoma and its variants
- Endometrial stromal tumors
  - Endometrial stromal nodule
  - Endometrial stromal sarcoma
- Mixed endometrial stromal tumors and mixed müllerian tumors
  - Adenofibroma
  - Adenosarcoma
  - Carcinofibroma
  - Carcinosarcoma
- Lesions arising from the myometrium
  - Submucous leiomyoma
  - Leiomyosarcoma
- Undifferentiated uterine sarcoma
- Endometrial metastasis from extrauterine tumors
- Gestation related lesions
  - Placental site nodule and plaque
  - Placental site trophoblastic tumor
  - Epithelioid trophoblastic tumor
  - Choriocarcinoma

Table 1.2: Pathological situations usually not detected by hysteroscopical examination without biopsy

- Endometrial epithelial metaplasias (except squamous metaplasia)
- Some stromal metaplasias
- Disordered proliferation and focal hyperplasia
- Intraepithelial endometrial carcinoma
- Infections and inflammatory pathology

UTERINE PATHOLOGY EPITHELIAL ENDOMETRIAL LESIONS

Endometrial Metaplasia

Replacement of the normal endometrium by another type of non-neoplastic epithelium. These metaplasias include squamous cell, ciliated cell, papillary syncytial change, mucinous metaplasia, eosinophilic change, hobnail and clear cell, intestinal and stromal metaplasia. They can be present together with endometrial hyperplasia or without it.

Endometrial Polyps

Endometrial polyps are benign, localized over-growths of endometrial tissue covered by epithelium and containing a variable amount of glands, stroma and blood vessels. On gross examination, polyps are usually solitary, but they can be multiple. They can be either pedunculated or sessile and occur anywhere on the endometrium. Occasionally they can fill the entire endometrial cavity and even extend down through the external cervical os. The surface is smooth and it can have foci of hemorrhage and necrosis.

The endometrial polyps have an endometrial epithelial lining on three sides, and a prominent stalk with thick-walled vessels (FIGURE 1.1). Often small fragments from endometrial polyp are often submitted to the laboratory for complete processing. These samples may show a proliferation of irregular, stellate, non-secretory glands and fibrotic stroma. Occasionally, these lesions have smooth muscle fibers (adenomyomatous polyps). A variant of adeno-myoma is the atypical polypoid adenomyoma. This is constituted by glands with varying grades of hyperplasia and atypia, sometimes approaching the appearance of carcinoma *in situ*, between endometrial stroma and smooth muscle fibers.

The hysteroscopic diagnosis of the endometrial polyps is further discussed in Chapter 12.

Endometrial Hyperplasia

Endometrial hyperplasia is defined as a proliferation of glands of irregular size and shape with an increase

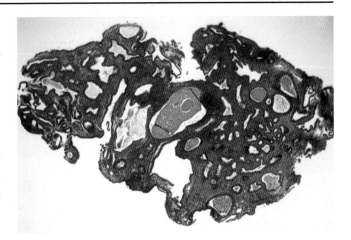

Figure 1.1: Endometrial polyp. The polyp has a fibrotic stroma, cystically dilated glands and vessels in the stalk

in the gland/stroma ratio compared with proliferative endometrium. The endometrium is increased in size, is soft and velvety. The hyperplasia may be either diffuse or localized. Endometrial hyperplasia has numerous classification systems. The most common categorizes the hyperplasias by both architecture and nuclear atypia (WHO, 1994). Glandular architecture may be either simple or complex. Simple consists of a minimal to mild increase in the gland: stroma ratio with cystic dilatation and occasional outpouching of glands. Complex describes more severe degrees of glandular crowding. Atypia describes the presence of atypical glandular epithelial nuclei. The nuclei are larger and rounder, with clumping and margination of the chromatin. There are four patterns of hyperplasia by this classification: Simple or complex without atypia (Non atypical hyperplasia) and simple or complex with atypia (Atypical hyperplasia) (WHO, 2002) (FIGURE 1.2).

Only atypical hyperplasia has a high likelihood of being associated with either concomitant carcinoma in the hysterectomy or the development of carcinoma in the follow-up. If the endometrial biopsy is very little, may be difficult to distinguish some well-differentiated carcinomas from atypical hyperplasia. Microscopic features favoring carcinoma include glandular confluence with a solid or cribriform pattern, extensive complex papillary formations, and desmoplastic stroma.

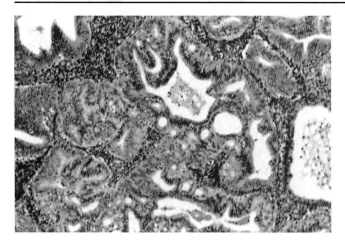

Figure 1.2: Atypical complex hyperplasia. Severe degree of glandular crowding. The stroma is scant. Nuclei are large and round, with clumping and margination of the chromatin

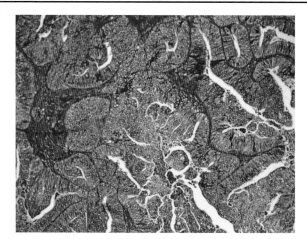

Figure 1.3: Endometrioid adenocarcinoma. The tumor is composed of well-formed glands with small foci of squamous differentiation

Endometrial Carcinoma

Endometrial carcinoma is the most common invasive neoplasm of the female genital tract in developed countries. Several lines of epidemiologic and clinicopathological evidence support the hypothesis that there are two distinct types of endometrial carcinoma. One type that occurs in perimenopausal women as a result of excess estrogenic stimulation, and tends to be low grade. In the second type hormonal risk factors have not been identified, and occurs in older postmenopausal women. These tumors have a very aggressive clinical course.

Grossly, carcinoma of endometrium is seen as a broad based polypoid mass or as diffused thickening of endometrium that infiltrates into the myometrium. The mass has an irregular surface, focally ulcerated with a soft white-grey tissue.

Approximately 70-80% of endometrial carcinomas are conventional endometrioid adenocarcinomas and arise in a background of endometrial hyperplasia. Microscopically, the tumor shows a glandular or papillary pattern (FIGURE 1.3). The grading system is based primarily upon architectural features: grade 1 is no more than 5% solid; grade 2 is 6-50%, and grade 3 is over 50% solid. Areas of squamous differentiation are not considered as solid tumor growth only on the glandular component. Marked differences in architectural grade can be seen within a tumor. The heterogeneity in differentiation accounts for the differences in grade that can be observed between the endometrial curettings and the hysterectomy specimen. The tumor increases their grade by one for significant nuclear atypia. They are cells with markedly enlarged, pleomorphic nuclei with large prominent nucleoli. Numerous variants of endometrioid adenocarcinoma have been described (Endometrioid carcinoma with squamous differentiation, villoglandular carcinoma, secretory carcinoma, ciliated carcinoma).

The remaining epithelial tumors of the endometrium are non-endometrioid adenocarcinoma (serous carcinoma and clear cell carcinoma). The serous carcinoma may contain papillae, glands and solid areas (FIGURE 1.4). The clear cell carcinoma displays tubulocystic, papillary or solid pattern. These tumors, frequently, deeply invade the myometrium and have vascular invasion. Multiple studies have found that most cases of serous carcinoma are related to a malignant transformation of the endometrial surface epithelium (endometrial intraepithelial carcinoma, EIC).

Now, the decision whether to perform lymph node sampling at the time of hysterectomy often depends on the tumor grade assigned in the biopsy and depth of myometrial invasion by transvaginal ultrasonography. Although not commonly used in staging endometrial carcinoma, hysteroscopy may assist in detecting lesions involving the cervix.

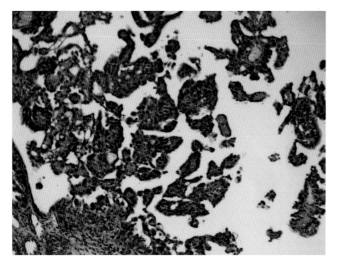

Figure 1.4: Serous carcinoma of the endometrium. A complex papillary architecture with many cells showing marked nuclear atypia

More detailed discussion of the hysteroscopic view of Endometrial Hyperplasia and Carcinoma is considered in Chapter 6.

MESENCHYMAL TUMORS

The mesenchymal tumors of the uterus form a big and heterogeneous group of tumors, benign and malignant.

Leiomyoma

The leiomyoma, the benign smooth muscle tumor, is the most common of all uterine neoplasms. It may occur in any position within the myometrium, preferably in the body of the uterus. This may protrude into the uterine cavity and may lead to atrophy or erosion of the endometrial surface. Occasionally, they may be pedunculated and may present at the external cervical os, often with an infarcted area. By means of hysteroscopic examination only submucous leiomyoma may be detected. Microscopically, leiomyoma are composed of interlacing bundles of smooth muscle cells, usually with a sharp demarcation from the surrounding myometrium. There are not nuclear atypia and mitotic figures are absent or sparse. Some degenerative changes (hyaline, cystic, myxoid and "red" degeneration and calcification) are found especially in large leiomyoma. There are some variants of leiomyoma, with distinctive features: cellular leiomyoma (with a bigger number of cells than the surrounding myometrium), epithelioid leiomyoma (tumor composed of round cells with eosinophilic or clear cytoplasm), atypical, symplastic or bizarre leiomyoma (composed of giant cells with multiple or atypical nuclei with lack of or few mitotic figures and without atypical mitosis) and myxoid leiomyoma (extensive myxoid changes in the intercellular substance). The hysteroscopic approach of the submucosal leiomyoma is seen in Chapter 10.

Leiomyosarcoma

Leiomyosarcoma is the malignant variant of smooth muscle tumor, and is the most frequent malignant non-epithelial tumor in the uterus. The leiomyosarcomas can arise in a pre-existing leiomyoma. On gross examination, may be similar to leiomyoma or may show necrosis, hemorrhagic areas and extra-uterine extension. On microscopic examination, leiomyosarcomas are generally more densely cellular, more atypical and contain mitotic figures. There is coagulative tumor cell necrosis. The degree of muscular differentiation is variable. In a small hysteroscopy-endometrial biopsy can be impossible to distinguish between a benign and a malignant smooth muscle tumor (FIGURE 1.5).

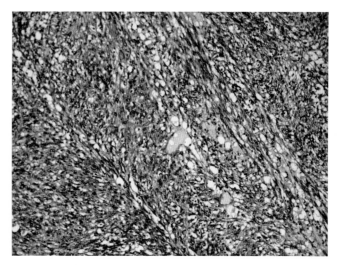

Figure 1.5: Leiomyosarcoma. The tumor is hypercellular, significant nuclear atypia and mitotic figures

Endometrial Stromal Tumors

Endometrial stromal tumors are neoplasms composed of stromal cells like those of the proliferative phase of endometrium. The cells are small, with scanty cytoplasm. A rich vascular pattern of small arterioles is characteristic. The benign variant, the endometrial stromal nodule is the most infrequent and is composed of endometrial stromal cells arranged as a well-circumscribed nodule, without invasive margins. This lesion usually arises in the myometrium, but can involve the endometrium or both, and may form a polyp in the uterine cavity.

The endometrial stromal sarcoma is similar in aspect, but has irregular and infiltrating margins, and can show more mitotic figures. Some stromal tumors contain prominent smooth muscle elements. Their gross aspect does not differ from stromal tumors without muscular elements.

Stromal tumors containing endometrial glands and tumors resembling the ovarian sex-cord tumor have been described. They are uncommon and have the same gross appearance as endometrial stromal nodules and sarcomas.

Undifferentiated Uterine Sarcoma

This a rare malignant tumor composed of pleomorphic mesenchymal cells that neither do not resemble the cells of the endometrial stroma nor is of muscular origin. It has a poor prognosis. On gross examination, the tumor is usually polypoid with apparent necrosis and infiltrates extensively into the myometrium. The cells are large, pleomorphic, with marked variation in size and shape. Mitotic figures are numerous and necrosis is always present.

MIXED MÜLLERIAN TUMORS

A peculiar group of uterine neoplasms that contain both mesenchymal and epithelial elements. They are benign or malignant.

Adenofibroma/Adenosarcoma

Adenofibroma is a very uncommon tumor of uterine cavity or of the cervix composed of both epithelial and mesenchymal benign elements. Adenosarcoma is the counterpart with epithelial elements of similar appearance but sarcomatous, usually low-grade, stromal elements. Both on gross examination are tumors which occupy and distend the endometrial cavity, depending on the size. They are soft, rubbery or firm, lobulated or polypoid masses. The cut surface of both tumors may be firm or soft and spongy or clearly cystic. In the malignant variant there is often hemorrhage and necrosis.

On microscopic examination, adenofibroma is composed of bland epithelial elements, usually of endometrial type. Stromal elements are fibroblasts and endometrial stromal cells. Nuclear atypia and mitotic figures are absent. In adenosarcoma, the stromal elements predominate over epithelial elements and stromal cells are concentrated around of the epithelial elements. There are nuclear atypia and mitotic figures.

Some adenosarcomas contain heterologous elements as rhabdomyomatous, chondrosarcomatous or liposarcomatous elements. The distinction between adenofibroma and adenosarcoma can be impossible on small hysteroscopy biopsy specimen or in curettage specimens because adenosarcoma cannot be excluded unless the whole tumor is sampled. A hysterectomy is necessary to know for certain that the lesion is benign.

Carcinofibroma/Carcinosarcoma

Carcinofibroma is a tumor composed of malignant epithelial elements and a benign but neoplastic stromal component. Its existence is uncertain and not all the authors accept it.

Carcinosarcoma (with old designations of malignant mixed mesodermal tumor and malignant mixed müllerian tumor) is the most common tumor in this group and is composed of malignant epithelial glands and malignant estromal elements. It is a tumor of post-menopausal women, has a bad prognosis.

On macroscopic examination, carcinosarcoma usually forms a broad-based polyp that takes up and expands the endometrial cavity, but can cause diffuse enlargement of the uterus, infiltrating and expanding its wall. The cut surface is usually heterogeneous and show necrosis and hemorrhage. On microscopic examination, the malignant epithelial component is nearly always of endometrioid pattern, usually poorly differentiated, with or without squamous component. Serous, clear cell or mucinous carcinomas are other frequent epithelial components. The proportion of epithelial and sarcomatous component is greatly variable. Stromal component can be homologous, resembling endometrial stromal sarcoma, fibrosarcoma, leiomyosarcoma or undifferentiated sarcoma. Heterologous component included rhabdomyosarcoma, chondrosarcoma and, rarely, osteosarcoma.

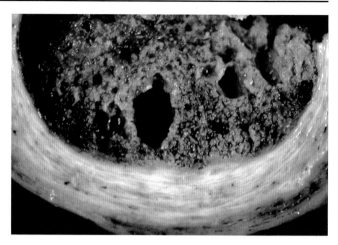

Figure 1.6: Macroscopic appearance of a hydatidiform mole

ENDOMETRIAL METASTASIS FROM EXTRAUTERINE TUMORS

The myometrium is more often involved than the endometrium. Mammary and gastrointestinal carcinomas are the most frequent. Occasionally the tumor can be diagnosed by an endometrial study, especially in cases of lobular carcinoma of the breast.

Pregnancy Related Lesions

Hydatidiform Mole

There are two trophoblastic lesions that contain chorionic villi. Complete and partial hydatidiform mole unusually warrants a hysteroscopic examination, because ultrasonography and serum monitoring of β-human chorionic gonadotropin (β-hCG) are sufficient to establish a diagnostic of molar pregnancy. Curettage is the election treatment and the pathologist made the diagnosis of one or other entity. The presence or absence of embryo or fetus, the size and contour of villi, the presence of cisterns and pseudo-inclusions, and the grade of trophoblastic proliferation, as well as the karyotype knowledge are useful to distinguish between both. It can be difficult to diagnose less than 14 weeks of gestation (FIGURE 1.6).

Placental Site Nodule and Placental Site Plaque

These are infrequent lesions that may be found by hysteroscopic examination. Both consist of nodules of intermediate trophoblast cells associated with dense hyaline stroma. They are single or multiple well-circumscribed small nodules or big plaques. The antecedent of pregnancy is not always recorded, and could have occurred months or years before.

Placental Site Trophoblastic Tumor

A malignant counterpart of intermediate trophoblastic cells is the placental site trophoblastic tumor. These tumors occur in women in the reproductive age, and follow a normal pregnancy or abortion, sometimes a hydatidiform mole. Their diagnosis is difficult if not impossible in small specimens, because an overlap exists with exaggerated placental site reaction and the tumoral cells that invade the myometrium without destroying it, as normal implantation site trophoblast. The appearance of trophoblastic cells is variable but usually forms monotonous sheets of large cells with eosinophilic cytoplasm. Mitotic activity is variable and atypical mitosis are not infrequent. It is usual to see extensive tumoral necrosis. One variant of this tumor is the epithelioid trophoblastic tumor.

Choriocarcinoma

Choriocarcinoma is a malignant tumor composed of a mixture of cytotrophoblast, intermediate trophoblast and syncytiotrophoblast. Frequently, it is preceded by complete hydatidiform mole, but can occur following a normal pregnancy or a spontaneous abortion. It can occur in a normal term placenta. On gross and microscopic examinations, choriocarcinoma is a large hemorrhagic mass with a small amount of tumor cells. They have biphasic pattern (mononuclear and multinucleated syncitial cells). Large areas of necrosis are often seen and vascular involvement is also usually extensive. Excepting in a term placenta, choriocarcinoma never contain chorionic villi.

Diagnosis of choriocarcinoma in uterine curetting or in hysteroscopy specimens may be difficult. Immunohistochemical studies may be useful.

BIBLIOGRAPHY

1. Fox H, Wells M (Eds). Haynes and Taylor Obstetrical & Gynecological Pathology (5th edn). Churchill Livingstone, London, 2002.
2. Kurman RJ (Ed). Blaustein's pathology of the female genital tract. 5th edition. Springer-Verlag. 2002.
3. Robboy SJ, Anderson MC, Russell P (Eds). Pathology of the female reproductive tract. Churchill Livingstone, London, 2002.
4. Silverberg SG, Kurman RJ. Tumors of the uterine corpus and gestational trophoblastic disease. Atlas of tumor pathology. Third Series. Fascicle 3. Washington, D.C. AFIP.1992.
5. Sternberg SS (Ed). Histology for pathologists. Second Edition. Lippincott-Raven publishers. Philadelphia, New York. 1997.
6. Tavassoli FA, Devilee P (Eds). WHO Classification of Tumors. Tumors of the breast and female genital organs. IARC Press, Lyon, 2003.

2

Maintenance of the Set of the Hysteroscopic Instruments

The Care of the Endoscopy Material: Theoretical and Practical Knowledges Guarantee of Quality in the Hysteroscopy Technology

Concepción García-Zarza
Pilar Arranz-García
Nuria de Argila Fernandez-Durán

INTRODUCTION

The central nucleus of all the activities of the infirmary must be the patient. Nevertheless, due to the fact that we have to work with a complex technology, with the utilization of an extremely delicate, very expensive material and with a limited usefulness, this chapter will approach only the technical aspects of the work to achieve. In fact, on this work depends to avoid the subsequent complications derived from one possible interruption of the surgical intervention. A deficient functioning of the set of instruments and an incorrect cleanliness and sterilization of these ones can do that the patient contracts a nosocomial infection.

After observing the different protocols that follow in the centers in which the hysteroscopy technology is practised, we deduce that there is no consensus on the treatment of the material to use.

In this Chapter, there will be detailed the fundamental processes that are in use in the managing and treatment of the endoscopy material. The efficiency of these processes has been corroborated by numerous publications and guides of hospitable hygiene edited by the Services of Preventive Medicine of a great number of institutions.

The present work develops in two blocks. The first one studies the summary, checking of the correct functioning and managing of the set of the hysteroscopy instruments that is in use in the operating room, as well as the own tasks of the postsurgical moment such as the disassembly and cleanliness, the disinfection and the movement of the reusable material.

The second block refers to the managing of the set of the hysteroscopy instruments in the sterilization center and describes the stages of the processes of sterilization, storage and transport.

Finally, it is necessary to mention that the election of the different procedures that here are described will depend on the professional nurse responsible for the material to using. For this reason, a good training of the whole personnel involved in the managing of the set of instruments and equipment, as well as a suitable planning, is indispensable to guarantee the success in the achieved work.

THE FIRST PHASE OF THE MANAGING OF THE SET OF HYSTEROSCOPY INSTRUMENTS IN THE OPERATING ROOM

Presurgical Time

Once known the surgical programming, it is necessary to take the following actions:
- Request of the set of instruments and of the available optics.
- In case of not having sufficient set of instruments for each of the hysteroscopy interventions, one must choose a sterilization method thinking in the necessary time for this process.
- Disposition of additional material in anticipation of possible complications (uterine perforation)
- Review and checking of the functioning of the equipments.

If the procedure is made in an operating room, with the corresponding integral elements (AIDA System, Central Computer, Endoscopy Tower and Monitors), it is necessary to follow the corresponding sequence, as this one:
- Open the personalized configuration of the surgeon
- Place the screens depending on the procedure to continue
- Place lamps
- Place the pedal in the suitable position
- Prepare the fluids of expansion to the corporal temperature.

Surgical Time

For practical reasons that allow us to unify criteria, the different devices used in the hysteroscopy surgery can qualify of the following way:
- Equipment/optical systems
- Set of instruments
- Electrical systems
- Systems of perfusion of fluids.

Equipment/ Optical Systems

The optical system of the hysteroscopy surgery is made up of:
- Television monitor
- Video camera
- Hysteroscopy or optics
- Light source of cold light
- Optical fiber

Considerations to having in account/precaution of the equipments

Video camera:
- The compress of the camera must adapt to the ocular piece of the optics, which diameter is standard.
- In the ocular piece of the optics, there is placed a protective sterile case that covers the compress of the camera and the cable, allowing its managing of sterile form.
- Make the balance of white colors in the control unit of the video camera, so that it allows an adjustment to the intensity of color or wave length of the used source. The balance of white color needs to direct the camera connected to the optical, towards a white surface, avoiding other colors in the setting. Later, there must be pushed the key of white balance in its control unit, indicating on the screen if it has been made correctly.
- Fix the camera in the sterile field and support it with stability in order to avoid a possible fall due to the position changes of the patient.
- Avoid the orientation of the camera towards a light source of high intensity (as the lights of the operating room), because this can damage the sensor element of light.
- Avoid placing solutions near of the control unit, because they might pour out accidental or splashing the unit, with the subsequent deterioration of the same one.
- Once finished the intervention, what we must gather first is the camera, taking the sterile cover away and putting the protector of the camera. This one has to be left in a sure place.
- The cable is gathered avoiding possible pulls, specially in the union point of the cable with the

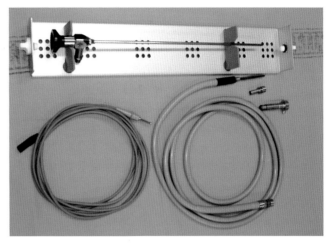

Figure 2.1: Optics, optical fiber and electric wire

camera, which could cause interferences or loss of brightness in the image.
- The integrity of the cable isolation has to be watched in order to avoid its deterioration.

Hysteroscopy or optics
- The optics (panoramic hysteroscopy) adapted to make the surgical hysteroscopy has an angle of vision that can be of 0° or of 12°. It is an instrument that is made up of lenses of increase. For being the most delicate instrument of the intervention, it needs to remain in a box for its move to the sterilization center and for its conservation.
- The optics must be placed in a sure place in the instrumentation table, avoiding the contact with other instruments that could break or scratch it.
- It is very important to verify the adequacy of the optics to the procedure and to check the compatibility with the resectoscopy. Also we have to arrange of adapters for the optical fiber (FIGURE 2.1).

Light Source
- The endoscopy procedures need an intensity of light adjusted to the procedure. The regulation of the light can be made of *manual* or *automatic* way.
- The automatic regulation depends on the diameter of the used optics and allows the adjustment of different types of optics.

- The exit orifice of the light and the end of the optical fiber do not have always the same caliber, therefore it is necessary to arrange of adapters to guarantee a perfect adjustment.
- In the surgical interventions, the light source has to be the last thing to activate and the first one in going out. When the equipment is not in use, the light source has to be put in position *standby*. The repeated connection and disconnection of the light source in the same surgical session spoils the lamp.
- The cold light source has to be in use with the minimal adjustment of light that is needed.
- It is necessary to arrange of a bulb which duration ranges between 300 and 600 hours.

Optical fiber

- The optical fiber (or the light cable) connects the optics to the light source. It is made up of fibers (optical material), which have the possibility to reflect light.
- The contact with the free end of a light cable can produce burns in its ends and in the final of the endoscopy. These ends never have to settle either on inflammable objects or on the patients.
- The optical fiber has to be prevented from doubling in excess, because it might break its fibers (The density of the optical fiber has to be proportional to the intensity of the light source, in order to prolong its useful life).
- The optical fiber has to be manipulated avoiding the contact with sharp instruments, both in the surgery and in its sending to the sterilization center.

Set of Instruments

In general terms, the realization of the surgical hysteroscopy needs surgical basic set of instruments to practise the hysterometry and the cervical dilatation (FIGURE 2.2) and the *resectoscopy*. This one is made up of double operative sheath (introduced with shutter) and of the work element (FIGURE 2.3).

Considerations to having in account/ precaution of the equipment

- The movements used for the assembly of the resectoscopy have to be soft.

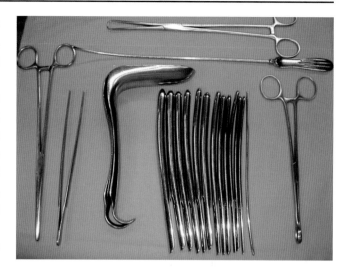

Figure 2.2: Surgical basic set of instruments

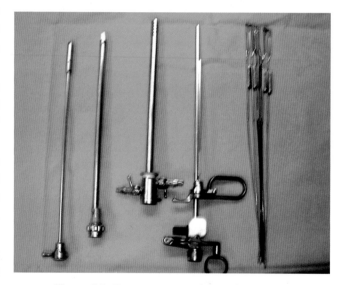

Figure 2.3: Resectoscopy and resection handles

- It is necessary to assemble and fit pivots and valves (the system of adjustment has the direction of the clock needles).

Electrical Systems

It is possible to use different electrical systems to make the endometrial resection-ablation (monopolar energy, two-pole system type Versapoint, laser YAG or others). Here we are going to describe the use of the generator for monopolar use. The wave used, in general, for the hysteroscopy electroresection is the type *cut-bend*.

Considerations to having in account/precautions of the equipment

- *Be vigilant with the cables*: We must check the integrity of the cable that connects to the generator of monopolar current of high frequency. Also it is necessary to arrange of supply cables, due to its continuous deterioration for the permanent sterilization processes. Any tear or break in the cables isolation can produce burns.
- *The resection handles*: The inlays in the electrode reduce the efficiency producing current lacks. An indication of this isolation failure can be the need of a higher power able to produce the electrical wished effect (FIGURE 2.4).
- *Thermic diffusion*: It is possible to produce thermic transmission of the monopolar electric power to the next organs, especially in the *tubaric ostium* (detectable complication in the postoperatory).
- *Involuntary activation of the high frequency generator*: It takes place when the switch of the pedal is touched involuntary. Also, it can owe to a short-circuit inside a cable or to the penetration of electricity conductive liquids in the control of the electrode or in the switch of the pedal.
- *Pedal position*: We must place the pedal in an accessible position to the surgeon and monitor the integrity of the cable, so that it is not pinzed. It is necessary to isolate it of the dampness.
- *Correct position of the neutral electrode or scalpel plate*:
  - The neutral electrode must hold on the arm (or thigh) more close to the operation field. Generally, it holds itself on the area with more electrical conductivity as the muscles.
  - It is necessary to avoid fats, down or sudoration. The surface where it sticks fast has to be clean and dry.
  - The surgical field has to be kept dry and it is necessary to avoid, specially, liquids accumulate in the surface of contact between the patient skin and the table of the operating room (disinfectants and fluids of irrigation), due to the electrical conductivity that they have.
  - The longest end of the scalpel plate has to be orientated towards the operative field.

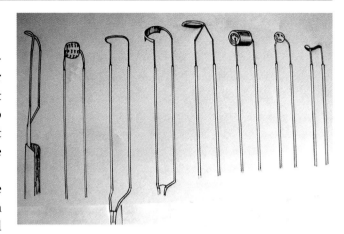

Figure 2.4: Resection handles

  - The patient cannot have anything metallically and even his/her body cannot touch any electricity conductive object.
  - It is possible to use electrical scalpel if the patient has metallic prosthesis fixed of titanium or of surgical steel, though the precautions carrying to extremes (as for the minimal adjustment of powers, utilization of scalpel plates of high safety and its position as close as possible to the application place of the active electrode).
  - It is important to use systems with high levels of safety that are inactivated when the plate of the neutral electrode is not in touch with the patient.

Systems of Perfusion of Fluids

In the surgical hysteroscopy, a way of expansion is necessary to have a suitable visualization of the uterine cavity. In case of using monopolar energy, it is necessary to use liquids of low molecular weight, which do not contain electrolytes and of null conductance, in order to allow the electrocoagulation and the resection. Currently, the most used liquid is Glicine's solution to 1.5%. It is necessary to warm it without exceeding the corporal temperature.

This liquid has low viscosity, for what its permanency in the uterine cavity is short and it is mixed by the blood too, forcing to use constant flow.

*Considerations to having in
account/precautions of the equipment*

It is recommended the use of *automatic bombs* that allow the flow control and the irrigation pressure, as well as *the pressure of the fluids suction* that are used in this surgery, in order to do the procedure with more safety.

It is indispensable the careful valuation of the quantity of absorbed flow (with balance of the instilated liquid and of the recovered one) during the whole procedure, due to the risk of a syndrome of an hydric retention (FIGURE 2.5).

Postsurgical Immediate Time

The first phase of the material maintenance begins when the operative act has finished. It is desirable to make this process as soon as possible, for what we recommend to do it inside the own operating room. By this way, once dismantled the material, this one must be cleaned of the macroscopic remnants of organic material.

Disassembly and Macroscopic Cleanliness

We explain each of the parts of the hysteroscopy material, in order to specify the need to make the cleanliness adequately:

Optics or hysteroscopy

An enzymatic product and water is applied, recommended by the guides of hospitable hygiene (according to instructions). It is necessary to use cotton material, because the gauzes can scratch the optics. In order to avoid harmful effects in the endoscopy parts, it is recommended to use demineralized water. Later, it is necessary to catch on and to dry off.

Before the sterilization, it is advisable to clean the optical glasses with a small stick impregnated in alcohol of 70%. The surfaces must be clean and brilliant so that the vision can be clear. Sediment can provoke a blurry vision so, to eliminate it, it is possible to use a cream commercialized by the manufacturer. It keeps in a specific casing for the hysteroscopy.

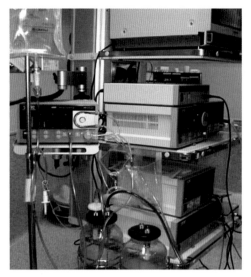

Figure 2.5: System of perfusion of fluids

Optical fiber or cable of light

They are cleaned by a humid cloth and a disinfectant. It is necessary to prevent it from doubling, in order not to spoil the transmission light fibers.

Electrical cables

It is cleaned by a humid cloth and by disinfectant. Normally, the sending to the sterilization center of the optical fiber and of the electrical cables, is done separately of the metallic set of instruments.

Metallic set of hysteroscopy instruments

The different parts of the hysteroscopy are dismounted: The pods, resection handles, element of work (FIGURE 2.3), and the surgical basic set of instruments (FIGURE 2.6).

It is necessary to verify the existence of the connections and valves to avoid losses, and the delicate material must be protected (resection handles and sharp instruments as Pozzi tenaculum).

Inspection and Register

The material must be inspected and registered. The effects are annotated with regard to the functioning of the material.

Moves to the Sterilization Center

First of all, it is necessary to be sure that the equipments are complete. The movement must be done as soon as possible, in order to avoid adherences of the organic matter and in closed containers in which it is necessary to separate metallic set of instruments, optical material, electrical cables and resection handles.

The Second Phase of the Managing of the Set of Instruments

- Service of sterilization
- Stages in the processing of the material
- Sterilization
- Storage and transport.

Generalities in the Process of Disinfection and Sterilization

The service of sterilization is responsible of the processing of the materials in the hospitals, which is in charge to provide to all the departments with sterile material (FIGURE 2.6).

The centralization of all the processes is the most effective and sure system because it allows the supervision, the uniform criterion and the rational managing of the resources.

The receipt and movement of the materials is done to facilitate the processes and to avoid the deterioration. A register system must exist to know and to evaluate the materials and the processes.

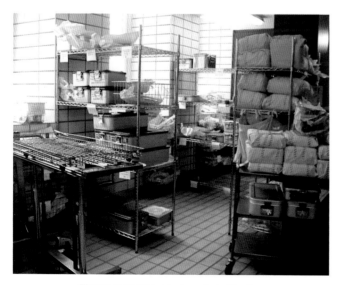

Figure 2.6: The service of sterilization

According to the characteristics of the material and to the use to which it is destined, they will be necessary different measures for its treatment. Depending on the risk of infection derived from the use of the clinical material, this one can divide in three categories.

Spaulding's Classification

Category	Maternal	Contact With	Maternal Treatment
Critic	Surgical set of instruments Arthroscopy Biopsy punches Resection handles	Sterile fabrics Sterile cavities Mucous membranes Vascular system	Sterilization
Semicritic	Bronchoscope Gastroscope Laryngoscope Vaginal speculum	Mucous membranes Mucous Not intact skin	High-level disinfection
No critic	Thermometers Wedges Fonendoscopes	Intact skin	Disinfection of interval or low level

Current Problems in Relation with Spaulding's with Classification

The selection of the Spaulding's method, in which the endoscopies are qualified in "*semicritics*", does not turn out to be completely adapted at present due to other factors like:

- *The design and the nature of the endoscopic material,* which makes difficult the wash and the safety of having eliminated completely the organic matter. In addition to this, the disinfection of high level is difficult to control, by which the procedure does not have total guarantee.
- *The emergent microorganisms,* on which there are not known the effects of the methods of sterilization, the chemical agents used as disinfectants of high level or the necessary time for its elimination. Some examples of these microorganisms are the Prione and the Mycobacteria.
- *Type of intervention*: The endoscopies, inside the Spaulding's classification, when they were contacting with the mucous ones were considered as *semicritics*, for what they had to undergo a

disinfection of high level. Nowadays, the material that contacts with sterile cavities is considered as *critic* and, therefore, this one needs of a sterilization degree.

In the diagnostic and surgical hysteroscopy sterile cavities are reached and, therefore, the whole used material is considered as *critic* and has to be submitted to a sterilization process.

Stages in the Processing of the Material

The set of the hysteroscopy instruments, once received by the sterilization unit, has to surrender to the following procedures:

Cleanliness

Manual cleanliness: The cleanliness is the previous indispensable step in the whole process of disinfection and sterilization so that, if the set of instruments is not totally clean, there will no be an effective sterilization of the hysteroscopy material. The wash of the set of instruments can qualify in:

- *Manual wash specific of the optical material and cable*:
  - Cleanliness with a cloth wetted in pure enzymatic liquid, supporting it during five minutes
  - Careful rinsed
  - Dried.
- *Manual wash of the metallic set of instruments*. This process includes the following steps:
  - Make a dragging wash using the shower of the sink or the water pistol for the hysteroscopy cannulated material. This cleanliness is very important because it eliminates 85% of dirtiness.
  - Introduce material in an enzymatic bath during 5 minutes. With this disinfectant one manages to emulsify the fats and to hydrolyze the proteins and the glucide.
  - Brush the biopsy channel. The brush of cleanliness must introduce for the entry of the valve suction until it goes out for the distal top, for three occasions.
  - Rinse the resector with water, external and internally.
  - Pass compressed air by the channels to dry and to expel the remains of organic material.

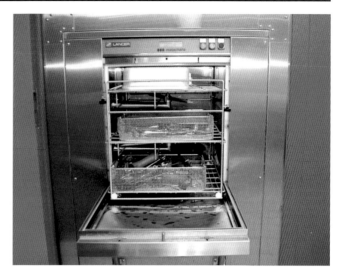

Figure 2.7: Washing machine

Once finished any of the previous steps, the responsible nurse will proceed to the set of instruments review, in order to detect problems of functioning, blunt or rusty instruments.

Mechanical cleanliness (FIGURE 2.7): It consists of making a cleanliness using wash machines destined to this purpose. These present the advantage of having controls that verify the appropriate process of cleanliness.

The whole hysteroscopy material, except the optical material (optics and fiber) and the electrical cable, is submitted to a mechanical cleanliness. For this purpose, they are introduced in the automated machines.

- The whole set of instruments, used or not, must be introduced, because during the intervention it can have been splashed inadvertently for blood or saline solution.
- All the joints must be opened and their components dismantled.
- The free, light or small material must be placed in special baskets.
- Introduce the baskets in the washer so that the arms remain free and do not touch the set of instruments.
- Select the program and start the washer according to instructions.
- The washers submit with several cycles programmed of factory. The warning screen

indicates the number of cycles selected the temperature of the water or of the air in the vat and the name of the function in course.

- The electrical washers are made up, generally, of several programs. The principal ones are five:
  - Prewashing
  - Wash, generally to less than 45° C, in order to avoid the albumens coagulation that was remaining adhered to the surface of the material, with its consequent deterioration.
  - Clarified. The temperature ranges between 75 and 90° C.
  - Thermal disinfection to 90° C during 10 minutes, to prevent the professional diseases in the manipulated set of instruments.
  - Dried of the set of instruments.
- There must be respected the dosing of the detergent recommended by the manufacturer, knowing that a minor dose will make it ineffective and a major one will increase its corrosive power.
- It is necessary to avoid any opening of the door during the cycle.
- Once finished the cycle, the supports, the baskets, the accessories and the washed objects have to cool before manipulating them.
- Finished the process, the washer disburdens, verifying that the material is clean and dry. It is suitable to pass the air pistol for the cannulated pieces.

Review and preparation of the material

After the dried process and in order to guarantee a perfect sterilization, it is necessary to check the material because in spite of the cleanliness of blood and debris, there can be mineral deposits and other impurities that would impede its later use. The aspects to have in count are the following:

- Perfect cleanliness of the set of instruments
- Absence of blemishes
- Correct functioning of the articulations: It must be perfectly clean, without blemishes and with the soft joints in order to assure an effective sterilization
- Oiling, if necessary.

Assembly of a container of set of hysteroscopy instruments

The whole hysteroscopy material puts in a box, except the optics, which is sterilized packed in double paper and preserved in the specific casing for it.

- Wash and dried of set of instruments and container
- Place of green cloth or crepped paper in the box
- Change filter of the lid
- Review and inventory of the set of instruments, according to protocol
- Introduction of strip of chemical control
- Checking of the hermetic closing of the container
- Place of the binding with signature of the one who makes the assembly
- Stick in the seal the control etiquette.

Sterilization

The sterilization consists of the destruction of any form of bacterial life, including the spores. The sterility of an object refers to the probability of which such object is not contaminated. The European pharmacopeia has fixed as maximum limit of not sterility in 10^6 (UNE Norm-EU 556). This means that we can find a not sterile object between a million objects submitted to the sterilization. The difficulty of demonstrating it does that, in the practice, an object is sterile considered when it has been submitted to the diverse processes of sterilization and the nurse has validated all the controls made in the process.

It is very important to consider the recommendations of the manufacturer about the material sterilization, as well as the fulfillment of the regulation corresponding CEE, eliminating the whole material of an alone utilization that has already been used.

Methods of Sterilization

The fundamental methods of sterilization are grouped as it is going to be described, although here only two of them are explained, because they are the most used for the sterilization of the hysteroscopy material.

Physical	Water steam to pressure Dry heat Ionizing radiations
Chemical	*Gases:* Oxide of ethylene, peroxide of hydrogen, gas takes form *Liquids:* They act only as disinfectants with minor exhibition times (peracetic acid, peroxide of hydrogen)

Physical Method: Sterilization for Water Steam to Pressure

The humid heat in the shape of saturated steam to pressure is very effective for the destruction of any form of microbial life, included the spores. The sterilizing action is produced by the double effect of the heat and of the dampness.

The sterilization for water steam is the most rapid, efficient and safe procedure of the existing ones to hospitable level. It is cheap and does not produce toxic residues. It is provided with programs that include the operations that the sterilizer makes such as the temperature reached, the exhibition time of the sterilized product and the dried time.

This sterilization method acts by the coagulation effect to the level of cellular protoplasm of the microorganisms. It must reach temperatures from 12° until 134° and must be verified if the optical ones support this treatment.

The hysteroscopy material is suitable for this type of sterilization (FIGURE 2.8).

Controls/Registers of Sterilization Parameters in Steam Autokeys

Bowie and Dick Test

This control is used to verify the sterilization functioning daily. It is used in the steam sterilizers with pre-empty, in order to value its capacity of air elimination and to verify if fugues exist in the camera. It has to be verified if the elimination of the air has been sufficiently good and if the penetration of the steam in the product is the correct one. The parameters of the cycle of proof are: 132-134°C and time of plateau 3.5 minutes.

On the sheet of proof verified, it is necessary to estimate a change of color in all its extension (FIGURE 2.9).

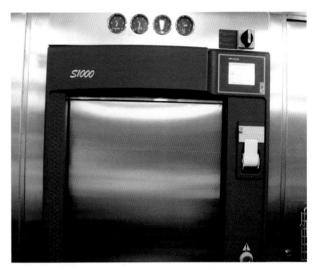

Figure 2.8: Steam autokey

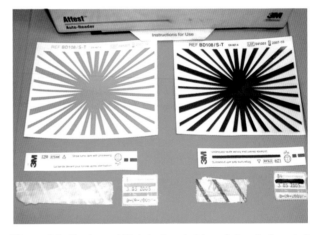

Figure 2.9: Bowie and Dick test and strips of chemical control

Physical Controls

They are made by external instruments with which the autokeys are provided and which allow the follow-up of the cycle and the continuous observation of the process using graphical records, barometers, etc.

The temperature and the pressure in the sterilizer camera are monitored during the whole process. The sterilizer is provided with a printer and a graphical recorder, which allow to obtain the digital and/or analogical register of the process (FIGURE 2.10).

Chemical Controls

They confirm that certain necessary conditions have been fulfilled for the correct sterilization. They are

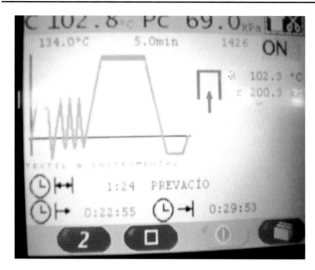

Figure 2.10: Physical control of sterilization

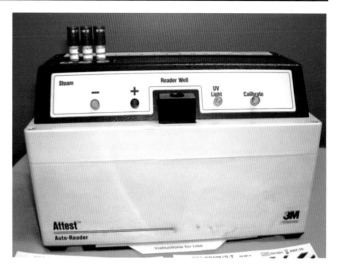

Figure 2.11: Sterilization center

special compounds impregnated with chemical products, sensitive to the fulfillment of the parameters of sterilization: Time, pressure and temperature, changing color in case they are fulfilled.

- *External or process indicators:* They serve to confirm if an article has been or not sterilized. They will be in use in all the packages. They must be printed in the external side of the bags or the self-adhesive tapes. The turn to the color indicated will be verified at the end of the sterilization process and before the material distribution.

- *Internal or integrators:* They indicate that the interior of the packages has reached the necessary conditions for the correct sterilization, according to the fulfillment of the sterilization parameters (time, pressure and temperature) by the color change of the reactivate inks. They place inside the container or package in the point of more difficult access to the steam. They appear, generally, in the shape of paper strips. These indicators cannot move back without altering the sterility conditions. The nurse of operating room will make her validation before proceeding to use the material.

Biological Controls

They serve to verify the efficiency of the different sterilization systems with the most resistant mechanisms for each method, simulating the most

adverse conditions that could be given in the process. They place in packages of proof that impede the steam penetration.

The bacilli used in the steam sterilization are the Bacillus stearothermophilus, contained in a blister with built-in culture medium, which incubation is made in the sterilization center (FIGURE 2.11).

Chemical Method: Liquid Peracetic Acid

This is a chemical way that allows a low temperature sterilization. Combined with a corrosion neutralizer turns out to be an excellent method to sterilize hysteroscopy material. It is necessary that all the elements remain immersed in the liquid during approximately 25 minutes to a temperature between 50 and 56°C. There exist machines that use this product in closed camera, so that the liquid sterilizing agent flows for all the channels, lumens and surfaces of the devices. This method has been the chosen one for several institutions because it allows a rapid re-utilization of the material without need to proceed to the packing. Nowadays, its efficiency is being evaluated.

Storage and Transport

Once finished with the cycles of the sterilizers, one proceeds to the opening of the same ones and to the exhaust of the material, remaining in the car until they cool. There must be verified physical and chemical controls of the cycles, annotating the result in the corresponding *cards of daily control of autokeys*. Also the biological controls move from the sterilizers away, registering in the control card cycle in the one that has been tried.

The transport is made by trolley and containers dedicated specially to this purpose. It is qualified allowing accessibility. There have to be verified integrity of the bundles, the process controls and the dates of caducity, before being used in the operating room.

ACKNOWLEDGMENTS

We thankfully acknowledge to:

- Pilar García Zarza, Licensed in Philosophy, Magister in Translation and Interpretation of the German language, for her aid in the preparation of this manuscript.
- Montserrat Doncel Gallego. Qualified in Infirmary. Nurse of the Sterilization Unit. University Hospital Santa Cristina. Madrid.
- To the whole personnel of the Sterilization Unit and of the Ambulatory Major Surgery of the University Hospital Santa Cristina, who has collaborated in the accomplishment of this chapter.
- To supervisors, nurses and assistants of different sanitary public institutions of the Community of Madrid (Virgen de la Torre Hospital, San Carlos' Clinical Hospital, Ramony Cajal Hospital) for their generous contribution of manuals on standardized procedures.

BIBLIOGRAPHY

1. 2° Congreso Nacional de Enfermería en Cirugía Endoscópica. Libro de Ponencias. Barcelona. Noviembre 2001.
2. ALVARADO CARLA, M.S. "Revisiting *the Spaulding Classification Scheme*" In: Chemical Germicidas in Health Care Edited by William Rutala: Internacional Symposium May 1994 (203-209).
3. AORN: *Prácticas Recomendadas para el Cuidado del Instrumental Quirúrgico y Endoscópico.* Edic MMISA.
4. AUCCASI ROJAS, MARCELINO. *Enfermería en Control de Infecciones Intrahospitalarias.* http://www. members. fortunecy.es/marcear/EN enfermería en control infecciones. html. Consultada 2/6/2005.
5. BROTO DELOR. *Instrumentación quirúrgica.* Técnicas en cirugía general. Volumen 1. E. Panamericana. 2000. Buenos Aires.
6. CASIELLES ELISABETH. PERALTA. SANDRA *Esterilización y desinfección del instrumental y equipo laparoscópico.*
7. CORTÉS RIDAURA, L. *Limpieza, desinfección y esterilización del material quirúrgico.* Hospital General Universitario de Valencia.
8. FULLER JOANNA RUTH. *Instrumentación Quirúrgica.* Principios y Práctica. 3ª Edición. Editorial Panamericana.
9. GARCÍA ZARZA, CONCEPCION, ARRANZ GARCÍA PILAR, PEREZ MEDINA TIRSO. Enfermería en cirugía endoscópica I. Excelencia enfermera 2005;12:1-60.
10. GARCÍA ZARZA, CONCEPCION, ARRANZ GARCÍA PILAR, PEREZ MEDINA TIRSO. Enfermería en cirugía endoscópica II. Excelencia enfermera 2006;13:1-78.
11. http://www.obgyn.net.Hysteroscopy and Fluid Management. Peter Dragonas, MD Interviews OBGYN.net. Consultada 28/06/04.
12. *Instrucciones de uso de endoscopios.* Tecno-medical. Optik Chirurgie GMBH & Co.KG. Tuttlingen/Germany.
13. LEJARÍN ABELLÁN, CARMEN. Estudio sobre variaciones de la temperatura corporal en pacientes sometidos a resección transuretral de próstata (4° Congreso Nacional de Enfermería Quirúrgica).
14. *Manual de Esterilización.* Hospital Universitario Santa Cristina. Madrid.
15. *Manual de Funcionamiento.* Lancer. 910 UP DIN.
16. *Manual de Instrucciones de operación. Esterilizadores a Vapor. S 1000.* Matachana.
17. *Manual de Procesos.* Central de Esterilización "Hospital Virgen de la Torre."
18. Matachana. Dep. Estudios Antonio Matachana, SA.
19. PAEZ R. OSCAR. *Desinfección de equipos y accesorios.* Guía de manejo en Gastroenterología. Profesor Asociado. Clínica Los Andes, ISS, Barranquilla.
20. *Pautas para la limpieza y desinfección en endoscopia gastrointestinal.* (European Society of gastrointestinal endoscopy).
21. PRIETO ESPIGA, Elsa. *Esterilización por Ácido peracético en cámara cerrada.* EL AUTOCLAVE. Año 16. N° 1. Mayo 2004.
22. *Protocolo de desinfección y esterilización.* Servicio de Medicina Preventiva. Hospital Ramón y Cajal 2003.
23. SEGO. *Documentos de consenso.*2.001.Editorial Meditex, Madrid.
24. SODRESTROM, R. *Cirugía Laparoscópica en Ginecología.* Ediciones Marban, Madrid.
25. SPAULDING, EH. *"Chemical sterilization of medical and surgical materials"* In CA Block, SS (Eds) Disinfection, Sterilization and Preservation. Philadelphia: Lea & Febiger, 1968:517-31.
26. VELASCO VALVERDE, Emilia. *Limpieza y Desinfección del Instrumental Quirúrgico.* El Autoclave. Año 15. N° 1. Abril 2003.

3

Office Hysteroscopy: Indications and Contraindications

Tirso Pérez-Medina
Enrique Iglesias Goy

INTRODUCTION

Diagnostic office hysteroscopy has revolutionized the gynecology and the management of many gynecologic conditions. Cost, convenience, accuracy, and patient acceptability of these procedures are clearly superior to traditional D & C. Nowadays, hysteroscopy is the gold standard for endometrial evaluation. To make a pathological diagnosis is not intended, but to alert the physician that intracavitary pathology is present, and to guide for surgical therapy and treatment.

Office hysteroscopy became practical with the introduction of small-caliber endoscopes allowing their use in an office setting without the need for cervical dilatation. The small-caliber hysteroscope simplifies examination and allows an easy and safe investigation of the uterine cavity. Office hysteroscopy is a simple procedure that can be undertaken in a short period of time with minimal morbidity and inconvenience to the patient. Bradley[1] documented a high patient acceptability, diagnostic accuracy, and cost-effectiveness in 417 patients undergoing office hysteroscopy.

Today, office hysteroscopy is no longer considered as a plain diagnostic procedure as was the case for diagnostic laparoscopy. The evolution of the instruments has made possible the philosophic approach of *see and treat*, and a lot of different pathologies can be managed in the same moment of the procedure, thus improving the acceptability and satisfaction of patients that, otherwise, should have to wait for a preoperative evaluation and an anesthetic and surgical procedure in the theater.[2]

The advantages of hysteroscopic visualization include direct visualization of the endometrium and endocervix with immediate evaluation, the ability to detect minor focal endometrial pathology, and the ability to perform directed endometrial biopsies.

The disadvantages of office hysteroscopy include the need for expensive office equipment (camera, insufflator, hysteroscope, and video equipment), a skilful and experienced hysteroscopist, and the cost of the procedure.

TECHNIQUE

Although the procedure of hysteroscopy is relatively simple, a very important factor is to decrease patient anxiety and concern by adequate previous instructions. The procedure and the informed consent have to be clearly explained to the patient. Patients should be put at ease as much as possible, by having the different options and the expected results of the procedure explained. Ideally, an electrically driven comfortable examining table should be used to tilt or elevate the patient as required.

It is important, therefore, to have the appropriate instrumentation displayed, a knowledgeable assistant, appropriate informed consent, and equipment for treatment of hypotension or other unwanted side effects or problems requiring resuscitation measures.

Vaginoscopic Hysteroscopy

This procedure was first proposed by Bettocchi in 1995.[3] It is performed without cervical dilatation, use of vaginal speculum or cervical tenaculum. The only instrumentation required is a small-diameter, continuous flow hysteroscope, that allows semirigid 5 Fr. instruments through its channel, that can be used to grasp, cut, biopsy, vaporize, or coagulate (More information about the appropriate instruments in Chapter 8).

The patient selected for hysteroscopy requires a bimanual pelvic examination to assess the position, size and shape of the uterus as well as the characteristics of the cervix (consistency, position).

The vagina and cervix are disinfected with an antiseptic solution such as clorhexidine. No systemic sedatives or medications are required as the procedure is practically painless.

The hysteroscope is introduced into the vagina until the external cervical os is seen and then, gently advanced through the cervical canal into the uterine cavity. The uterine distention is maintained by the pressure exerted by two connected 3-liters bags of saline situated 1 meter above the level of the vagina, achieving a pressure around 70 mm Hg approximately. The examination begins by slowly and systematically following the small microcavity produced by the liquid in front of the endoscope. Once the endocervical canal is completely explored, the endoscope is advanced in the internal cervical os to allow a panoramic evaluation of the uterine cavity, including the uterotubal cornua and tubal ostia. The endocervical canal is examined during the withdrawal of the instrument. The findings can be explained to the patient observing the video monitor.

Office procedures should be simple, expeditious and comfortable to the patient to achieve the full value of the technique—decreasing costs and inconveniences to the patient and to the gynecologist, allowing better utilization of resources.

Failure rates of vaginoscopic approach range from 0 to 2.4% and most of them are due to failure of the technique. Even cervical stenosis can be easily managed by means of the endoscopic scissors or graspers to find the right way.

Anesthesia for Diagnostic Procedures

The use of a rigid hysteroscope for outpatient hysteroscopy has very good optical properties, requires little time for the procedure, and has an excellent success rate. However, women experience more discomfort with rigid hysteroscopes. Comparing normal saline with CO_2 as distending media, resulted in similar pain during the procedure, less pain immediately after the procedure, greater patient satisfaction and a trend towards lower risk of vasovagal reaction. Diagnostic outpatient hysteroscopy using 4-5 mm diameter hysteroscopes has a 96-98% success rate. The most common complaint responsible for failure is severe pain. This is the cause, by which several authors report improved rates of office hysteroscopic feasibility using paracervical block.[4]

Pain can be alleviated by a variety of medications and techniques including analgesics, local anesthetics, conscious sedation and general anesthesia (Chapter 18).

Local Anesthesia

The reduction of pain in the conscious patient can be achieved by a variety of perioperative medications (TABLE 3.1). Analgesia for the cervix and uterus can

Table 3.1: Perioperative medications in diagnostic hysteroscopy

- Non-steroidal anti-inflammatory drugs
  - Indomethacin 100 mg rectal suppository 1 hours preoperatively
  - Ketorolac 10 mg IM or 30 mg IV intraoperatively
- Anxiolytics
  - Midazolam 7.5 mg VO preoperatively
- Analgesics
  - Paracetamol 1 g VO
  - Petidine 100 mg IV

be achieved by several gels and sprays. Lignocaine gel applied to the cervix did not reduce pain associated with hysteroscopy, while lidocaine aerosol spray in the cervix was effective in reducing pain and discomfort. Pain was not alleviated in patients receiving 5 mL of 2% intrauterine lidocaine for outpatient diagnostic hysteroscopy or endometrial biopsy. In addition, lidocaine did not prevent the occurrence of vasovagal reactions.[5]

The advantages of paracervical analgesia in hysteroscopic surgery remain in doubt. Unlike the uterine wall, the endometrium and endometrial polyps are insensitive to pain. Dilatation of the cervix is usually painful. A recent review of available evidence concluded that, it is reasonable to use nonsteroidal antiinflammatory drugs 1 hour before the procedure, if not, otherwise contraindicated and topical analgesia before the insertion of the hysteroscope.

Anyway, it must be remembered that the most important prophylactic measure for the pain is the prior correct explanation of the procedure, and the gentle manipulation of the cervix.

Cervical Priming

In some cases, especially in cervical atrophy, scarring or anatomic stenosis, when diagnostic hysteroscopy has not been possible, it is wise to schedule the patient for another diagnostic exploration with the prior application of some agents or cervical primers that can facilitate the procedure. This is the case for misoprostol, a prostaglandin analog that, mediated through the liberation of the nitric oxide that is produced, softens the cervix and facilitates the access to the cavity.

The use of oral misoprostol, 400 μg, given 12 hours prior to diagnostic hysteroscopy was shown to be beneficial over placebo in the ease of cervical dilatation.[6] This benefit was seen in both premenopausal and postmenopausal women, and in those pretreated with gonadotrophin-releasing hormone (GnRH-α).

Vaginal misoprostol, 200 μg, given 9-10 hours prior to hysteroscopy in premenopausal women, increased ease of cervical dilation, facilitated the procedure and resulted in fewer complications compared with placebo.[7] It should be taken into account that, when an endometrial polyp is present, the uterine contractions make the polyp congestive and bleeds, thus difficulty the vision.

The most frequent adverse effects of misoprostol are gastrointestinal events, diarrhea and mild abdominal pain. Less common are nausea and/or vomiting, flatulence, cramps in the lower abdomen, vaginal bleeding, headache, or fever. All these adverse effects are dose-related and often resolve after misoprostol discontinuation. As the vaginal route is associated with fewer complications, this is our preferred route. The tablets must be moistened, and divided prior to the insertion to achieve a better absorption.

Office Electrical Procedures

A major innovation in hysteroscopic surgery, used to minimize the risk of electrical burns, has been the introduction of bipolar electrosurgery.

Intrauterine surgery using a versatile coaxial bipolar electrode (VersaPoint, Gynecare Inc., Somerville, NJ, USA) in normal saline solution was introduced in 1997.[8] The electrosurgical system consists of a high-frequency electrosurgical generator and coaxial bipolar electrodes designed to either cut, desiccate (coagulate), or vaporize tissue. The 1.7 mm diameter (5 Fr), 36 cm long, flexible bipolar electrodes can be used through any operating hysteroscope.[9] There are three electrode tips available: A spring to vaporize, a twizzle to cut, and a ball to coagulate tissue. These *wise* electrodes are preset to a determined output of energy each, so the mistakes in the current

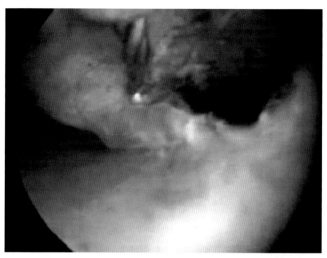

Figure 3.1: The Versapoint twizzle electrode (cutting)

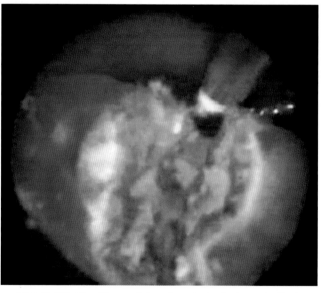

Figure 3.2: The Versapoint spring electrode (vaporization)

selection are minimized and can only function in a normal saline environment (FIGURES 3.1 and 3.2).

The VersaPoint system can be used to treat a variety of intrauterine lesions. The correct place of this attractive instrument is the one between the procedures that can be accomplished with the semi-rigid scissors and graspers (endometrial biopsies, small polyps, mild adhesions or small septa), and the ones that are to be performed in the theatre (big polyps, submucous myomas, total septa, Asherman's syndrome). A summary of the characteristics and advantages of the VersaPoint system are described in the TABLE 3.2.

Table 3.2: Characteristics and advantages of the VersaPoint system

- Requires no additional dilatation (5.5 mm)
- Office surgery, "see and treat"
- "Touch" technique
- Uses normal (0.9%) saline solution
- Low voltage, bipolar current
- Preset "intelligent" electrodes
- Vaporizes tissue, eliminating the necessity for tissue removal

SPECIFIC COMPLICATIONS

Vasovagal Syndrome (Chapter 15)

Vasovagal syndrome was reported in 15 of 2079 (0.72%) women undergoing outpatient hysteroscopy without analgesia. Severe pain was often associated with vasovagal reactions. The risk was higher with the use of a rigid hysteroscope (1.85%) and CO_2 as the distending media (2.3%), regardless of the indication for hysteroscopy. Other studies have reported rates of vasovagal syndrome during office hysteroscopy ranging from 1.0 to 1.7%.[10]

Topical anesthesia and smaller hysteroscopes (3.5 mm) decrease the risk of vasovagal syndrome. The office should have an established emergency protocol for all patients scheduled for invasive procedures, such as hysteroscopy. The office staff should know the protocol, location of an emergency cart, and ensure that emergency equipment is readily available and working. Most patients with a vasovagal reaction recover simply by stopping the procedure. Others may require steep Trendelenburg's position. If the vasovagal reaction is persistent, 1 ampule of subcutaneous atropine helps for a rapid recovery. If severe, the atropine must be administered intravenously.

Uterine Perforation

A prospective multicenter study involving 13600 hysteroscopic procedures reported perforation rate during diagnostic hysteroscopy of 0.13%. A survey of physicians learning and performing endometrial resection reported that 52% of uterine perforations occurred during the first five cases and 33% occurred during the first case.[11]

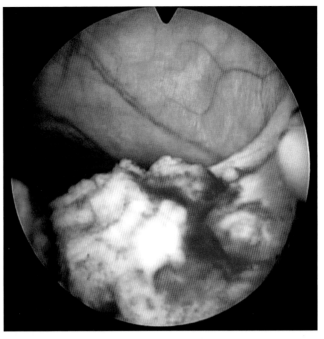

Figure 3.3: Uterine perforation

When this occurs, the patient must be admitted and observed carefully. Antibiotics and analgesics as well as total diet restriction must be ordered (FIGURE 3.3). As most of the perforations in diagnostic hysteroscopy occur during dilation, no electric current is involved in the accident, and an expectant management can be sufficient. If the patient worsens, a diagnostic laparoscopy should be considered.

Cancer Cells Dissemination

The prevalence of endometrial carcinoma in women presenting with abnormal uterine bleeding is 10-15%. Diagnostic hysteroscopy with tissue sampling is a feasible and widely accepted procedure for the assessment of abnormal uterine bleeding (FIGURE 3.4).

Recently, the safety of diagnostic hysteroscopy preceding surgical treatment of endometrial carcinoma has raised concern.[12] Several studies[13,14] indicate that the risk of positive peritoneal washings in patients with endometrial carcinoma, is higher after diagnostic hysteroscopy has been performed, suggesting that hysteroscopy can cause abdominal dissemination of malignant cells in patients with endometrial carcinoma. A higher risk (up to 17%) of positive peritoneal washings after hysteroscopy was described

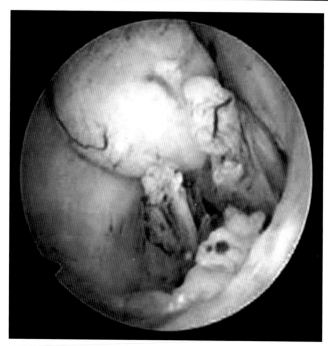

Figure 3.4: Focal adenocarcinoma in the left ostium

Table 3.3: Indications for diagnostic hysteroscopy

- Evaluate unexplained abnormal uterine bleeding in premenopausal patients
- Evaluate recurrent uterine bleeding in postmenopausal patients with atrophic endometrium
- Diagnosis and stratification of endocervical and endometrial carcinoma
- Diagnose intrauterine pathology suspected in other image techniques (TVUS, SIS, MRI)
- Evaluate infertile patients who have abnormal hysterosalpingogram
- Recurrent pregnancy wastage
- Infertility in cases of repeated failed IVF cycles
- Follow-up after hysteroscopic surgery
- Follow-up after hormonal treatment for hyperplasia
- Preoperatively in hysteroscopic surgery
- Persistent postpartum or post-abortion bleeding
- Detection and extraction of foreign bodies in vagina (atrophic, children)
- Extraction of IUD in pregnant women

after a prolonged interval to surgery in several studies, but was not confirmed in other studies. Obermair[14] found a higher disease-free survival rate in patients with FIGO stage I, difference in prognosis was shown.

Anyway, the studies are not conclusive and, until more evidence is available, there is no reason to avoid diagnostic hysteroscopy.[15] Meanwhile, it is wise to reduce the intrauterine pressure during the diagnostic hysteroscopy to a minimum and to leave the outflow channel of the hysteroscope continuously open during the procedure, to avoid the opening of the tubal ostia.

INDICATIONS FOR OFFICE HYSTEROSCOPY

In order to perform hysteroscopy, the surgeon must have a correct indication for the procedure, obtain informed consent, access and distend the uterine cavity, and use appropriate instruments to guide surgery. Adequate training and surgical expertise, including complete knowledge of endoscopic surgical principles and equipment are of paramount importance.[16] The gynecologist must also understand the serious complications of hysteroscopy to facilitate

prevention, fast recognition and appropriate management, when complications occur.

During the last years, there have been refinements, innovations and advancements in surgical techniques, instrumentation and indications of hysteroscopy. These were designed to minimize patient discomfort and inconvenience, reduce complications, and optimize patient safety and clinical outcomes.[17]

The following clinical situations account for the majority of the indications for office hysteroscopy (TABLE 3.3).

- Unexplained uterine bleeding in either premenopausal ovulatory women, premenopausal anovulatory women who fail medical therapy, and postmenopausal bleeding
- Infertility evaluation: Routine triage, pre-IVF evaluation, follow-up evaluation for an abnormal hysterosalpingogram or indeterminate saline infusion sonography (SIS), recurrent IVF failures, or evaluation of recurrent miscarriage
- Evaluation of congenital uterine malformations including unicollate uterus, uterus didelphys, and septate or bicornuate uteri.
- Postoperative evaluation of myomectomy (abdominal and hysteroscopic) or evaluation of cesarean section scars (FIGURE 3.5).

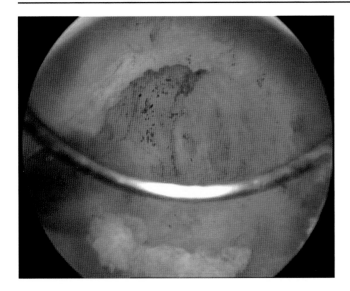

Figure 3.5: The myometrial "bed" after hysteroscopic myomectomy

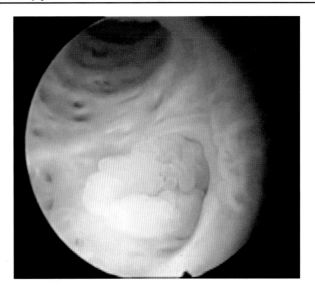

Figure 3.6: Early endocervical carcinoma

• Preoperative endometrial evaluation of women undergoing abdominal myomectomy, endometrial ablation, or adhesiolysis
• Preoperative office hysteroscopy is useful in evaluating the extent of disease (FIGURE 3.6) or follow-up after treatment in women with suspected endometrial hyperplasia (FIGURE 3.7)
• Persistent postpartum, postmolar, or postabortion bleeding
  – Extraction of foreign bodies in stenotic vaginas, as children, virgins
  – Extraction of IUD in pregnant women.

The procedures that can be performed in an office setting during hysteroscopy are shown in TABLE 3.4.

Abnormal Uterine Bleeding

Patients frequently visit gynecologists because of abnormal uterine bleeding. About one-third of

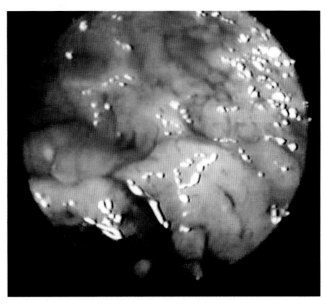

Figure 3.7: Stromal hypervascularization after progestogen therapy

Table 3.4: Office procedures in diagnostic hysteroscopy

• Directed biopsies
• Remove endometrial polyps
• Locate and retrieve "lost" intrauterine devices and other foreign bodies
• Correction of endocervical canal stenosis
• Resect uterine septum
• Resect mild intrauterine adhesions
• Hysteroscopic sterilization

gynecological patients have this problem; among peri- and postmenopausal patients, it accounts for 69% of gynecological consultations. A decade ago, the diagnostic measure most frequently applied in the treatment of bleeding disorders was D & C. According to different reports, the accuracy of findings on curettage is between 10 and 25%, since some of the lesions are small (e.g. polyps, submucosal myoma, early neoplastic processes), even an experienced surgeon, finds difficult to remove no more than 50% of the endometrium during curettage.[18] Sampling by hysteroscopy eliminates the false negatives of these blind techniques.

Abnormal uterine bleeding is the main indication for hysteroscopy, particularly in premenopausal women with persistent abnormal bleeding, and bleeding in peri- and postmenopausal patients. Direct visualization of the uterine cavity increases the accuracy of diagnoses of suspected intrauterine pathology by offering the opportunity to obtain selected biopsies of abnormal or suspicious areas of endometrium (FIGURE 3.8). Although suction aspiration of the endometrium is used routinely in the evaluation of patients with abnormal uterine bleeding, the accuracy and completeness of this evaluation may be limited in the presence of submucous leiomyomas or endometrial polyps and focal areas of endometrium, particularly at the uterotubal junctions.[19]

Endometrial polyps and fibroids are common causes of abnormal uterine bleeding. Patients evaluated with TVUS measurements of the endometrium, may have altered endometrial echoes due to the intracavitary mass. In addition, false negative sampling errors occur in such patients.[20,21]

Hysteroscopy allows targeted biopsies of abnormal or suspicious areas of endometrium to be taken. Direct visualization of the uterine cavity enhances evaluation of architectural distortions, allowing visual exploration of the entire uterine cavity. Because visualization alone cannot adequately distinguish between benign and malignant, or premalignant endometrial lesions, biopsies of these lesions are particularly important (FIGURE 3.9).

When the endometrial biopsy is insufficient, indeterminate, or cannot be performed, there are two additional ways to evaluate the patient with an underlying risk of neoplasia. Therefore, it is imperative that patients with persistent, unexplained bleeding obtain an accurate diagnosis.

To diagnose endometrial cancer, which occurs in 10% of women with postmenopausal bleeding, diagnostic testing is essential. However, its detection rate increases with age, especially in women greater

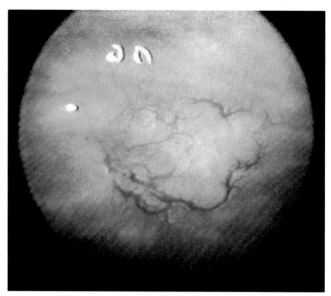

Figure 3.8: Endometrial intraepithelial neoplasia (in situ pre-invasive state of the uterine serous carcinoma)

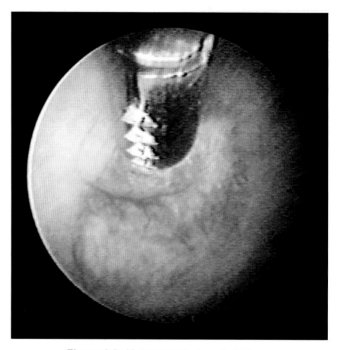

Figure 3.9: Hysteroscopic targeted biopsy

than 60 years. It can present as a variegated, multifocal lesion, or an isolated lesion within a polyp.[22]

The usefulness of TVUS in managing bleeding disorders is related to menopausal status. TVUS is an excellent initial diagnostic method for ruling out endometrial abnormalities in postmenopausal patients with bleeding because of the well defined and narrow range of normal endometrial echo. It is of limited use in premenopausal women with irregular bleeding because of the wide range of normal endometrial thickness.

Several studies have shown that endometrial thickness, as measured by TVUS, is related to endometrial pathology in postmenopausal women.[23-25] Measuring the thickness of the endometrial echo is important in postmenopausal women because it correlates with potential abnormalities of the endometrium. During the menopause, the endometrium is primarily composed of a thin, basalis layer.

Measurement of the endometrial echo represents the apposition of the two basal layers. A normal postmenopausal endometrium is rather monotonous, rarely changes in appearance or thickness. Granberg[23] evaluated 205 patients with postmenopausal bleeding utilizing TVUS and endometrial biopsy. Patients with endometrial atrophy diagnosed by endometrial biopsy had a mean endometrial thickness of 3.4 +/-1.2 mm, while those with endometrial cancer, had a mean endometrial thickness of 18.2 +/-6.2 mm. Using a cutoff of 5 mm, they found a positive predictive value for hyperplasia or neoplasia of 87.3%.

The Nordic trial, published by Karlsson,[24] involving 1168 women with postmenopausal bleeding is one of the largest to analyze the sensitivity and specificity of transvaginal endometrial thickness (from 1 to 72 mm) against histologic findings obtained by D & C. In postmenopausal women, TVUS had a sensitivity of 94% in diagnosing an endometrial abnormality and a specificity of 78% using a cutoff of 5 mm for the endometrial echo.

When a focal lesion is detected by TVUS in a symptomatic patient, it may be more appropriate to perform operative hysteroscopy in order to remove a focal lesion, rather than relying on the report of a "blind biopsy".

The patients with postmenopausal bleeding must be evaluated by TVUS in the first place. When the endometrium is 5 mm or thinner in TVUS and is the first episode, there is no need for further evaluation (FIGURE 3.10). When the endometrium is abnormally thicker, or is technically immeasurable, further

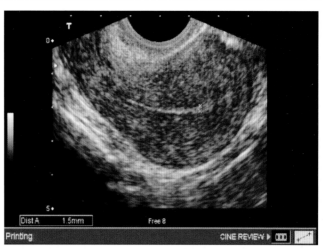

Figure 3.10: Sonographic atrophic endometrium

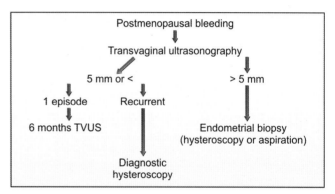

Figure 3.11: Algorithm for postmenopausal bleeding

evaluation is required.[25] If an intracavitary polyp or fibroid is found, hysteroscopic removal is recommended. If there is a focal thickening of the endometrium, diagnostic hysteroscopy or endometrial sampling with an aspiration cannula is required. In patients with a negative TVUS and recurrent bleeding, an office hysteroscopy would be the method of choice (FIGURE 3.11).

The prevalence of menstrual complaints increases every decade after age 20, and peaks in the mid 40's to 50's. Increasingly, as women live longer and electively utilize hormone replacement therapy (HRT) or tamoxifen (FIGURE 3.12), the prevalence of postmenopausal bleeding will increase and require evaluation.[26] The etiology of abnormal bleeding requires vigilant assessment, despite the fact that benign or normal findings will be generally encountered. Nagele reported abnormal findings in only 48% of 2500 outpatient diagnostic

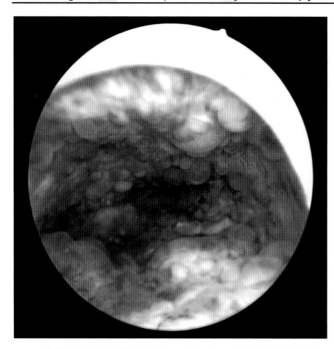

Figure 3.12: Effect of tamoxifen in endometrium

hysteroscopies performed.[27] However, if benign pathology such as polyps and submucosal or intramural fibroids are identified and treated hysteroscopically, high patient satisfaction is achieved.

Hysteroscopy for Fertility Disorders

A prospective randomized study concluded that office hysteroscopy, SIS and HSG were statistically equivalent regarding evaluation of the uterine cavity in infertile women (Chapter 5). However, in view of the low complication rates, minimal time require-ment, and negligible effect on the postoperative course associated with hysteroscopy, it should become a routine procedure in all infertile women undergoing diagnostic laparoscopy. A significant percentage of women have intracavitary lesions that may impair the success of fertility treatments.

Uterine Septum (Chapter 11)

Hysteroscopy with concomitant laparoscopy is considered to be the gold standard for diagnosis and treatment of the septate uterus. Incidental finding of a septate uterus is not an indication for surgical

intervention in the absence of infertility or adverse obstetrical outcome. The septum can be divided by hysteroscopic scissors, electrosurgery (monopolar or bipolar) or laser fibres under local, general or no anesthesia at all. A residual septum of less than 1 cm does not appear to have an adverse effect on reproductive outcomes.[28]

Intrauterine Adhesions

Intrauterine adhesions may occur after trauma to the basalis layer of the endometrium by vigorous diagnostic or postpartum curettage, endomyo-metritis, multiple myomectomies, endometrial ablation, and pelvic radiation (Chapter 17). The occurrence of such adhesions may result in decrease or absence of menstruation, infertility and pregnancy disorders such as recurrent pregnancy loss, placenta accreta and intrauterine growth restriction. The risk of uterine perforation during operative hysteroscopy for adhesiolysis has been reported as 7.5%. Hysteroscopic adhesiolysis requires the use of small diameter hysteroscopes. The procedure can be performed using scissors, laser fibres or the VersaPoint electrode.[29]

Hysteroembryoscopy

Investigations following unexplained fetal demise in early pregnancy include imaging as well as tissue and biochemical examination, postevacuation (Chapter 16). Frequently, the cause of fetal death remains elusive and becomes a major source of frustration and guilt for parents and healthcare providers. Anatomical fetal deformities, surface skin lesions and cord accidents can be identified, and selective targeted embryo biopsies undertaken.[30]

Proximal Tubal Sterilization

Hysteroscopic methods of tubal occlusion were explored in the 1970s. They included the use of formed-in-place silicon plugs, hydrogelic devices, laser fibres or radiofrequency electrodes to coagulate the tubal ostia. Office hysteroscopic sterilization was accomplished in approximately 90% of women and no significant complications were noted.

The Essure System

A permanent, irreversible sterilization device, Essure™ (Conceptus Inc., San Carlos, CA, USA) is a dynamically expanding micro-insert coil that is placed in the proximal section of the fallopian tube using a hysteroscopic approach (Chapter 14). By 3 months, fibrosis completely occludes the fallopian tube.[31]

The Adiana System

The Adiana catheter system is another hysteroscopic tubal sterilization procedure currently undergoing evaluation. During the procedure, low-power (<1 W) bipolar energy is delivered to the superficial endosalpinx and a porous matrix is left in the lumen. Tubal occlusion by fibrosis is completed within 3 months. An advantage of this system is the need to cannulate only 1 cm of the intramural fallopian tube. The bilateral first-attempt access rate for this procedure was 94.5% (241/255 women), and over 50% of patients were treated using local anesthesia without sedation. The mean total hysteroscopy time was 14 minutes. In 1000 women, months of exposure to intercourse, there have been no pregnancies and no significant complications related to the procedure or the device.[32]

REFERENCES

1. Bradley L, Widrich T. State-of-the flexible hysteroscopy for office gynecologic evaluation. J Am Assoc Gynecol Laparosc 1995;3:263-7.
2. Pérez-Medina T, Bajo JM, Martinez-Cortés L, Castellanos P, Perez de Avila I. Six thousand office diagnostic-operative hysteroscopies. Int J Gynecol Obstet 2000;71:33-8.
3. Bettocchi S, Selvaggi L. A vaginoscopic approach to reduce the pain of office hysteroscopy. J Am Assoc Gynecol Laparosc 1997;4:255-8.
4. Readman E, Maher PJ. Pain relief and outpatient hysteroscopy: A literature review. J Am Assoc Gynecol Laparosc 2004;11:315-9.
5. Hitchings S. Paracervical anesthesia in outpatient hysteroscopy: A randomized double-blind placebo controlled trial. BJOG 2000;107:143-4.
6. Valente EP, de Amorim MM, Costa AA, de Miranda DV. Vaginal misoprostol prior to diagnostic hysteroscopy in patients in reproductive age: A randomized clinical trial. J Minim Invasive Gynecol 2008;15:452-8.
7. Darwish AM, Ahmad AM, Mohammad AM. Cervical priming prior to operative hysteroscopy: A randomized comparison of laminaria versus misoprostol. Hum Reprod 2004;19:2391-4.
8. Bettocchi S, Nappi L, Ceci O, Selvaggi L. What does 'diagnostic hysteroscopy' mean today? The role of the new techniques. J Am Assoc Gynecol Laparosc 1997;4:255-8.
9. Cicinelli E. Diagnostic minihysteroscopy with vaginoscopic approach: Rationale and advantages. J Minim Invasive Gynecol 2005;12:396-400.
10. Agostini A, Bretelle F, Ronda I, Roger V, Cravello L, Blanc B. Risk of vasovagal syndrome during outpatient hysteroscopy. J Am Gynecol Laparosc 2004;11:245-7.
11. Bradley LD. Complications in hysteroscopy: Prevention, treatment and legal risk. Curr Opin Obstet Gynecol 2002;14:409-15.
12. Solima E, Brusati V, Ditto A, Kusamura S, Martinelli F, Hazonet F, Carcangiu ML, Maccauro M, Raspagliesi F. Hysteroscopy in endo1metrial cancer: New method to evaluate transtubal leakage of saline distension medium. Am J Obstet Gynecol 2008;198:214-14.
13. Yazbeck C, Dhainaut C, Batallan A, Benifla JL, Thoury A, Madelenat P. Diagnostic hysteroscopy and risk of peritoneal dissemination of tumor cells. Gynecol Obstet Fertil 2005;33:247-52.
14. Obermair A, Geramou M, Gucer F, Demison U, Graf AH, Kapshammer E, Neunteufel W, Frech I, Kaider A, Kainz C. Does hysteroscopy facilitate tumor cell dissemination? Incidence of peritoneal cytology from patients with early stage endometrial carcinoma following dilatation and curettage (D&C) versus hysteroscopy and D&C. Cancer 2000;88:139-43.
15. Biewenga P, de Block S, Birnie E. Does diagnostic hysteroscopy in patients with stage I endometrial carcinoma cause positive peritoneal washings? Gynecol Oncol 2004;93:194-8.
16. Black JE, Hudson HJ, Duffy SR. Standard setting for outpatient gynecology procedures: A multidisciplinary framework for implementation. Best Pract Res Clin Obstet Gynecol 2005;19:793-806.
17. Vilos GA, Abu-Rafea B. New developments in ambulatory hysteroscopic surgery. Best Pract Res Clin Obstet Gynecol 2005;19:724-42.
18. Neuwirth RS. Hysteroscopy. Major Problems in Obstetrics and Gynecology 1975;8:103-13.
19. Weber A, Belinson J, Bradley LD, Piedmonte M. Vaginal ultrasound versus endometrial biopsy in women with postmenopausal bleeding. Am J Obstet Gynecol 1997;4:924-9.
20. Emanuel MH, Verdel MJ, Wamsteker K, Lammes FB. A prospective comparison of transvaginal ultrasonography and diagnostic hysteroscopy in the evaluation of patients with abnormal uterine bleeding: clinical implications. Am J Obstet Gynecol 1995; 172:547-52.
21. Bradley LD, Falcone T, Magen AB. Radiographic Imaging Techniques for the Diagnosis of Abnormal Uterine Bleeding. Obstet Gynecol Clin North Am 2000;27:245-76.
22. Triolo O, Antico F, Palmara V, Benedetto V, Panama S, Nicotina PA. Hysteroscopic findings of endometrial carcinoma. Evaluation of 104 cases. Eur J Gynecol Oncol 2005;26:434-6.
23. Granberg S, Wikland M, Karlsson B, Norstrom A, Friberg LG. Endometrial thickness as measured by endovaginal ultrasonography for identifying endometrial abnormality. Am J Obstet Gynecol 1991;64:47-52.
24. Karlsson B, Granberg S, Wikland M, Ylostalo P, Torvid K, Marshal K. Transvaginal ultrasonography of the endometrium in women with postmenopausal bleeding. A Nordic multicenter study. Am J Obstet Gynecol 1995;172:1488-94.

25. Dijkhuizen FP, Brolmann HA, Potters AE, Bongers MY, Heintz AP. The accuracy of transvaginal ultrasonography in the diagnosis of endometrial abnormalities. Obstet Gynecol 1996; 87:345-9.

26. Nand SL, Webster MA, Baber R. et al. Bleeding pattern and endometrial changes during continuous combined hormone replacement therapy. Obstet Gynecol 1998;91:678-84.

27. Nagele F, O'Connor H, Davies A, Badawy A, Mohamed H, Magos A: 2500 Outpatient Diagnostic Hysteroscopies, Obstet Gynecol 1996;88:87-92.

28. Bettocchi S, Ceci O, Nappi L, Di Venere R, Masciopinto V, Pansini V, Pinto L, Santoro A, Cormio G. Operative office hysteroscopy without anesthesia: Analysis of 4863 cases performed with mechanical instruments. J Am Assoc Gynecol Laparosc. 2004;11:59-61.

29. Valle RF. Intrauterine Adhesions (Asherman's Syndrome). In, Office and Operative Hysteroscopy. Marty R, Blanc B, deMontgolfier R (Eds). Springer-Verlag. New York. 2002;229-42.

30. Ferro J, Martinez MC, Lara C, Pellicer A, Remohi J, Serra V. Improved accuracy of hysteroembryoscopic biopsies for karyotyping early missed abortions. Fertil Steril 2003;80:1260-4.

31. Kerin JF, Cooper JM, Price T, Herendael BJ, Cayuela-Font E, Cher D, Carignan CS. Hysteroscopic sterilization using a micro-insert device: Results of a multicentre Phase II study. Hum Reprod 2003;18:1223-30.

32. Abbot J. Transcervical sterilization. Curr Opin Obstet Gynecol 2007;19:325-30.

4

The Role of Ultrasonography, Doppler Ultrasonography, 3D Ultrasonography, Hysterosonography, Magnetic Resonance Imaging and Hysterosalpingography in the Detection of Intrauterine Anomalies

Tirso Pérez-Medina
Francisco Salazar Arquero
Miguel-Angel Huertas

The advantages and disadvantages of each imaging technique to be used in it the appropriate clinical setting must be known. For instance, hysterosalpingography (HSG) evaluates correctly the patency and architecture of fallopian tubes, the uterine cavity suboptimally, and poorly the myometrium. Magnetic resonance imaging (MRI) does not evaluate tubal patency, but provides superb visualization of the uterine cavity and myometrium, particularly in women with large uterus.

In this chapter, the findings of uterine lesions assessed with conventional, Doppler and 3D transvaginal ultrasound, hysterosonography, MRI, and hysterosalpingography are discussed.

TRANSVAGINAL ULTRASONOGRAPHY

Fibroids

The sonographic aspect of uterine fibroids is quite varied depending on their location. Fibroids are difficult to locate because they transmit the sound poorly, attenuate the sound beam, and have ill-defined borders. Fibroids may obscure endometrial measurements when transvaginal ultrasonography (TVUS) is used, because they create an irregular interface between the endometrium and myometrium. In addition, fibroids may vary in appearance, having calcified, hypoechoic, echogenic, isoechoic, and mixed echogenic patterns.

The aspect also depends on, if they have caused secondary changes or not, and the relative quantity of muscle fibers and stroma that they are formed of. They may appear as iso, hyper or hypoechogenic.[1] When isoechogenic, they may be identified when they deform the uterine contour (subserous) or when they displace the endometrium (submucous). If they are intramural they may be difficult to identify and color Doppler may be used for this purpose (FIGURE 4.1). If they are hypoechogenic they are easier to see because they are differentiated from the healthy myometrium, even when they are small (FIGURE 4.2). When hyperechogenic, they are very homogenous and are clearly identified from the rest of the myometrium. The acoustic transmission is poor. In most cases fibromyomas are heterogeneous, with variable echogenicity, but always with precise limits.

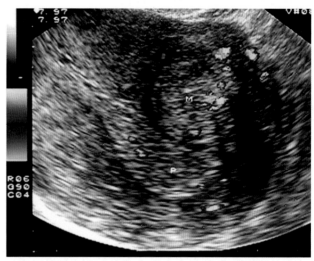

Figure 4.1: Classical TVUS intramural myoma

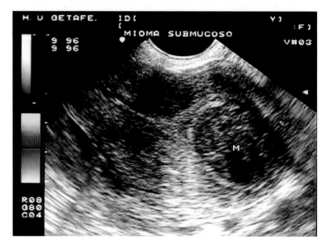

Figure 4.2: Submucous myoma displacing the endometrial midline

Sometimes a pseudocapsule may be seen, which is a sign that the lesion is benign and helps the sonographer and the gynecologist with differential diagnosis.[2] Hyperechogenicity usually corresponds to regions of fibrosis. Generally, the larger the myoma, the more heterogeneous is its structure due to areas of degeneration and necrosis which show sonoluscent images.

With TVUS the number of false positive diagnoses has decreased.[3] Years ago, the confusion between diagnoses of fibromyomas and ovarian pathology were frequent. Nowadays, the exact number and delimitation of the tumors is easier. This helps prepare for surgery, decreasing unexpected surgical situations. Sonography also helps in visualizing different types of uterine fibroid tumor degeneration that appears when they grow and are not removed.[4] Sonoluscent areas appear in the interior (haline degeneration or fat) or echorefringent areas of the periphery of the tumors (calcification of the fibromyoma).

Adenomyosis

The most exact diagnostic criteria for adenomyosis with sonography is the presence of a thickened uterus, asymmetric with heterogeneous myometrium, spotted with heterogeneous echogenicity, although mostly hypoechogenic. Sometimes adenomyosis is associated with the presence of small intramyometrial cystic images (FIGURE 4.3). These cystic images correspond to intramyometrial endometrial glands that become visible due to focal hemorrhages. In 4% of the cases, adenomyosis is seen as a heterogeneous intramyometrial zone without hypoechogenic areas.

Adenomyosis produces an alteration in the area between the basal myometrium and the endometrium. This alteration causes distortion of the subendometrial line that does not allow the sonographic distinction between the endometrium and the subjacent myometrium.[4] Depending on the extension of the adenomyosis, the alteration of the myometrium-endometrium junction can oscillate between the erasing of the junction limits to the presence of linear furrows in the area, or loosely limited echogenic nodes. Atri et al, in a sonographic study on uteri obtained from hysterectomies, assessed the echostructure of the myometrium-endometrium junction and they found the presence of undefined borders or subendometrial lineal furrows were more frequent in uteri with adenomyosis increasing the positive predictive value of sonography.[5]

Endometrial Polyps

The diagnosis of endometrial polyps (EP) is of fundamental importance because they cannot be diagnosed by physical exploration, and curettage may be unsuccessful which implicates persistence or repeated symptoms.

Transvaginal ultrasonography has meant an important advancement in non-invasive diagnosis of EP which show a series of characteristic signs.[5]

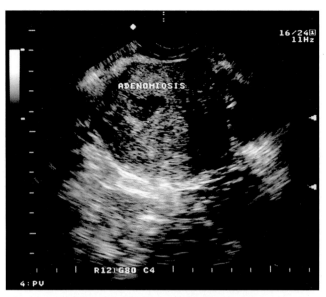

Figure 4.3: Hypoechogenic adenomyoma deep in the myometrium

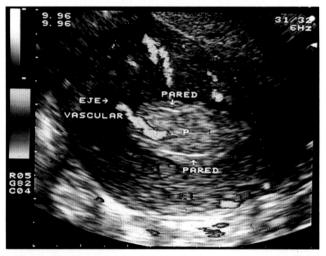

Figure 4.4: Endometrial polyp. The hyperechogenic endometrial line acts as a "trigger" for the diagnosis (arrows)

A diagnosis of EP is suspected when a hyperechogenic image with regular contours, occupying the uterine lumen either partly or in full, outlining the endometrial walls on which it rested, surrounded by a small hypoechogenic halo is observed (FIGURE 4.4). EP widen the endometrial echo and create the appearance of increased endometrial thickness with TVUS. EP appear well defined and are uniformly homogeneous or hyperechoic.

A thin, hyperechogenic line, reflecting the interface between the endometrium and the polyp, translating the displacement of the endometrial line, acts as a trigger for the diagnosis and states the diagnosis of EP. The sensitivity of TVUS in the diagnosis of the EP is 92.3%; the specificity 90.2% the positive predictive value 64.2%, and the negative predictive value 98.4%.[6]

Uterine Malformations

Sonography is useful in evaluating internal and external uterine morphology as is magnetic resonance imaging. Sonography is less expensive, faster and more readily available, and so it is the indicated first election method.

Sonographic study of uterine abnormalities should begin with an abdominal scan, with the bladder partially full because if the bladder is too full the morphology of the uterus may vary. The contour and fundus of the uterus is examined to screen lateral masses that could correspond to rudimentary or to a contralateral uterus. The endometrial cavity and its contents may also be visualized as well as the possible existence of another complete cavity as in a didelphys uterus or partial division as a bicornuate or arcuate uterus (FIGURE 4.5).

In case of endometrial cavity assessment, TVUS almost always allows us better resolution and delimitation, especially with minimally rudimentary uteri with little endometrium that could lead to a missed image in an abdominal scan.[7]

Intrauterine Synechiae (Adhesions)

Destruction of the basal layer of the endometrium may result in scarring and development of bands of scar tissue (synechiae) in the uterine cavity. This damage of endometrium may occur, as a result, in a too vigorous curettage of an advanced pregnancy. Tuberculosis may also cause uterine adhesions. Menstrual pattern is characterized by amenorrhea or hypomenorrhea. Ultrasound scan of a patient with Asherman's syndrome shows a mixed picture: In some parts of uterine cavity no endometrium can be visualized; and in others; the endometrium appears normal. If there are adhesions in the uterine cavity, they are visualized as hyperechoic bridges (FIGURE 4.6). Intrauterine adhesions do not display increased vascularity on color Doppler examination.

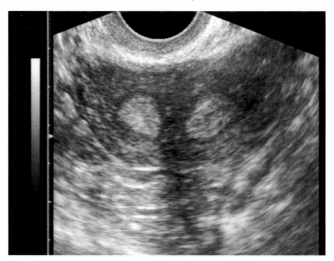

Figure 4.5: Double cavity uterus. It is not possible to distinguish between a bicornuate and a septate uterus

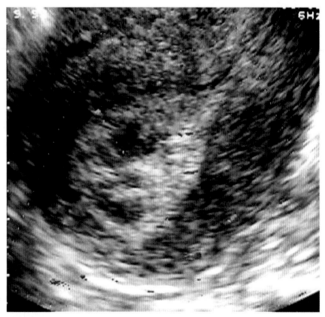

Figure 4.6: Ultrasound scan of a patient with Asherman's syndrome. Adhesions in the uterine cavity are visualized as hyperechoic bridges and do not display increased vascularity on color Doppler examination

They are better visualized during menstruation when intracavitary fluid outlines them.

Endometrial Carcinoma

The ultrasonographic measure of the endometrial thickness is a determination easy to perform, objective, and able to establish a cut off point, corresponding to the atrophic endometrium, below which it does not appear malignant pathology. There are many studies in the bibliography that show a high accuracy for this sonographic parameter, with rates of sensitivity that varies between a 68 and 100% and specificity between 43 and 89%.[8]

In the classical study by Karlsson,[9] a multicentric Nordic study, TVUS and D&C are compared in 1168 women with postmenopausal bleeding. Establishing as cut point, an endometrial thickness < 4 mm, 96% of sensitivity and 68% of specificity in the diagnosis of endometrial pathology is obtained. If the cut point is set as < 5 mm the specificity raises to 78% but the sensitivity achieved is just 94%, with two false negatives of carcinomas. This study concludes that, in postmenopausal bleeding and endometrial thickness < 4 mm seems reasonable to abstain to perform D&C.

The evaluation of the ecostructure of the endometrium allows collecting more data than the single determination of its thickness (FIGURE 4.7). The determination of the homogeneity, the presence of symmetrical central echo and the absence of hyperechogenicity are excellent markers with good correlation with the histological results of normality in the endometrium between 3 and 10 mm (PPV of 99% and NPV of the 100%).[10]

DOPPLER ULTRASONOGRAPHY

Transvaginal ultrasonography (TVUS) has its limits. It is difficult to precisely differentiate between polyps and myomas, two formations with their own well-defined characteristics in hysteroscopy, which can present similar images in transvaginal sonography without color Doppler with false positive results decreasing specificity. Visualizing the stalk with color Doppler adds a sign to differentiate with submucous fibromyomas, that do not have a stalk but peripheral irregular blood flow sometimes in the shape of a circle. Color Doppler (2DPD) also helps in differential diagnosis with other pathological entities and defines which polyps need to be removed. Those with definite vascularization and those with a resistance index under 0.5 should be extracted due to the possibility of atypia.[11] This limit is arbitrary and is based on Kurjak's studies attaining a sensitivity of 92%, a

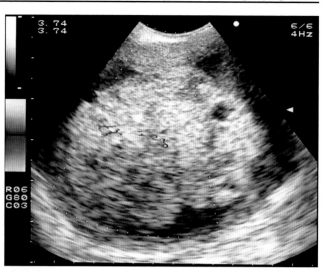

Figure 4.7: An hyperechogenic, thickened endometrium with diffuse limits are known characteristics of endometrial carcinoma

specificity of 97.8%, a positive predictive value of 68.6% and a negative predictive value of 98.6%.

Fibroids

Fibromyomas have a perivascular tumoral network which forms when the tumor grows on the myometrium and displaces the myometrium vessels. This network is visualized by color mapping (FIGURE 4.8). Not withstanding, not many vessels are visualized inside the tumor because fibroids are not highly vascularized and only a weak Doppler signal is perceived. In the periphery of the tumor vessel reorganization is observed, which connects the perivascular network with the large uterine vessels. The resistance index (RI) is usually high (above 0.5) in the interior of the fibroid but are difficult to evaluate because of the scarce vascularization.[12]

As seen before on the TVUS, the uterine leiomyomas may be represented with uterine enlargement, distortion of the uterine contour, and varying echogenicity depending on the amount of connective or smooth muscle tissue.

2DPD demonstrates vascularization on the periphery of the myoma of uterine origin, with the RI of 0.5, allowing better delineation of the tumor.[13]

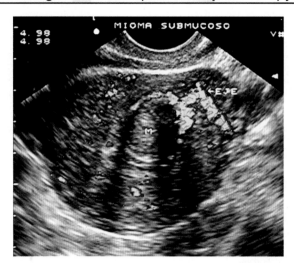

Figure 4.8: Transvaginal color Doppler scan of the uterus with a submucosal leiomyoma and the surrounding color Doppler vessels.

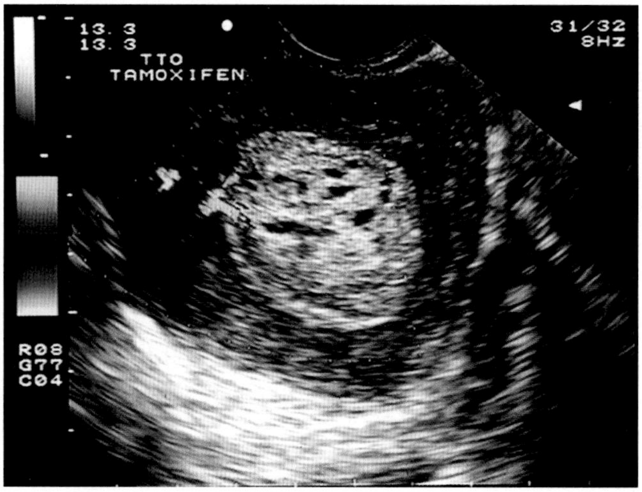

Figure 4.9: Tamoxifen polyp with its irrigating artery

Endometrial Polyps

EP develop as solitary or multiple, soft, sessile, and pedunculated tumors containing hyperplastic endometrium. Clinically, asymptomatic or symptoms like infertility, bleeding, infection, endometritis or pain are usually present in patients with EP. Ultrasonographic appearance of EP is best seen in the early proliferative phase.

Supported by already existing vessels originating from terminal branches of the uterine arteries assessed by transvaginal color Doppler ultrasound, it is possible to identify flow in regularly separated vessels and analyze the velocity of blood flow through them.[14]

The RI is moderate, usually higher than 0.5 (FIGURE 4.9). Infection or necrosis of polyps may lower the impedance to blood flow (RI < 0.4). The importance of EP lies in the fact that marked reduction in blood flow impedance noted on the periphery and/ or within the EP may lead an inexperienced ultrasonographer to a false-positive diagnosis of endometrial malignancy.

The data from Goldstein[15] suggest that the objective assessment of blood flow impedance (resistance index, pulsatility index) in EP and the size of these polyps cannot replace surgical removal and pathologic evaluation to predict histologic type. Patients with nonfunctional polyps were older, and less likely to have vaginal bleeding.

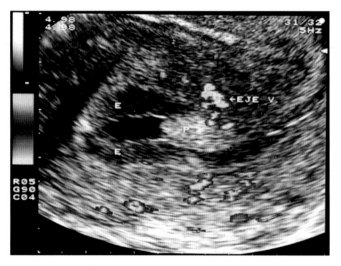

Figure 4.10: Color map inside the endometrial polyp, reflecting some kind of activity

Perez-Medina et al[16] evaluated the efficacy of color Doppler exploration for assessing atypia inside EP (polyp stalk). Thirty-five polyps (out of 106) with sonographic indications of atypia were pathologically confirmed. Sonographic indications of atypia inside 16 polyps were not confirmed. Three no questionable EP had atypia inside them. They conclude that low Doppler resistance (RI < 0.50) is highly predictive of atypia inside EP.

If color Doppler is used, a color signal is seen at the base of the stalk corresponding to the artery that feeds the polyp (FIGURE 4.10). The resistance index of the vessel is middle to high (FIGURE 4.11).

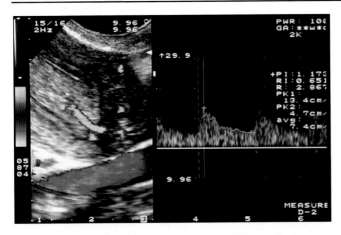

Figure 4.11: Measurable waveform at the stalk.
Resistance index can be obtained

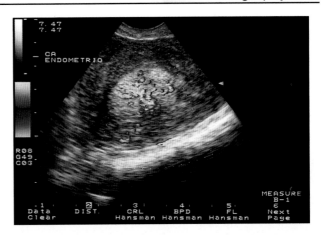

Figure 4.12: Exuberant color map in the context of an endometrial
neoplasia

Endometrial Carcinoma

The introduction in clinical practice of the pulsed
and color Doppler has improved the predictive ability
of TVUS; The color Doppler can identify the presence
of neoangiogenesis showing an increase of signals
of dispersed distribution; Even more, the pulsed
Doppler shows the characteristics of the wave flow
that, in case of neoformed vessels, appears as low RI
and PI.

At the moment, most of the authors agree in
admitting that in the uterine adenocarcinoma there
are many more signals than in the atrophic
endometrium or in benign pathology, but they do
not agree in admitting a cut of point in the RI and PI
values to confirm the diagnosis of adenocarcinoma.

In a study conducted in our Service in 1995[17] with
41 diagnosed postmenopausal women with histological diagnosis of uterine adenocarcinoma, a color
map with measurable wave form and low RI was
found (FIGURE 4.12).

The RI in the intramyometrial vessels is low. When
a cut-off value is set in 0.70 in the arcuate arteries
and 0.50 in basal endometrial vessels, a high predictive
value can be obtained in the diagnosis of malignancy
(sensitivity 92.3%; specificity 96.7%) (FIGURE 4.13).
The presence of irregular vessels in neoplasia is a
present finding in the 82.9% of the corpus carcinoma
in our series. This incidence is higher than the
reported in other studies.[18,19]

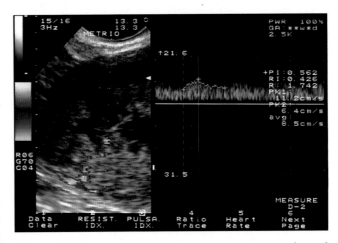

Figure 4.13: Low resistance index measured in the waveform of
an endometrial carcinoma

3D ULTRASONOGRAPHY

Three-dimensional ultrasound (3D-TVUS) is being
evaluated presently and may allow for both better
mapping of uterine leiomyomas, uterine contours,
and better visualization of the anatomy and patency
of the fallopian tubes.

It allows exploration of the outer and inner
contour of uterine cavity patency, improving the
visualization of the lesions and it also offers more
accurate volume estimation. Some recent studies have
compared the three-dimensional saline infusion
sonohysterography with the diagnostic hysteroscopy for the diagnosis and classification of submucous fibroids finding, that there is a good overall

agreement between these both techniques in classification of submucous fibroids, but this agreement is better in cases where a greater proportion of the fibroid is contained within the uterine cavity.

As well, new studies are carrying out to evaluate the clinical relevance of three-dimensional saline infusion sonography, in addition to conventional SIS in women with abnormal uterine bleeding suspected of having intrauterine abnormalities.

Great advances have recently been obtained in gynecology secondary to the development of high-performance TVUS probes. However, even this advanced technology can provide only two-dimensional views of three-dimensional structures. Although an experienced examiner can easily conform together different sequential 2D planes for building a mental 3D image, individual sectional planes cannot be achieved in a 2D image because of obvious difficulties. Today, 3D-TVUS can create not only individual image planes, it can also store complex tissue volumes which can be digitally manipulated to display a multiplanar view, allowing a systematic tomographic survey of any particular field of interest. The main advantage of 3D-TVUS is the addition of the coronal plane to the sagittal and longitudinal ones obtained with conventional ultrasonography. The same technology can also display surface rendering and transparency views, to provide a more realistic 3D portrayal of different structures and anomalies.[20]

Submucosal Leiomyoma

Using simultaneous display of three perpendicular planes assessed by 3D-TVUS, demonstrates the accurate location and size of myomas and, what is more important, is its relationship to the surrounding endometrium (FIGURE 4.14).[21]

One limitation of scanning the uterus with myomas by 3D-TVUS or 2D-TVUS is due to a significant shadowing from calcification.

Myomas are localized thickenings of the myometrium. The volume measurement is performed using longitudinal plane delineating the whole of the uterine cavity in a number of parallel longitudinal sections 1 to 2 mm apart. Then, the myoma volume

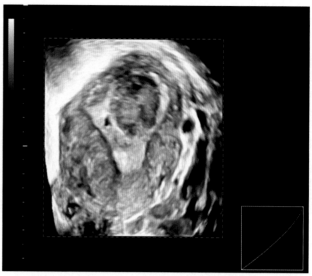

Figure 4.14: 3D aspect of an intramural myoma

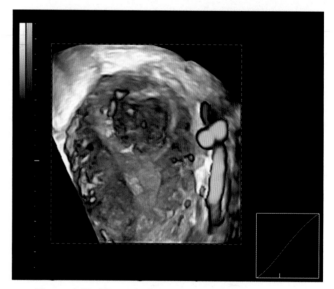

Figure 4.15: The typical appearance of the vasculature surrounding the myoma as seen with 3DPD

is calculated automatically by the inbuilt computer software programs.[21]

3DPD detected regular vascularity at the periphery (FIGURE 4.15); while in cases of secondary degenerative lesions; the findings were suggestive of neovascularity, irregular branching and chaotic vascular arrangement, because necrosis, inflammation and degeneration altered the leiomyoma vasculature. Because of the low-positive predictive value of 16.67%, this method should not be used as first line technique for the evaluation of myometrial pathology, both benign and malignant.

Endometrial Polyps

Using the multiplanar views, polypoid structures can be nicely visualized, allowing for the optimal plane to present their pedicle. Surface rendering mode can suppress undesirable echos allowing seeing the polypoid structure in continuity with the endometrial lining.

When comparing the endometrial thickness, their were similar patients with endometrial hyperplasia and endometrial polyps, but the endometrial volume in hyperplasia was significantly higher than the volume in patients with polyps. The difference between endometrial hyperplasia and polyps cannot be detected by the measurement of endometrial thickness, but with 3D volume measurement.[22]

Uterine Malformations

This is one of the most promising applications for this technique. As conventional ultrasonography, Doppler sonography, hysterosonography (SIS) and HSG can not reliably differentiate between septate uterus and bicornis uterus, only MRI and 3D-TVUS can perform an accurate diagnosis (FIGURE 4.16). This is very important because a perfect characterization of the malformation is mandatory prior to the surgery in order to avoid an unnecessary concomitant laparoscopy (FIGURES 4.17 and 4.18). As 3D-TVUS is more

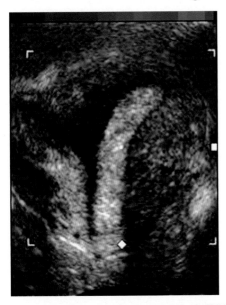

Figure 4.16: Uterine septum as seen in 3D-TVUS

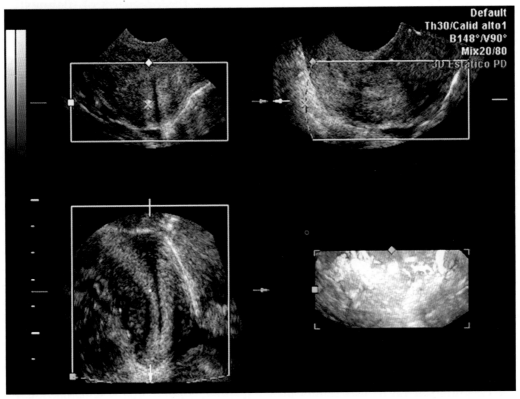

Figure 4.17: 3D-TUVS of a septate uterus. A round-shaped fundus can be seen in the coronal plane (bottom left)

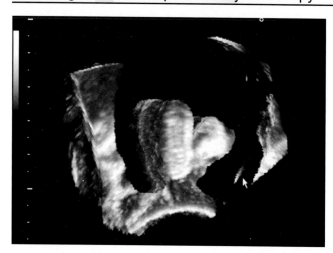

Figure 4.18: 3D vocal reconstruction of the septum

readily available than MRI, this should be the technique of choice in these cases.[23]

Intrauterine Adhesions

3D-TVUS is helpful in delineation of intracavitary adhesions and determination of their location which assists in surgical planning. In the cases of bridging adhesions, the degree of cavity obliteration is accurately assessed. Similarly, this technique is beneficial for differentiation between small polyps and adhesions.

Endometrial Carcinoma

Given the high efficacy of color Doppler ultrasonography in the diagnosis of endometrial carcinoma, the purpose of PD3D was to assess whether 3D power Doppler indexes can predict extension of the endometrial carcinoma. In a study by Mercé et al,[24] 84 women with uterine bleeding and a histopathologic diagnosis of endometrial malignancy were preoperatively examined by PD3D. Endometrial thickness, vascularization index (VI), flow index (FI), vascularization-flow index (VFI), and the intratumoral resistance index (RI) were measured.

The endometrial VI was significantly higher when the tumor stage was greater than I. All the 3D power Doppler indexes were significantly higher when the carcinoma infiltrated more than 50% of the myometrium. The intratumoral RI was significantly lower in cases with a high histologic grade, myo-metrial infiltration of more than 50%, and lymph node metastases, concluding that intratumoral blood flow evaluated by PD3D can effectively predict the spread of endometrial carcinoma.

HYSTEROSONOGRAPHY

The pursuit of endometrial histology is often prompted by postmenopausal or dysfunctional endometrial bleeding, a pathologically thickened central endometrial complex on ultrasound, infertility, or routine screening caused by risk factors for underlying pathology. If a focal endoluminal process is responsible, it can remain undiagnosed when a blind method of biopsy is used. TVUS coupled with hysterosonography can provide the necessary information to triage these patients to the most appropriate tissue sampling technique and avoid the common problem of a false negative biopsy result. In many circumstances, a focal process can be more specifically characterized and localized during SIS, information which could also help direct subsequent hysteroscopic biopsy, if needed.[25] The saline instillation to improve the precision of diagnostic ultrasound techniques is called sonohysterography (SIS). The econegative contrast produced through the use of a saline solution allows the enhancement of the image of the endometrium, making it possible to reveal the margins of an intrauterine mass, if this exists.

Thus, saline-infusion sonography is an extremely useful and easy-to-use technique, which has become a standard test in gynecological outpatient facilities. Standard TVUS is able to show endometrial thickness, distortion of the endometrial lining and abnormal constructions, while SIS allows the details of intrauterine abnormalities to be visualized. In addition, SIS can be used to provide a clinical diagnosis, such as endometrial polyps or submucosal leiomyoma, thus enabling further strategies to be devised. Because SIS has a potential to distinguish between diffuse endometrial thickening and focal intracavitary lesions, it is useful in determining whether subsequent hysteroscopic biopsy is necessary. If a focal lesion is observed using SIS, even if the imaging features suggest that it is benign, biopsy should be performed.

In premenopausal cases, SIS should be performed in the follicular phase of the menstrual cycle, after menstruation is completed to ensure accurate diagnosis. In postmenopausal patients with considerable hemorrhage, SIS should be avoided and the examination should not be performed until after the hemorrhage has stopped.

First of all, a standard TVUS should be carried out to assess the endometrial lining before SIS. A speculum is inserted into the vagina after removal of the transvaginal transducer, and the cervix is visualized. The external os of the cervix is cleansed fully with antiseptic solution and a catheter is then inserted into the external cervical os and introduced into the uterine cavity beyond the internal cervical os. The balloon is filled with as little air, or fluid, as possible to prevent a countercurrent of normal saline infusion. It is common to place the balloon just beyond the internal cervical os; however, intracervical placement of the balloon is less painful for the patient and allows observation of the lower part of the uterus. After the placement of the catheter, the inner introducer is removed. A syringe containing warm saline is connected to the catheter transducer and is reinserted to the catheter. After the air is released from the catheter, saline is slowly injected and the uterine cavity is carefully observed.

Submucosal Leiomyoma

Leiomyoma is visualized as a low echogenic shadow using TVUS, whereas SIS reveals the contours of the leiomyoma (FIGURE 4.19), allowing to see the degree of attachment to the myometrium, and so facilitating the plan of the hysteroscopic surgery. When deciding on an operative strategy, it is important to determine the size, location and rate of protrusion of the fibroid into the uterine cavity before operating. It is especially difficult to perform the hysteroscopic removal of a fibroid with an intracavitary portion below 50 percent. SIS can give a preoperative assessment of the submucosal grading; that is, the measurement of the degree of intracavitary development. A systematic review has demonstrated that SIS and

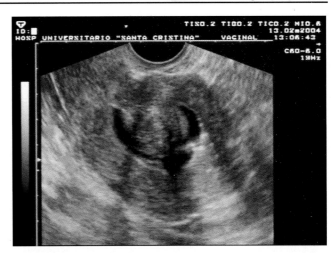

Figure 4.19: Submucosal leiomyoma have a sessile attachment to the posterior uterine wall, which is clearly enhanced in the hysterosonography

hysteroscopy show high accuracy in diagnosing submucosal fibroids.[26]

Saline infusion sonohysterography (SIS) performed with 3D-TVUS (3D-SIS) has some advantages over that with conventional 2D-TVUS in women with abnormal uterine bleeding suspected of having intrauterine abnormalities. It gives more accurate information about the location of abnormalities which is very important for preoperative assessment and distinguishing pathologies. Furthermore, the uterus is distended for shorter time compared to the time necessary for 2D examination which results in better patients' acceptance. 3D-SIS is valid and reliable in women suspected of having intrauterine abnormalities and may indeed have relevant clinical value in addition to conventional SIS.[27]

Visualization of the uterine cavity and endometrial thickness was better with 3D-SIS than with any of the other ultrasound techniques. The results with 3D-SIS corresponded to the findings observed with hysteroscopy.[28]

Endometrial Polyps

Routine TVUS evaluation detects intrauterine anomalies. EP are the most common focal lesions occurring in uterine cavities. In the clinical diagnosis of EP, SIS works better than standard TVUS and HSG (FIGURE 4.20).

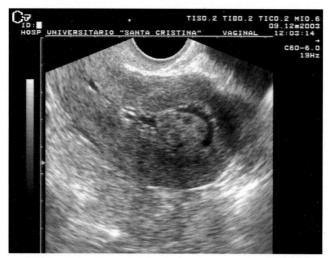

Figure 4.20: The saline produces a better appreciation of the polyp during saline infusion sonohysterography

Saline infusion sonohysterography can differentiate pedunculated from sessile polypoid masses. During fluid instillation, polyps undulate as the anechoic fluid surrounds them; their attachment, stalk size, and location are easily seen with SIS. Polyps typically do not distort the endomyometrial complex. A large EP is difficult to distinguish from a small pedunculated leiomyoma using SIS. It has been reported that color Doppler SIS might be useful in distinguishing polyps from submucosal fibroids based on the vascularity of the lesions; that is, polyps typically contain a single feeding vessel, whereas fibroids have several vessels.[29] However, there is no change in the treatment of hysteroscopic resection in either. The SHG alone is not sufficient for pathological diagnosis and additional studies are necessary for a complete treatment or hysteroscopic resection.[27]

Ryu et al compared conventional 2D and 3D scanning of the uterine cavity with and without saline contrast medium in the detection and evaluation of focal endometrial polyps. Twenty-three patients out of 642 women suggestive for intrauterine anomalies at routine TVUS were examined by 2D and 3D sonography before and after intrauterine saline contrast medium. Sonographic appearance was verified by hysteroscopic and histological evaluation.[30] TVUS diagnosed 23 polyps versus 16 confirmed at hysteroscopic and histologic examinations, revealing a specificity of 69.5%; SIS diagnosed 17 polyps, with a specificity of 94.1%; 3D-TVUS diagnosed 18 polyps, with a specificity of 88.8%; 3D SIS diagnosed 16 polyps according to hysteroscopic and histologic findings, with a specificity of 100%. SIS has been demonstrated to be an effective and suitable method in the detection of intrauterine anomalies, particularly with 3D sonography.[31]

Endometrial Hyperplasia

Endometrial hyperplasia cannot be diagnosed with SIS alone, because the ranges of endometrial thickness in hyperplasia and carcinoma overlap. A histologic diagnosis based on a hysteroscopically obtained or an endometrial office biopsy specimen is also required. Most endometrial hyperplasias are 0.6 to 1.3 cm thick in postmenopausal patients, with a mean thickness of 1 cm. In most endometrial cancer, the thickness is more than 4.7 mm. Most often, hyperplasia occurs diffusely; however, it can be focal or appear as a broad-based polyp. Saline infusion sonography may also reveal asymmetrical or multifocal areas of endometrial irregularities in endometrial hyperplasia. The endometrial-myometrial interface is intact.

Endometrial Carcinoma

Endometrial cancer is difficult to distinguish from hyperplasia except when the endometrium is irregular, has mixed echogenicity, has irregular borders, demonstrated endomyometrial interface disruption, or demonstrates "bridging of the endometrium". Most studies report that the endometrium is thicker in patients subsequently found to have malignant endometrial pathology, than in patients with benign conditions, although the range of thickness may overlap between the two conditions, as mentioned above. The postmenopausal patient not receiving hormonal replacement therapy usually has an endometrial echo less than 4 mm thick.[9] An endometrial echo of less than 5 mm is rarely associated with endometrial cancer. However, when the endometrial echo thickens, the positive predictive value of the test increases.

Intrauterine Adhesions

In cases of intrauterine adhesions, the use of SIS is particularly helpful as the acoustic window provided by the liquid helps in the distinction between scars, normal endometrium and fibrous bridges. Adhesions appear as thin or thick bridging bands that may distort the endometrium. The endometrium may be difficult to distend during saline infusion. During real time scanning, adhesion movement can easily be seen.

Even more, the use of echogenic contrast media is more accurate than saline-contrast 3D-SIS. Anyway, the proportions of failed SIS are high, especially when the synechia affects the endocervical canal, and saline cannot progress upwards.

MAGNETIC RESONANCE IMAGING

The routine use of MRI to evaluate disease of the female pelvis has been limited, despite the fact that there are several conditions that are better demonstrated by MRI than any other imaging modality. These conditions include congenital uterine anomalies, leiomyomas and adenomyosis. Limited access, perceived cost differentials and lack of physician awareness may account for some of the under used MRI. Indeed, there is some evidence that the use of MRI may decrease medical costs.[32] Benign diseases of the uterus can be evaluated by ultrasound, HSG, SIS, hysteroscopy, and magnetic resonance imaging (MRI). The use of MRI appears to be cost-effective in the diagnosis of complex müllerian abnormalities, endometrial thickening following treatment by tamoxifen, selection of candidates for selective myomectomy and the follow-up of medically treated adenomyosis.

Fibromyoma

MRI provides an excellent visualization of uterine leiomyomas. Using T_2-weighted images, the demarcation between the endometrium and myometrium can be visualized very well. The addition of gadolinium IV contrast medium allows for accurate assessment of the location of uterine leiomyomas and the degree of myometrial involvement.

Leiomyomas usually appear as well-defined, homogeneous, low signal-intensity uterine masses on T_2-weighted images. MRI has been demonstrated to be more accurate than ultrasonography in diagnosing leiomyomas and in correct assessment of uterine location.[33] This is especially helpful in preoperative planning. Also, MRI readily differentiates pedunculated submucosal leiomyomas from other solid pelvic masses, when ultrasound is indeterminate. MRI reliably identifies their number, size, and location. These features help triage patients to appropriate therapy. MRI can be recommended as the first choice modality for exact evaluation of submucous myomas before advanced minimal invasive treatment of myomas.[34]

As with ultrasound and CT, MRI cannot identify sarcomatous degeneration within a leiomyoma.

Adenomyosis

Adenomyosis can be difficult to diagnose clinically, ultrasonographically, and invasively. MRI has been shown to be superior to TVUS in the diagnosis of adenomyosis. Diffuse or focal thickening of the junctional zone of > 5 mm is the most common finding in adenomyosis. Occasionally, high signal intensity regions in the junctional or myometrial zones can also be identified. Particularly helpful is the differentiation between adenomyosis and leiomyomas in patients presenting with an enlarged uterus.

When the case is adenomyosis, MRI establishes the diagnosis in cases of equivocal or non-diagnostic ultrasounds. MRI also has been used to confirm an ultrasound diagnosis of adenomyosis when curative surgery is being considered. Intravenous gadolinium chelates are not necessary to make the diagnosis of either adenomyosis or leiomyomas,[35] but it provides useful information about vascularity of lesions, a factor that may impact the type of treatment undertaken.

Endometrial Polyps

TVUS only reached intermediate quality levels as a diagnostic tool for exclusion of uterine cavity abnormalities, and no data support that MRI, TVUS, or SIS may exclude hyperplasia without concomitant endometrial sampling. Hysteroscopy and SIS were equally effective and apparently better than TVUS, especially for identification of polyps. However, all techniques carried a significant number of false positive results. MRI does not satisfy current diagnostic demands for detection of endometrial abnormalities, but it is sufficiently accurate, as discussed above, for submucous myoma evaluation. TVUS, SIS, and hysteroscopy carry an elevated interobserver variation as opposed to MRI. In experienced hands TVUS should be a first choice modality, but its precision and consistency are low, and it should therefore be supplemented by other techniques. SIS or hysteroscopy performed by experienced clinicians should be used as supplements to TVUS for exclusion of polyps.

A central fibrous core (low signal intensity on T2-weighted images) and intratumoral cysts (high signal intensity on T2-weighted images) were seen more frequently in EP than in carcinomas; myometrial invasion and necrosis showed high predictive value for carcinomas. In a study, the readers' responses showed a mean sensitivity of 79%, specificity of 89%, accuracy of 86%, positive predictive value of 82%, and negative predictive value of 88% for diagnosis of carcinoma. The mean area under the receiver operating characteristic curve for the three readers was 0.87 for the diagnosis of carcinoma.[36] MR images can help to distinguish most polyps from endometrial carcinomas on the basis of morphologic features. Accuracy does not appear to be sufficient to obviate biopsy, partly because carcinomas and polyps frequently coexist, and the detection of EP was found to be 79% with MRI.

Uterine Malformations

Systematic analysis of MR images allows accurate morphologic demonstration and classification of uterovaginal anomalies, thereby indicating the appropriate treatment.[37] The multiplanar ability of MRI allows the routine display of coronal long-axis images of the uterus (FIGURE 4.21).

The following parameters are recorded in MR images: Uterine size, external fundal contour,

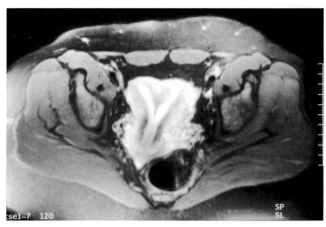

Figure 4.21: The anatomical image of a partially septate uterus as seen through MRI. Note the straight fundal edge as opposed to the bicornuate uterus

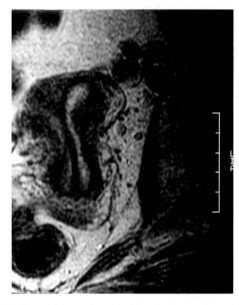

Figure 4.22: A complete septum involving the cervical canal is clearly seen in the MRI (Compare the similarity with Figures 4.12 and 4.13)

intercornual distance, zonal anatomy, and presence of uterine or vaginal septa. Another advantage is that associated pelvic lesions or renal anomalies, frequent in these cases, are reported.[38] MRI allows diagnosis of obstructive uterovaginal anomalies. Determining the site of obstruction is imperative for planning the proper surgical approach (FIGURE 4.22).[39,40] The main interest is the accuracy of MRI in differentiating a septate uterus which can be treated through the hysteroscope from the bicornuate uterus which cannot. MRI alone may be able to provide an accurate and adequate preoperative assessment in patients with uterine and vaginal septa.

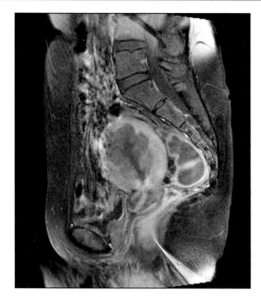

Figure 4.23: Magnetic resonance image of
a huge endometrial carcinoma

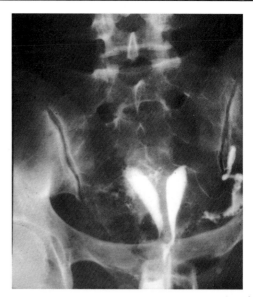

Figure 4.24: Classic image of a "double cavity" uterus in the HSG.
It is not possible to differentiate between septate or bicornuate uterus

Endometrial Carcinoma

Although abnormalities of the endometrium are demonstrated by MRI, the findings are nonspecific. Early endometrial carcinoma and endometrial hyperplasia have a similar appearance (endometrial thickness > 4 mm in postmenopausal women), and histological diagnosis is required.[41]

MRI has been successfully used in some centers to predict the invasion of myometrium and for local staging in cases of known endometrial carcinoma.[42] Loss of the junctional zone can be predictive of invasion into the underlying myometrium; MRI is 85% accurate in predicting the depth of such invasion and, furthermore, 91% for cervical invasion, a question frequently forgotten as cervical extension can modify the surgical approach (FIGURE 4.23).[43]

HYSTEROSALPINGOGRAPHY

Hysterosalpingography (HSG) consists of injecting radiopaque medium through the cervical canal in order to assess the uterine cavity and the fallopian tubes. This diagnostic method should be performed during the follicular phase in order to avoid the possibility of performing the study during early pregnancy.[44]

The primary indication of HSG is to evaluate fallopian tube patency, but can be also useful in

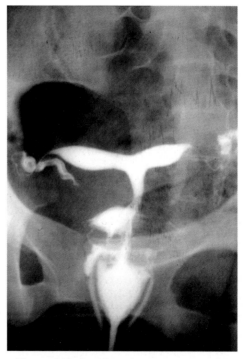

Figure 4.25: Double cavity uterus in the HSG

detecting unicornuate uterus, double uterus (FIGURE 4.24), uterus didelphys (FIGURE 4.25), T-shaped uterus, adenomyosis, EP, synechiae, endometrial hyperplasia/carcinoma, cervical incompetence, intrauterine adhesion, submucosal fibroid and endometrial polyposis.[45,46] HSG is 6-55% accurate in classifying uterine anomaly, whereas MRI and TVS are 96-100% and 85-92% accurate respectively. As far as assessment of the uterine cavity, if the HSG shows no abnormality, it is not probable that hysteroscopy will reveal any different.[40] Some kind of uterine anomaly has been found in 10-12% of women consulting for infertility such as adhesions, submucous fibromyomas, or septa.[47]

Although HSG is not the method of choice for the screening of uterine anomalies, it offers some information although inferior to that of MRI. Hysteroscopy is considered the gold standard in the identification of the uterine cavity pathology.

CONCLUSION

MRI extraordinarily delineates uterine leiomyomas, even in women with large tumors, and has the added advantage of identifying adenomyosis and adenomyoma more accurately than ultrasound, but it provides no information on tubal patency. Because of cost considerations, 2D-TVUS with and without fluid infusion remains the best alternative for mapping uterine leiomyomas in women, in whom the uterus is not excessively enlarged.

Although other methods of evaluating the female pelvis, including laparoscopy, hysteroscopy, colposcopy, and ultrasonography are often superior in both sensitivity and specificity to MRI, it is still incumbent for the gynecologist to understand these techniques. There are a few indications in which MRI are superior to other modalities. The global view provided by these modalities can be helpful in many confusing clinical settings. Furthermore, many patients undergo these studies for other reasons and are subsequently referred to the gynecologist because of the abnormalities of the female genital tract which are revealed. Understanding the value and limitations of the initial modality will enable the practitioner to proceed logically with further studies or treatment.

While MRI and TVUS are superior in demonstrating the zonal anatomy of the corpus, cervix and vagina, HSG is valuable in evaluating fallopian tubal patency, intrauterine adhesion and septa.

REFERENCES

1. Lawson TL, Albarelli Jn. Diagnosis of Gynecologic pelvic masses by scale gray ultrasonography: Analysis of specificity and accuracy. Am J Roetgenol 1977;128:1003.
2. Hall D, Yoder I. Ultrasound evaluation of the uterus. In: Ultrasonography in Obstetrics and Gynecology. Callen P (Eds): Saunders Company. New York, 1994;603-5.
3. Bazot M, Daraï E, Rouger J, Detchev R, Cortez A, Uzan S. Limitations of transvaginal sonography for the of adenomyosis, with histopathological correlation. Ultrasound Obstet Gynecol 2002;20:605-11.
4. Fedele L, Bianchi S, Dorta M, Brioschi D, Zanotti F, Vercellini P. Transvaginal ultrasonography versus hysteroscopy in the diagnosis of uterine submucous myomas. Obstet Gynecol 1991;77:745-53.
5. Atri M, Mazarnia S, Aldis AE, Reinhold C, Bret PM, Kintzen G. Transvaginal US appearance of endometrial abnormalities. Radiographics 1994;14:483.
6. Pérez-Medina T, Bajo J, Huertas MA, Rubio A. Predicting atypia inside endometrial polyps. J Ultrasound Med. 2002;21:125-8.
7. Puscheck EE, Cohen L. Congenital malformations of the uterus: The role of ultrasound. Semin Reprod Med 2008;26:223-31.
8. Gramberg 5, Wikland M, Karlsson B, Norstróm A, En-berg LG. Endometrial thickness as measured by endovaginal ultrasonography for identifying endome-trial abnormality Am J Obstet Gynecol 1991;164:47-52.
9. Karlsson B, Granberg 5, Wickland M, Ylóstalo P, Torvid K, Marsan K, Valentin L. Transvaginal ultrasonography of the endometrium in women with postmenopausal bleeding: A Nordic trial. Am J Obstet Gynecol 1995;172:1488-94.
10. Gull B, Karlsson B, Milsom I, Granberg S. Can ultrasound replace dilation and curettage? A longitudinal evaluation of postmenopausal bleeding and transvaginal sonographic measurement of the endometrium as predictors of endometrial cancer. Am J Obstet Gynecol 2003;188:401-8.
11. Carter J, Saltzman A, Hartenbach E et al. Flow characteristics in benign and malignant gynecologic tumours using transvaginal color flow Doppler. Obstet Gynecol 1994;83:125-30.
12. Kurjak A, Zalud I. The characterization of uterine tumors by transvaginal color Doppler. Ultrasound Obstet Gynecol 1991;1:50-2.
13. Sladkevicius P, Valentin L, Marsal K. Transvaginal Doppler examination for the differential diagnosis of solid pelvic tumors. J Ultrasound Med 1995;14:377-80.
14. Bakour SH, Khan KS, Gupta JK. The risk of premalignant and malignant pathology in endometrial polyps. Acta Obstet Gynecol Scand 2000;79:317-20.
15. Anastasiadis PG, Koutlaki NG, Skaphida PG, et al. Endometrial polyps: Prevalence, detection, and malignant potential in women with abnormal uterine bleeding. Eur J Gynaecol Oncol 2000;21:180-3.
16. Pérez-Medina T, Martínez O, Folgueira G, Bajo JM. Which endometrial polyps should be resected? J Am Assoc Gynaecol Laparosc 1999;6:71-4.
17. Huertas MA, Pérez Medina T, Zarauz R, Uguet C, Bajo JM. Utilidad del estudio transvaginal con Doppler color en el diagnóstico de adenocarcinoma de endometrio. Clin Invest Gin Obstet 1995; 22:152-7.

18. Kurjak A, Shalan H, Socic A. Benic S, Zudenigo D, Kupesic 5, Predanic M. Endometrial carcinoma in postmenopausal women: Evaluation by transvaginal color Doppler ultrasonography. Am J Obstet Gynecol 1993;169(6):1597-602.

19. Sladkevicius P, Valentin L, Marsál K. Endometrial thickness and Doppler velocimetry of the uterine arteries as discriminators of endometrial status in women with postmenopausal bleeding. A comparative study. Am J Obstet Gynecol 1994;171:722-8.

20. Maymon R, Herman A, Ariely S, Dreazen E, Buckovsky I, Weinraub Z. Three-dimensional vaginal sonography in obstetrics and gynaecology. Hum Reprod Update 2000;6:475-84.

21. Radoncik E, Funduk-Kurjak B. Three-dimensional ultrasound for routine check-up in in vitro fertilization patients. Croat Med J 2000;41:262-5.

22. La Torre R, De Felice C, De Angelis C, Coacci F, Mastrone M, Cosmi EV. Transvaginal sonographic evaluation of endometrial polyps: A comparison with two dimensional and three dimensional contrast sonography. Clin Exp Obstet Gynecol 1999;26(3-4):171-3.

23. Bonilla-Musoles F, Raga F, Osborne NG, Blanes J, Coelho F. Three-dimensional hysterosonography for the study of endometrial tumors: comparison with conventional transvaginal sonography, hysterosalpingography, and hysteroscopy. Gynecol Oncol 1997;65:245-52.

24. Merce L, Alcazar JL, Lopez C, Iglesias E, Bau S, Alvarez de los Heros JI, Bajo J. Clinical usefulness of 3-dimensional sonography and power Doppler angiography for diagnosis of endometrial carcinoma. J Ultrasound Med 2007;26:1279-87.

25. Dudiak KM. Hysterosonography: A key to what is inside the uterus. Ultrasound Q 2001;17(2):73-86.

26. Imm DD, Murphy CA, Rosensheim NB. Hysterosonography as an adjunct to transvaginal sonography in the evaluation of intraluminal lesions of the uterine cavity. Prim Care Update Ob Gyn 1998;5:194-8.

27. De Kroon CD, Louwe LA, Trimbos JB, Jansen FW. The clinical value of 3-dimensional saline infusion sonography in addition to 2-dimensional saline infusion sonography in women with abnormal uterine bleeding. J Ultrasound Med 2004;23:1433-40.

28. Brown SE, Coddington CC; Schnorr J, Toner JP, Gibbons W, Oehninger S. Evaluation of outpatient hysteroscopy, saline infusion hysterosonography, and hysterosalpingography in infertile women: A prospective, randomized study. Fertil Steril 2000;74:1029-34.

29. Syrop CH, Sahakian V. Transvaginal sonographic detection of endometrial polyps with fluid contrast augmentation. Obstet Gynecol 1992;79:1041-3.

30. Ryu JA, Kim B, Lee J, Kim S, Lee SH. Comparison of transvaginal ultrasonography with hysterosonography as a screening method in patients with abnormal uterine bleeding. Korean J Radiol 2004;5:39-46.

31. Rogerson L, Bates J, Weston M. Duffy S. A comparison of outpatient hysteroscopy with saline infusion hysterosonography. Br J Obs Gyn 2002;109:800-4.

32. Kinkel K, Vincent B, Balleyguier C, Helenon O, Moreau J. Value of MR imaging in the diagnosis of benign uterine conditions. J Radiol 2000;81(7):773-9.

33. Dueholm M, Lundforf E, Hansen ES, Ledertoug S, Olsen F. Evaluation of the uterine cavity with magnetic resonance imaging, transvaginal sonography, hysterosonographic examination, and diagnostic hysteroscopy. Fertil Steril 2001;76(2):350-7.

34. Celik O, Sarac K, Hascalik S, Alkan A, Mizrak B, Yologlu S. Magnetic resonance spectroscopy features of uterine leiomyomas. Gynecol Obstet Invest 2004;58(4):194-201.

35. Ascher SM, Jha RC, Reinhold C. Benign myometrial conditions: leiomyomas and adenomyosis. Top Magn Reson Imaging 2003;14(4):281-304.

36. Grasel RP, Outwater EK, Siegelman ES, Capuzzi D, Parker L, Hussain SM. Endometrial polyps: MR imaging features and distinction from endometrial carcinoma. Radiology 2000;214(1):47-52.

37. Saleem SN. MR imaging diagnosis of uterovaginal anomalies: Current state of the art. Radiographics 2003;23:e13.

38. Piu MH. Imaging diagnosis of congenital uterine malformation. Computerized Medical Imaging and Graphics 2004;28:425-33.

39. Mueller GC, Hussain HK, Smith YR, Quint EH, Carlos RC, Johnson TD, DeLancey JO. Müllerian ducts anomalies: comparison of MRI diagnosis and clinical diagnosis. AJR Am J Roentgenol 2007;189:1294-308.

40. Brown JJ, Thurnher S, Hricak H. MR imaging of the uterus: Low signal intensity abnormalities of the endometrium and endometrial cavity. Magn Reson Imaging 1990; 8(3): 309-13.

41. Posniak HV, Olson MC. Malignant diseases of the uterus. In Tempany CMC, ed. MR and imaging of the Female Pelvis. St Louis: Mosby 1995;155-84.

42. Cicinelli E, Marinaccio M, Barba B, Tinelli R, Colafiglio G, Pedote P, Rossi C, Pinto V. Reliability of diagnostic fluid hysteroscopy in the assessment of cervical invasion by endometrial carcinoma: A comparative study with transvaginal sonography and MRI. Gynecol Oncol 2008;111:55-61.

43. Pellerito JS, McCarthy SM, Doyle MB, Glickman MG, DeCherney AH. Diagnosis of uterine anomalies: Relative accuracy of MR imaging, endovaginal sonography, and hysterosalpingography. Radiology 1992;(3):795-800.

44. Azsarlak O, De Schepper AM, Valkenburg M, Delbeke L. Septate uterus: Hysterosalpingography and magnetic resonance findings. Eur J Radiol 1995;21(2):122-5.

45. Chang AS, Goldstein J, Moley KH, Odem RR, Dahan MH. Radiologic and surgical demonstration of uterine polyposis. Fertil Steril 2005;84:1742-3.

46. Baramki TA. Hysterosalpingography. Fertil Steril 2005;83:1595-606.

47. Golan A, Eilat E, Ron-El R, Herman A, Soffer Y, Bukivsky I. Hysteroscopy is superior to hysterosalpingography in infertility investigation. Acta Obstet Gynecol Scand 1996;75:654-6.

5

Hysteroscopy and Infertility

Tirso Pérez-Medina
Jennifer Rayward

INTRODUCTION

At present the tendency to use hysteroscopy in fertility is increasing. Its role has constantly changed since its introduction in the eighties, and while there is still controversy to its acceptance as a diagnostic tool, as costs lowers and technology improves its role is more and more important. It is not perhaps the gold standard in the evaluation of the endouterine cavity in patients with fertility problems however, there is greater penchant towards using hysteroscopy to diagnose and treat endouterine pathology. Pathological hysteroscopy findings in fertility patients with normal hysterosalpingography (HSG) show false negatives with widely ranging results. Different authors report between 8-62% false negative results.[1-3] The rate of false positives and false negatives in HSG give the technique high sensitivity (around 97%) and low specificity (23%).

When comparing studies reported to date that compare HSG with other diagnostic tests, such as the transvaginal ultrasonography (TVUS) or the hysterosonography (SIS), hysteroscopy is the gold standard in the diagnosis of intrauterine lesions.[4] HSG is no longer the procedure of choice because TVUS is more sensitive and specific. TVUS is not as specific as SIS and its sensitivity and specificity equals that of the hysteroscopy. Therefore, it has been reported in studies that TVUS and SIS can be used in the initial diagnosis of the lesions and alterations of the endouterine cavity.[5]

Generally speaking, performing HSG when endometrial cavity pathology is suspected is not needed. Whenever a HSG shows any modification of the uterine cavity, it is important to perform diagnostic hysteroscopy. Conversely, when HSG doesn't show any intracavitary changes this can be confirmed by TVUS and when in doubt, a SIS can be performed. Hysteroscopy will not only solve any doubts, it will also be therapeutic. One can say that at present HSG and hysteroscopy are complementary procedures in infertility evaluation. Different pathologies like endometrial polyps, cervical stenosis, myomas that deform the cavity, some Müllerian malformations, endometritis, intrauterine adhesions or Asherman's syndrome can be treated by this endoscopic method with excellent results. It is also useful in specific conditions in assisted reproduction such as the evaluation of the repeated failed IVF cycles or in proximal tubal occlusions (PTO).

Indications

Reproductive medicine reaps the benefits of hysteroscopy in two different ways: (1) In the precise diagnosis of any alteration of the endocervical canal or the uterine cavity in patients with fertility problems or in patients with repeated failed IVF cycles, and (2) in patients who have cervical pathology or a cavity susceptible to hysteroscopy correction and to provide a normal uterine cavity for embryonic transfer.

Lesions of the uterine cavity diagnosed in infertile patients by hysteroscopy have been reported in 19-62% of all patients. Most pathology is due to intrauterine synechiae, endometrial polyps, submucosal myomas, uterine malformations, endometritis and cervical stenosis.

There are indications for diagnostic hysteroscopy that compete with conventional HSG and with new sonographic techniques (Chapter 3).

Nowadays, hysteroscopy has left the operating room and now can be performed in an office setting without anesthesia, without a speculum, cervix graspers or cervical dilation. Besides the immediate diagnosis, it facilitates the immediate resolution of some small lesions (see and treat). The resectoscopy with anesthesia in the operating room allows the treatment of intrauterine lesions that, only a few years ago were resolved by complex abdominal techniques.

At present, we face revolutionary changes in hysteroscopy. Almost three decades of constant studies have gone by with continuous analysis and technology development, that have improved the technique with more reliable and successful applications. The conscientious assessment of the patients, together with the precise indication of the procedure, the correct evaluation of the possible problems that could arise, the use of an appropriate exploratory, and surgical technique together with the correct employment of this technology make hysteroscopy at the present time an ideal method with low morbidity.

HYSTEROSCOPY IN INFERTILITY

In the infertile patient hysteroscopy is selectively indicated by some groups and systematically by others. Nowadays, diagnostic hysteroscopy, even with a difficult cervix is perfectly feasible in the office without anesthesia by means of vaginoscopy, if a small caliber hysteroscopy is used.

In infertility evaluation, hysteroscopy is indicated in a wide group of patients including patients needing confirmation of suspected pathology found in HSG and/or hysterosalpingosonography, in tubal proximal pathology, confirmed by laparoscopy to visualize the ostiums and to recanalize them, and to perform selective chromopertubation, and also after repeated failed embryonic transfers post-IVF.

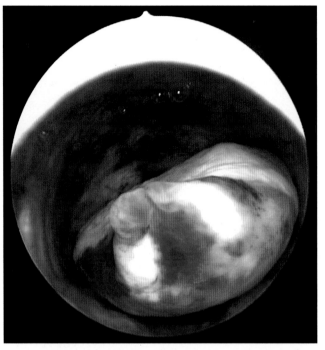

Figure 5.1: Endocervical polyp arising from the endocervical canal

Diagnostic Hysteroscopy

Cervix

In the evaluation of the cervical canal different types of pathology can be visualized. Even though cervical stenosis, polyps and synechiae (FIGURES 5.1 and 5.2) may not be strongly correlated to sterility, they may be also associated with other alterations. In general the cervical factor is easy to correct with simple hysterometry or with the hysteroscopy mechanical dilation, as used in endocervical polyps, cervical stenosis or intracervical synechiae.[6-8]

Endometritis

Chronic endometritis has been related to infertility and recurrent pregnancy loss. It is usually asymptomatic, and the diagnosis is rarely suspected clinically.

Endometritis represents a debatable entity because genital infectious disease is a contraindication of endoscopy. So, the diagnosis is rarely performed by hysteroscopy.[9] Two kinds of endometritis can be identified: Acute endometritis characterized by an edema and a bleeding endometrium, covered by abnormal mucus; and chronic endometritis with

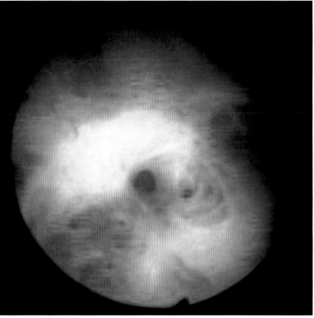

Figure 5.2: Intracervical synechia and cervical stenosis

areas of red endometrium, flushed, with a white central point, localized or scattered throughout the cavity. This is the called the "strawberry aspect" (FIGURE 5.3). The correlation between hysteroscopic aspect and histological or bacteriologic samples exists in only 35% of cases. According to R Frydman,[10]

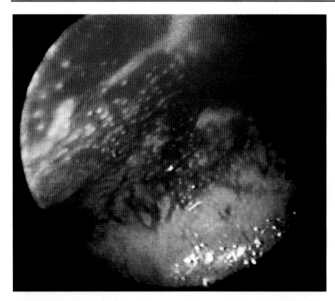

Figure 5.3: The strawberry image of the chronic endometritis. It is due to a congestive, hypervascularized stromal base and white glandular openings

chronic endometritis appears in 22% of patients in IVF programs, in 14% of cases with unexplained infertility, and 23.6% of women with a history of first trimester miscarriages. Chlamydia and ureaplasma are the most frequent germs. Thus, in cases of unexplained infertility hysteroscopy diagnosis of chronic endometritis can be treated with antibiotics.[11]

In a study conducted to evaluate the feasibility of hysteroscopy in the diagnosis of endometritis, with the endometrial biopsy for histopathological study as gold standard, the hysteroscopy sensitivity was 16.7%, the specificity was 93.2%, the positive predictive value was 25%, and the negative predictive value was 89.1%.[12] This suggests that hysteroscopy is not useful in the screening of chronic endometritis in asymptomatic infertile women.

Tubal Ostium Membranes

In 1990, Van der Pas and Siegler separately described the visualization by hysteroscopy of membranous formations in the tubal ostia, possibly functional in origin.[13] They did not believe they were pathological. Five years later, Coeman[14] reported the presence of these membranes in 10% of his sterile patient's and in only 2% of fertile women. There is no later study to confirm these findings.

In Vitro Fertilization (IVF)

The evaluation of the uterine cavity by hysteroscopy in repeated failed IVF cycles has been proven useful, and therefore is highly recommended in these cases. Studies such as the one reported by Golan where in, up to 50% of the patients were found to have intrauterine pathology in failed IVF cycles with high quality embryos transferred, conclude that routine hysteroscopy before IVF should be seriously considered.[15] Shamma et al found 45% of the anomalies to be endocervical or intrauterine showing that these lesions can produce a statistically significant decrease in pregnancy rates compared to those patients who had a normal hysteroscopy.[16]

Goldbemberg et al found that 19% of patients with at least 2 failed IVF cycles presented some type of anomaly in hysteroscopy and of those, 24% were due to cervical pathology. This suggests that hysteroscopy should be used as a routine procedure before IVF/ET.[17]

These reports have made some groups perform hysteroscopy before any type of assisted reproduction technologies (ART) even if it is doubtful uterine or cervical pathology exists. Diagnostic office hysteroscopy without anesthesia need not keep the patient from immediately going back to their daily activities. All authors believe in hysteroscopy if any endocavitary pathology that causes symptoms. Controversy arises when there is "small endocavitary pathology", because it is not fully demonstrated that this causes infertility. The inclusion of hysteroscopy in ART shows that these patients have higher endocavitary pathology.

Dicker (1992) studied the incidence of unsuspected endouterine abnormalities in IVF patients who failed to conceive during three or more cycles. They underwent repeated hysteroscopy evaluation and he found pathology in 18% of the patients. This pathology was generally new endometrial lesions, i.e. hyperplasia, polyps, endometritis, and synechiae. After hysteroscopy correction in 43 IVF cycles studied, 14 pregnancies were achieved.[18]

These results indicate that repeated hysteroscopy evaluation in cases of recurrent IVF failure is an important adjunctive tool for further evaluating and possibly optimizing IVF procedure. The role of hysteroscopy in the evaluation of the endometrial cavity, especially in the unexplained infertility before IVF, is generally accepted. However, there are controversies in the literature. We believe that the hysteroscopy evaluation of endometrial cavity in the unexplained infertility before an IVF program improves the pregnancy outcome, because it detects lesions such as chronic endometritis, osseous metaplasia, and other entities that are not diagnosed accurately with other diagnostic methods.

Operative

As well as in the tubal-peritoneal factor, the benefits of the endoscopic surgery like shorter hospitalization, less postoperatory pain and the possibility of resuming normal life quickly are advantages obtained at lower costs. The effectiveness is the same so the type of uterine pathology that is tributary to hysteroscopy surgery must be defined.

Endometrial Polyps

Endometrial polyps (EP) are frequently found during routine TVUS or infertility testing. Although the precise mechanism by which intrauterine polyps may cause infertility is unclear, their removal has been reported to increase fertility, and their extraction significantly improves the chance for pregnancy (FIGURE 5.4). The cause for this pathology is unknown. Richlin demonstrated an increase in glycodelin levels in the periovulatory period in women with EP. Glycodelin is a protein that facilitates implantation by decreasing NK cell activity. During the normal periovulatory phase during a functional cycle, glycodelin decreases because it inhibits the sperm-oocyte binding. In this situation EP produce significant amounts of glycodelin, and thus make implantation difficult.[19]

Studies in the literature concerning infertility and EP are scant and in none, clear conclusions are reached in any of them. Sillo-Seidl reports finding, 10.8% of the patients in a study of 1000 sterile patients had EP.[20] Pregnancy was obtained after polypectomy

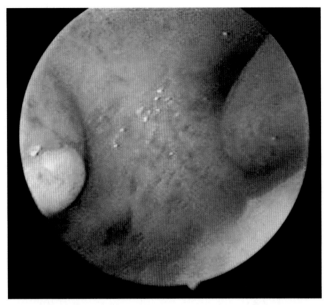

Figure 5.4: Endometrial polyps filling the uterine cavity

in 8 patients. Conversely, Hereter, in a study which included 33 patients with EP compared to 280 patients without EP, found no difference in implantation and abortion rates in the 2 groups after undergoing IVF.[21]

In the study by Varastéh in a series of 23 sterile women, the correlation between polypectomy and the accumulated pregnancy rate was 65.2%. The shortcoming of this report was that polyps and myomas were mixed and the study was not randomized so their conclusions raise questions.[22] In the series by Spiewanciewicz, 19 out of 25 infertile patients (76%) in whom polypectomy was performed conceived in a 12 months period.[23]

Our group conducted a clinical trial,[24] in a study on 204 women scheduled for intrauterine insemination (IUI). There were 103 patients in the control group where no polypectomy was performed and 101 patients in the control group where hysteroscopy polypectomy was performed. A total of 93 pregnancies were achieved: 64 in the study group and 29 in the control group. Women in the study group had a greater probability of achieving pregnancy after polypectomy with a relative risk of 2.1 (CI 95% 1, 5-2, 9). The survival analysis showed that, after 4 cycles, the pregnancy rate was 51.4% in the study group and 25.4% in the control group ($p < 0.001$). Interestingly, pregnancies in the study group were obtained before the first IUI in 65% of cases. The rest were obtained over 4 IUI cycles without a clear predominance of any cycle.

We think polypectomy should be performed in infertile women with the only known problem is EP as stated by Spiewanciewicz, Oliveira and Mooney[23,25,26] in their studies in ART patients.

After polypectomy, pregnancies are frequently obtained spontaneously while waiting for the treatment, suggesting a strong cause-effect of the polyp in the implantation process. This leads us to recommend postponing the first IUI to three menstrual cycles after polypectomy is performed.

Proximal Tubal Obstruction

Tubal disease accounts for 25-35% of all infertility cases. Salpingitis is believed to account for more than 50% of these cases. Although it is seen occasionally in multiple sites, tubal blockage usually involves the proximal, mid, or distal portion. Proximal blockage of the fallopian tube occurs in 10-25% of women with tubal disease and is mainly due to *salpingitis isthmica nodosa* (SIN), chronic salpingitis, intratubal endometriosis, amorphous material (e.g. mucus plugs), or spasm.[27]

In 1954, Rubin discussed the difference between tubal obstruction and tubal occlusion: Obstruction is a time-limited process that may be reversible, such as tubal spasm or plugging by amorphous material, and occlusion is organic pathology that is permanent, such as SIN. The lesions of SIN occur primarily around the intramural and proximal isthmic endosalpinx. The etiology remains controversial; inflammation, mechanical factors, hormonal factors, and congenital predisposition are possible causes. Most researchers favor an infectious or inflammatory etiology, but this is unresolved and pelvic inflammatory disease, polypoid lesions or endometriosis as possible agents have been suggested.

Proximal tubal blockage, suggested by failure of contrast medium to enter the intramural or isthmic portion of either tube, is diagnosed in 10-20% of HSGs performed for infertility (FIGURE 5.5). There are no pathognomonic radiographic findings to confirm the presence of tubal obstruction or

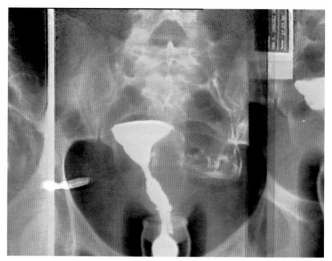

Figure 5.5: Hysterosalpingogram in a case of proximal tubal obstruction

occlusion. Characteristic findings are seen only in SIN, where a stippled or honeycombed appearance on HSG indicates retained contrast medium in small diverticular projections.

The significance of intermittent obstruction at HSG has been questioned. Spasm can be induced by excessive pressure at injection, but in the absence of using high pressure, intermittent obstruction at HSG suggests genuine tubal disease. Confirmation of proximal blockage requires the performance of a second HSG or laparoscopy. In patients with spasm, the contrast medium may pass the functional block with time. Repeated examination with spasmolytic agents, such as glucagon, has been suggested, but its efficacy has not been established.

Selective salpingography and transcervical cannulation under fluoroscopic guidance are effective at establishing patency in appropriately selected patients, and are less invasive and costly than the surgical alternatives.[28] While uterotubal chromopertubations were performed early in the 1970s, with the introduction of hysteroscopy, cornual cannulation was extended and adapted to fluoroscopy. The disadvantages of fluoroscopy include the difficulty in ruling out tubal spasm, inability to evaluate distal tubal disease, and other pelvic abnormalities. Hysteroscopy tubal cannulation is an excellent alternative to treat patients with cornual obstruction. While cannulation with coaxial catheters began under fluoroscopy, the use of the hysteroscope simplifies the technique.

Daniell and Miller[29] reported the first at term birth after hysteroscopy correction of cornual occlusion, in 1987. In the same month, Sulak et al published a report of two patients who were treated by hysteroscopy cannulation.[30] Both patients had bilateral proximal blockage documented by HSG and laparoscopy. One became pregnant 2 months after operation and was delivered at term; the other was lost in follow-up.

The procedure is performed under general anesthesia and laparoscopic guidance. With vaginoscopic approach, a 5.5 mm diagnostic hysteroscope with a 5 French working channel is introduced with saline as distention medium. The tubal ostia are visualized. The Novy coaxial catheter is introduced through the working channel and placed near the tubal ostium. The tip of the guide wire is placed at the tubal ostium and gentle pressure is applied until patency is achieved under direct laparoscopic imaging. The inner catheter is then introduced and the guide wire retired (FIGURE 5.6). Methylene blue contrast is now passed to laparoscopically confirm the resolution of the obstruction (FIGURE 5.7). The simplicity of coaxial catheters makes this approach appealing and with the hysteroscope, one can avoid exposure to radiation. Serious complications are rare.[31]

A report of proximal blockage by Ransom and Garcia gave total, ongoing, and ectopic PRs after hysteroscopic cannulation of 59%, 47%, and 5.9%, respectively.[32] These are similar to the total and ongoing PRs of 52% and 38%, respectively after microsurgery provided in the same report. A report by Das[33] cited an ongoing PR of 57% and an ectopic PR of 3.6% in 21 patients who were treated by hysteroscopic cannulation and concurrent laparoscopy. Sakumoto et al reported a total PR of 43% in a series of 25 patients who were treated by hysteroscopy with simultaneous laparoscopy.[34] The average ongoing PR for hysteroscopic transcervical cannulation was 49% in this study.

The results obtained with tubal cannulation are encouraging, and this procedure should be offered as the initial method to attempt treatment of tubal cornual obstruction. It can represent an excellent

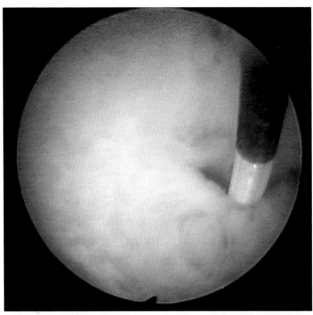

Figure 5.6: The novy flexible catheter is introduced in the tubal ostium

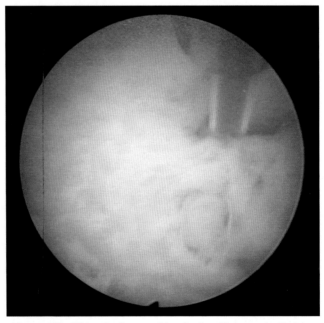

Figure 5.7: When the inner guide wire is withdrawn, methylene blue is passed to test the permeability of the tubes

alternative to microsurgical tubal anastomosis or prior to IVF procedures.

Intrauterine Adhesions

Intrauterine adhesions are scars that result from anything from trauma to a recently pregnant uterus. In 1894, Fritseh described the case of post curettage amenorrhea. In 1948, Asherman[35] reported 29 cases defining the syndrome that bears his name.

Over 90% of the cases are caused by curettage. Usually the trauma has occurred because of excessive bleeding requiring curettage, 1-4 weeks after delivery of an at term or preterm pregnancy or an abortion. During this vulnerable phase of the endometrium any trauma may denude or remove the basalis endometrium causing the uterine walls to coapt each other and form a permanent bridge between them.[36,37]

In other cases, procedures affecting the uterine lumen such as abdominal metroplasty or abdominal myomectomies may cause intrauterine adhesions. These adhesions are usually due to suture materials rather than the true coaptation of denuded areas of myometrium that occur following postpartum or post-miscarriage curettage. The type and consistency of these adhesions varies; some are focal, some extensive, some mild and filmy, and some thickened and dense, with extensive fibromuscular or connective tissue components. The extent and type of uterine cavity occlusion correlates with the extent of trauma during the vulnerable phase of the endometrium following a recent pregnancy. Fibrosis usually follows the longevity and duration of these adhesions, the adhesions become thickened and dense and form connective tissue.

Its true incidence is unknown, as most of them are asymptomatic. It has been stated that adhesions are present in 5% of recurrent pregnancy loss patients and in 23% of postpartum curettages.

Intrauterine adhesions frequently result in menstrual abnormalities like hypomenorrhea or even amenorrhea, depending upon the extent of uterine cavity occlusion. Patients with long-standing intra-uterine adhesions may also develop dysmenorrhea. Over 75% of women with moderate and severe adhesions will have either amenorrhea or hypomenorrhea. Defects in the phase of placentation may produce *placenta accreta* or *increta*.

The relationship with the sterility and infertility is greater than the more extensive and fibrous adhesions. Their pathogenesis is more related to the defective vascularization at the implantation site, than to the reduced uterine room. It is not always possible to correlate miscarriages and adhesions and to identify if they are the cause or the consequence. What is certain is, once adhesions exist miscarriage is a possibility.

Hysterography is a good diagnostic method. Polyedric, well-defined images are visualized. When adhesions fill the cavity or the inner cervical orifice is affected, only the endocervical canal can be seen. As in these cases, when TVUS can know the remaining endometrium and distinguish between partial and total occlusion, although hysteroscopy is the best diagnostic method when determining the exact extent and consistency of adhesions.

The management of adhesions varies based upon the degree of severity. The transparent or mild endometrial adhesions can be easily broken with the tip of the hysteroscope. Fibromuscular or connective synechiae require more complex operative procedures and special instruments as rigid or semirigid endoscopic scissors that produce less thermal lesion and scarification in the endometrium as the surgeon is opening the small cavities with less risk of perforation than with monopole electrodes (FIGURE 5.8).

It is advisable to prescribe continuous estrogen therapy for 3 weeks prior to surgery with the aim of ultrasonographically determining the amount of remaining endometrium before the procedure. The

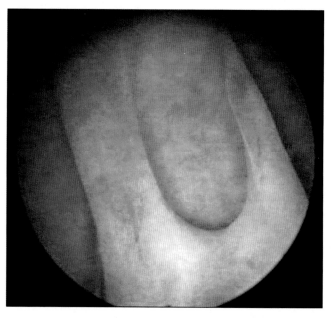

Figure 5.8: Fibromuscular intrauterine adhesions

prognostic is directly related to it. In second place TVUS provides information to guide the surgeon during the lysis of dense adhesions, when the little nests of proliferated red endometrium are found decreasing the risk of perforation.

The laparoscopic observation during the procedure is not useful and cannot predict the probability of perforation. Contrarily, the sonographic control will guide the surgeon precisely when the image of the echorefringent element contrasts with the normal endometrium and the sonoluscent distending fluid. In severe cases a postoperative IUD insertion is recommended.

Postoperatively, broad-spectrum antibiotics are prescribed along with high dose conjugated estrogens for 21 days and adding medroxy-progesterone acetate the last 10 days. More prolonged treatments are not required, as the basic healing period and endometrial reparation occurs in that time. When an IUD is left in place it must be extracted after menstruation at the end of this cycle, when the follow-up hysteroscopy is performed. Some cases require a second intervention.

The results of hysteroscopy treatment of intrauterine adhesions correlate well with the extent of uterine cavity occlusion and the type of adhesions present. Schlaff[38] informs of no pregnancy when endometrial tissue is not sonographically demonstrated before the lysis. Contrarily, March[39] obtains a 90% of regular menses after the hysteroscopic lysis in previously amenorrhea patients.

Obstetric results are excellent for Valle.[40] Normal menstruation is restored in over 90% of the patients. Of 187 patients treated hysteroscopically by Valle and Sciarra, removal of mild, filmy adhesions in 43 cases gave the best results, with 35 (81%) term pregnancies; in 97 moderate cases of fibromuscular adhesions, 64 (66%) term pregnancies occurred and in 47 severe cases of connective tissue adhesions, 65 (32%) at term pregnancies occurred. Overall restoration of menses occurred in 90% of the patients, and the overall at term pregnancy rate was 79.7%. These results demonstrate a much better reproductive outcome than was previously obtained with blind methods of therapy (Chapter 17).

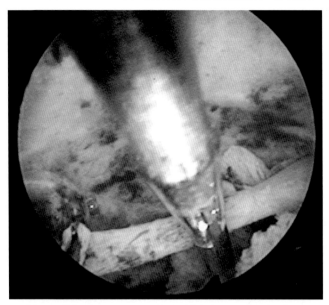

Figure 5.9: Osseous metaplasia. This long trabecular bony structure, is pathognomonic of the condition

Osseous Metaplasia

The intrauterine structures are not suspected clinically because they remain asymptomatic, and in TVUS usually appear like an IUD. In some cases, the retained fetal bones are visualized as filling defects on hysterosalpingogram.

The hysteroscopic appearance of this form of the disorder is easily recognizable. Osseous lamellae are white and either fan- or disk-shaped and are reticulated, deeply embedded in the mucosa and may have the appearance of a flat coral (FIGURE 5.9). They have the same effects as an IUD. When examined histologically the lesion is osseous tissue that is distinguishable from the normal surrounding endometrium.

Two main hypotheses have been proposed to account for their formation. The main hypothesis suggests the presence of osseous fetal tissue after an abortion that has occurred at 3 months' gestation. Metaplasias encountered in the nulliparous patient must represent true osseous metaplasia, that is similar to what occurs after the calcification of myomata or abscesses.[41] Endometrial ossification may be associated with acute or chronic inflammation that leads to ossification by metaplasia rather than retention of bone tissue at the time of abortion.

Many women with retained fetal bone will have symptoms of menometrorrhagia, dysmenorrhea, vaginal discharge, pelvic pain, and spontaneous elimination of bony fragments in the menses. If no other cause of infertility exists, pregnancy almost invariably follows removal, as was also the case in the current report.

Osseous metaplasia causes subfertility by changing the milieu of the uterine cavity through the increase in production of prostaglandins. The menstrual volume and total prostaglandin concentration decreased 50% after the retained bone was removed. It is also possible that reactive endometritis caused by the bone fragments interferes with blastocyst implantation.[42]

Over the past few decades, there have been several case reports describing endometrial ossification. It is most commonly believed to be due to retained fetal bone fragments, but in some cases may be due to metaplasia of mature endometrial stromal cells in response to chronic inflammation or trauma. Recently, it has been suggested that the incidence of this complication after pregnancy termination or spontaneous abortion has been underestimated in the literature.

In the early 1990's Melius et al found 50 cases in the literature.[43] Eighty percent of the cases occur after pregnancy. Retrospective research revealed a case of favorable pregnancy outcome in a woman with osseous metaplasia of the uterus. In this case the mass was embedded in the myometrium, with only a small spicule lying within the uterine cavity. The degree to which the uterine cavity is involved is of particular clinical relevance. The inability of the endometrium to permit implantation, retention and development of the embryo is one cause of failed implantation in an IVF cycle and secondary infertility in these patients. Extensive or endocervical forms are generally so deeply embedded that they are inaccessible to surgical hysteroscopy management.[44]

Notwithstanding the above controversies, the optimum method of treatment of osseous metaplasia is by hysteroscopy. In 1993, Acharya et al claimed to make the first report of the endoscopic resectoscope being used to diagnose and treat a woman with osseous metaplasia.[45] Since then, numerous reports have appeared in the literature on successful hysteroscopy management of osseous metaplasia.

To conclude, endometrial ossification, because it is a rare finding, can be misdiagnosed. An infertility physician must be alert if a scan shows an intrauterine structure that resembles an IUD. The final diagnosis is revealed by hysteroscopy. Furthermore, osseous metaplasia treated by hysteroscopy restores the ability of endometrium to achieve implantation.

HYSTEROSCOPY IN RECURRENT PREGNANCY LOSS

Diagnostic Hysteroscopy

Although in the infertile patient diagnostic hysteroscopy is very useful but not always indicated, in recurrent pregnancy loss the technique is mandatory. In woman with recurrent pregnancy loss when the state of the tubes is not important diagnostic hysteroscopy should be systematic as it contributes more information and produce the same discomfort as HSG. Although the TVUS has been effective in the diagnosis of uterine malformations, intrauterine adhesions, submucosal myoma and endometrial polyps, the direct vision of these pathologies gives diagnostic precision. On the other hand, conventional surgery has been displaced by the hysteroscopy surgery in the treatment of these pathologies when the gynecologist has mastered the surgical technique.

Embryoscopy

Morphological alterations are very difficult to diagnose in the embryos between the fourth and the sixth week unless they are very evident as in an embryonic sac.

Philipp and Kalousek[46] described and documented a series of embryonic neural tube defects in ten selected cases, concluding that transcervical embryoscopy (TE) is able to accurately diagnose development defects in cases of early pregnancy loss.

The embryo's morphology changes quickly. This process is very dynamic, and when correctly understood, allows to conclude that in some cases, when studying a detained pregnancy, some changes are observed in those embryos in which the only alteration seems to correspond to a delay of the development of just some corporal segments with regard to other segments of the same embryo or even compared with the development of other structures of the sac that have continued its development in-spite of having a dead embryo.[47]

It is from 7th week when a diagnosis of a craniofacial, branchial arches, vertebrae or limb defects can be observed. Even sex can be observed (FIGURE 5.10). These alterations can be clearly demonstrated when dating the embryo or if all segments have developed synchronously.[21] There are other morphological alterations with a well-described presentation like myelomeningocele, anencephaly, encephalocele, leporine lip, palatine fissure, polydactyly, the cord cysts and the evident pathologies beginning at week 7-8.[48]

There is no doubt of the value of TE in twin or multiple gestations, in which the technique allows to obtain independent samples of each of the embryos and membranes.[49]

It is important to remember that independent samples of the embryo and villus must be performed since as stated in many studies, chromosomal discrepancies between fetus and placenta may exist. These biopsies will be able to be studied in morphological, cytogenetic and immunohisto-chemical research.[50]

At present, the sonographic diagnosis of embryo-nic anomalies in early gestations, especially those under 10 weeks is not possible.[51]

TE in cases of missed abortion could thus reveal morphological abnormalities undetectable by TVUS.[25] It could increase the diagnoses spectrum and posterior evaluation of the pregnancy loss. This technique could establish a favorably characterized cohort of abortion specimens with seemingly normal chromosomes as a starting point for extensive detailed genetic studies. Such studies are needed to reach a better understanding of the embryopathogenesis and consequently early pregnancy loss.

It is still debatable if TE and cytogenetic studies should be offered to every woman with missed abor-

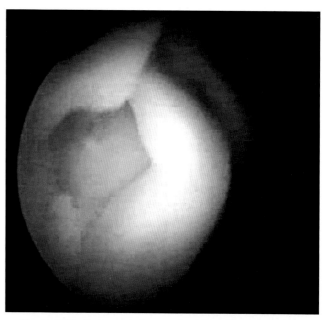

Figure 5.10: Endoscopic image of a 10 weeks male embryo

tion. These examinations provide etiologic data, but it is an invasive procedure and extra costs are requi-red in addressing a condition with a low recurrence risk rate. However, a detailed embryoscopic examination of the deceased embryo could prove to be useful in couples suffering recurrent abortion. In these cases chromosomal analysis is generally recommended.[52] TE could be indicated prior to the D&C in these patients to carry out chromosomal analysis in order to achieve a better understanding and diagnosis of the etiology of this entity.

Another potential application for the TE is the chorionic villus sampling under direct visual control. Some authors have explored this possibility and suggest that the number of abortions equals the number produced by classical ultrasonographic CVS, but the number of inconclusive diagnosis or placental mosaicism are reduced (This technique is explained in Chapter 16).

Operative Hysteroscopy

Submucosal Myoma

The actual involvement of myomas in sterility-infertility problems is not known. In 1-4% of all cases myomas are the only apparent cause of sterility.[53]

Different mechanisms have been postulated to explain the negative effect on fertility associated with myomas. These include irregularities in spermatic and embryonic transport, endometrial abnormalities that interfere with implantation, irregularities in uterine contractility, and interference with expansion and growth during pregnancy.

There are no well-designed studies comparing women with or without myomas, and desire for reproduction. At present, based on indirect studies in patients who underwent IVF, we can state that only submucosal or intramural myomas that affect the uterine cavity decrease or worsen the implantation and pregnancy rates. Their removal improves fertility. Therefore, these myomas should only be treated in young asymptomatic women who want to get pregnant.[54,55]

Nowadays, whereas SIS provides adequate information of the suspected affected cavity (specially of the intramural portion and the distance from the capsule to the serosa), only diagnostic hysteroscopy will determine the percentage of the cavity affected as well as the possibility of hysteroscopic resection.

Subserous fibromas create very few reproductive problems. Submucosal fibromas can cause methrorraghias that cause miscarriage due to placentation problems. In hysteroscopy it is rare to find submucosal fibromas that do not cause pathology. The finding of fibromas in this localization has increased because of greater diagnostic power with hysteroscopy, between 2-22% of the cases studied.

This relationship is more evident in the case of submucosal fibromas and in large intramural fibromas that make placentation difficult by altering the vascular bed or inducing uterine contractions (FIGURE 5.11). In 1063 pregnancies in women diagnosed with fibromas, 41% ended in miscarriage or the delivery of an unviable fetus. After myomectomy the risk was reduced to 19%. If we refer to submucosal fibromas over 5 cm, after myomectomy there were only 61% live newborns.[56]

Large intramural fibromas sometime cause chronic pain, preterm delivery, abruptio placenta and alterations in uterine dynamics during delivery or

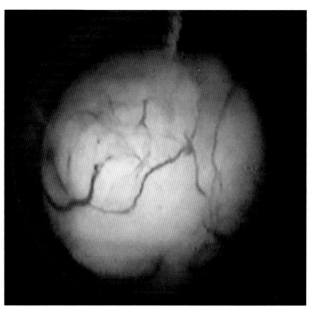

Figure 5.11: Type 0 submucous myoma filling the uterine cavity

postpartum hemorrhaging. Sonographic diagnosis identifies these high-risk cases and reduces fetal morbimortality.

Transvaginal sonography diagnoses with precision, the size and characteristics of fibromas, but also it distinguishes a fibroma from a polyp and the degree of penetration into the endometrial cavity (FIGURE 5.12). The introduction of saline solution via the cervical canal improves the sonographic images and competes with hysteroscopy in precision. When diagnostic hysteroscopy is essential to indicate surgery, the information that transvaginal sonography gives is very important too when informing about the depth of healthy myometrium that exists between the fibroma and uterine serosa.

The conduct to be followed in uterine fibroma depends also on the symptoms associated to sterility or infertility, on the number of tumors and their localization.

In asymptomatic sterile patients, myomectomy is performed only when other more frequent causes of sterility have been discarded or when the size or localization indicated that surgery would be beneficial.

Myomectomy by hysteroscopy was first described by Neuwirth in 1976 and a diathermal loop similar to a urological resector was used. It is the frequently used method. Other methods such as Nd-YAG laser

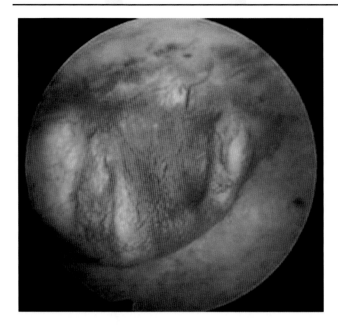

Figure 5.12: Three centimeters type I submucous myoma

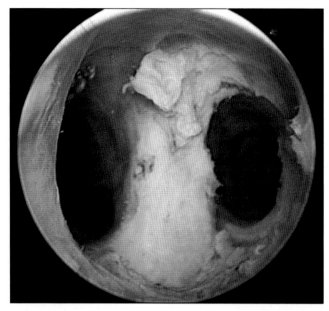

Figure 5.13: Uterine septum as seen from the isthmus

or just simple resection with scissors due to cost or difficulty are not extended practices.[57] Multiple submucosa fibromas are susceptible to this technique but the potential benefit must be carefully studied because post-resection synechiae may result more easily than if only one fibroma is removed. This is due to endometrial re-epithelialization.

At present, GnRH may be administered for two to three months to reduce the size, and the vascularization of the submucosal fibroids to make surgical resection easier. GnRH also atrophies the endometrium that helps with resection, decreasing the intensity of the hemorrhage although the inconvenience lies in cervical dilation prior to the introduction of the resector. Results are spectacular in abnormal uterine hemorrhaging.

Uterine Malformations

The reproductive outcome following hysteroscopy of symptomatic septate uteri has not only equaled but has surpassed the results obtained with traditional abdominal metroplasties. Viable pregnancies are achieved in 85-90% of patients with a history of recurrent pregnancy loss.[58] Furthermore, the patient has not had to undergo laparotomy and a hysterotomy, eliminating the potential for pelvic

adhesions and secondary infertility as well as the associated pain, disability, and expense to occur. Patients treated by hysteroscopy need to wait only four weeks to attempt conception, and do not require a mandatory cesarean section.[59]

Uterine malformations can be present in patients with normal fertility, with infertility or with recurrent pregnancy loss. The estimated incidence in recurrent pregnancy loss is about 2% in the general population.

The uterine septum is due to a lack of reabsorption of an original septum that results from a fusion of the two Müllerian ducts in the mid-portion to form the uterus (FIGURE 5.13). Because the remaining septum is usually avascular and composed of fibrotic tissue, when implantation occurs at this site, the blastocyst may not have sufficient nutrients and eventually is aborted. Furthermore, the compromised distending ability of a hemiuterus can cause irritability and premature labor.

HSG is 6-55% accurate in classifying uterine anomaly, whereas MRI and TVS are 96-100% and 85-92% accurate respectively. The main interest is the accuracy of MRI in reliably diagnosing a septate uterus that can be treated through the hysteroscope in order to avoid laparoscopy and general anesthesia. The 3-D ultrasonography is reliable too.

In the case of asymptomatic women, particularly those who require expensive treatments for ovulation induction, insemination, or in vitro fertilization and embryo transfer methods, may benefit from prophylactic removal of a uterine septum. The routine treatment of a uterine septum in patients who have proven fertility does not seem to be warranted (more information on this topic in Chapter 11).

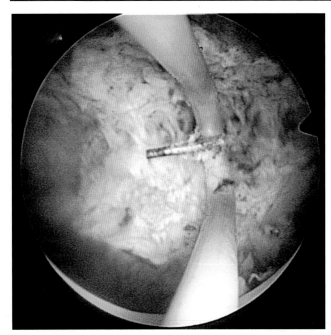

Figure 5.14: Collin's electrode for the hysteroscopic section of a uterine septum

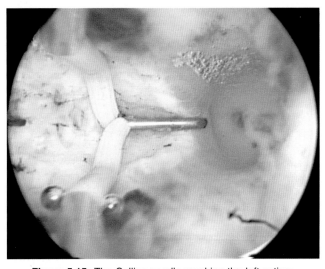

Figure 5.15: The Collins needle reaching the left ostium

The hysteroscopic resection of the septum or septolysis by means of mechanical or electrosurgical instruments has no significant differences in results and depends more on the personal preferences of the surgeon (FIGURES 5.14 and 5.15).[60-62] A 21-day administration of combined hormone therapy is advisable postoperatively. Follow-up office hysteroscopy is scheduled after the menstruation following hysteroscopy and remaining small adhesions can then be easily cut.

REFERENCES

1. Baramki TA. Hysterosalpingography. Fertil Steril 2005;83:1595-606.
2. Golan A, Eilat E, Ron-El R, Herman A, Soffer Y, Bukivsky I. Hysteroscopy is superior to hysterosalpingography in infertility investigation. Acta Obstet Gynecol Scand 1996;75:654-6.
3. Preutthipan S, Linasmita V. A prospective comparative study between hysterosalpingography and hysteroscopy in the detection of intrauterine pathology in patients with infertility. J Obstet Gynecol Res 2003;29:33-7.
4. Fedele L, Bianchi S, Dorta M, Brioschi D, Zanotti F, Vercellini P. Transvaginal ultrasonography versus hysteroscopy in the diagnosis of uterine submucous myomas. Obstet Gynecol 1991;77:745-53.
5. Dudiak KM. Hysterosonography: A key to what is inside the uterus. Ultrasound Q 2001;17(2):73-86.
6. Noyes N. Hysteroscopic cervical canal shaving: A new therapy for cervical stenosis before embryo transfer in patients undergoing in vitro fertilization. Fertil Steril 1999;71(5):965-6.
7. Seoud M, Awwad J, Adra A, Usta I, Khalil A, Nassar A. Primary infertility associated with isolated cervical collecting diverticulum. Fertil Steril 2002;77(1):179-82.
8. Pabuccu R, Ceyhan ST, Onalan G, Goktola U, Ercan CM, Selam B. Successful treatment of cervical stenosis with hysteroscopic canalization before embryo transfer in patients undergoing IVF: A case series. JMIG 2005;12:436-8.
9. Polisseni F, Bambirra EA, Camargos AF. Detection of chronic endometritis by diagnostic hysteroscopy in asymptomatic infertile patients. Gynecol Obstet Invest 2003;55(4):205-10.
10. Frydman R, Eibschitz I, Belaisch-Allart JC, Hazout A, Hamou JE. In vitro fertilization in tuberculous infertility. J In Vitro Fert Embryo Transf 1985;2(4):184-9.
11. La Sala GB, Montanari R, Dessanti L, Cigarini C, Sartori F. The role of diagnostic hysteroscopy and endometrial biopsy in assisted reproductive technologies. Fertil Steril 1998;70(2):378-80.
12. Cravello L, Porcu G, D'Ercole C, Roger V, Blanc B. Identification and treatment of endometritis. Contracep Fertil Sex 1997;25(7-8):585-6.
13. Siegler AM. Uterine causes of infertility. Curr Opin Obstet Gynecol 1990;2(2):173-81.
14. Coeman D, Van Belle Y, Vanderick G. Tubal ostium membranes and their relation to infertility. Fertil Steril 1995;63(3):666-8.
15. Golan A, Ron-El R, Herman A, Soffer Y, Bukovsky I, Caspi E. Diagnostic hysteroscopy: Its value in an in vitro fertilization/embryo transfer unit. Hum Reprod 1992;7(10): 1433-4.

16. Shamma FN, Lee G, Gutmann JN, Lavy G. The role of office hysteroscopy in in vitro fertilization. Fertil Steril 1992;58(6):1237-9.

17. Goldenberg M, Bider D, Ben-Rafael Z, Dor J, Levran D, Oelsner G, Mashiach S. Hysteroscopy in a program of in vitro fertilization. J in vitro Fert Embryo Transf 1991;8(6):336-8.

18. Dicker D, Ashkenazi J, Feldberg D, Farhi J, Shalev J, Ben-Rafael Z. The value of repeat hysteroscopic evaluation in patients with failed in vitro fertilization transfer cycles. Fertil Steril 1992;58(4):833-5.

19. Richlin S, Ramachandran S, Shanti A, Murphy AA, Parthasarathy S. Glycodelin levels in uterine flushings and in plasma of patients with leiomyomas and polyps: Implications and implantation. Hum Rep 2002;17,2742-7.

20. Sillo-Seidl G. The analysis of the endometrium of 1000 sterile women. Hormones 1971;2:70.

21. Hereter L, Carreras O, Pascual MA. Repercusión de la presencia de pólipos endometriales en un ciclo de FIV. Prog Obstet Ginecol 1998;41:5-7.

22. Varasteh NN, Neuwirth RS, Levin B, Keltz MD. Pregnancy rates after hysteroscopic polypectomy and myomectomy in infertile women. Obstet Gynecol 1999;94:168-71.

23. Spiewankiewicz B, Stelmachóv J, Sawicki W, Cedrowski K, Wypych P, Swiderska K. The effectiveness of hysteroscopic polypectomy in cases of female infertility. Clin Exp Obst & Gyn 2003;30:23-5.

24. Pérez-Medina T, Bajo-Arenas J, Salazar F, Redondo T, SanFrutos L, Alvarez P, Engels V. Endometrial polyps and their implication in the pregnancy rates of patients undergoing intrauterine insemination: A prospective, randomized study. Hum Reprod 2005;20:1632-5.

25. Oliveira F, Abdelmassih VG, Diamond MP, Dozortsev D, Nagy ZP, Abdelmassih R. Uterine cavity findings and hysteroscopic interventions in patients undergoing in vitro fertilization–embryo transfer who repeatedly cannot conceive. Fertil Steril 2003;80:1371-5.

26. Mooney SB, Milki AA. Effect of hysteroscopy performed in the cycle preceding controlled ovarian hyperstimulation on the outcome of in vitro fertilization. Fertil Steril 2003;79,637-8.

27. Deaton JL, Gibson M, Riddick DH, Brumsted JR. Diagnosis and treatment of cornual obstruction using a flexible tip guidewire. Fertil Steril 1990;53(2):232-6.

28. Honore GM, Holden AF, Schenken RS. Pathophysiology and management of proximal tubal blockage. Fertil Steril 1999;71:785-95.

29. Daniell JF, Miller W. Hysteroscopic correction of cornual occlusion with resultant term pregnancy. Fertil Steril 1987;48(3):490-2.

30. Sulak PJ, Letterie GS, Hayslip CC, Coddington CC, Klein TA. Hysteroscopic cannulation and lavage in the treatment of proximal tubal occlusion. Fertil Steril 1987;48(3):493-4.

31. Valle RF. Tubal cannulation. Obstet Gynecol Clin North Am 1995;22(3):519-40.

32. Ransom MX, Garcia AJ, Doherty K, Shelden R, Kemman F. Direct gamete uterine transfer in patients with tubal absence or occlusion. J Assist Reprod Genet 1997;14(1):35-8.

33. Das K, Nagel TC, Malo JW. Hysteroscopic cannulation for proximal tubal obstruction: A change for the better. Fertil Steril 1999;63(5):1009-15.

34. Sakumoto T, Shinkawa T, Izena H, Sakugawa M, Takamiyagi N, Inafuku K, Kanazawa K. Treatment of infertility associated with endometriosis by selective tubal catheterization under hysteroscopy and laparoscopy. Am J Obstet Gynecol 1993;169(3):744-7.

35. Asherman JG. Traumatic intrauterine adhesions. J Obstet Gynaecol Br Emp 1950;57:892-6.

36. Klein SM, Garcia CR. Asherman's syndrome: a critique and current review. Fertil Steril 1973;24:722-735.

37. Valle RF, Sciarra JJ. Intrauterine adhesions: Hysteroscopic diagnosis classification, treatment and reproductive outcome. Am J Obstet Gynecol 1988;158:1459-70.

38. Schlaff WD, Hurst BS. Preoperative sonographic measurement of endometrial pattern predicts outcome of surgical repair in patients with severe Asherman's syndrome. Fertil Steril 1995;63(2):410-3.

39. March CM. Intrauterine adhesions. Obstet Gynecol Clin North Am 1995;22(3):491-505.

40. Valle RF. Lysis of Intrauterine Adhesions (Asherman's Syndrome). In, Endoscopic Surgery for Gynaecologists. Sutton C, Diamond M (Eds): WB Saunders Company Ltd., London: Philadelphia. Toronto. Sydney Tokyo 1993;338-44.

41. Enrique Cayuela, Tirso Pérez-Medina. Osseous metaplasia: The bone is not from a fetus. Fertil Steril 2009;91:1293.e1-e4.

42. Lainas T, Zorzovilis I, Petsas G, Alexpoulou E, Lainas G, Loakimidis T. Osseous metaplasia: Case report and review. Fertil Steril 2004;82:1433-5.

43. Melius FA, Julian TM, Nagel TC. Prolonged retention of intrauterine bones. Obstet Gynecol 1991;78:919-21.

44. Onderoglu LS, Yarali H, Gultekin M, Katlan D. Endometrial osseous metaplasia; an evolving cause of secondary infertility. Fertil Steril 2008;90: 2013.e9-e11.

45. Acharya U, Pinion SB, Parkin DE, Hamilton MP. Osseous metaplasia of the endometrium treated by hysteroscopic resection. Br J Obstet Gynaecol 1993;100(4):391-2.

46. Kalousek DK. Anatomical and chromosomal abnormalities in specimens of early spontaneous abortions: Seven years experience. Birth Defects 1987;23:153-68.

47. Ferro J, Martinez MC, Lara C, Pellicer A, Remohi J, Serra V. Improved accuracy of hysteroembryoscopic biopsies for karyotyping early missed abortions. Fertil Steril 2003;80:1260-4.

48. Warburton D, Kline J, Stein Z, Hutzler M, Chin A, Hassold T. Does the Karyotype of a spontaneous abortion predict the karyotype of a subsequent abortion? Evidence from 273 women with two cariotipod spontaneous abortions. Am. J. Hum. Genet 1987;41:465-83.

49. Quintero RA, Romero R, Mahoney MJ, Abuhamad A, Vecchio M, Holden J, Hobbins JC. Embryoscopic demonstration of hemorrhagic lesions on the human embryo after placental trauma. Am J Obstet Gynecol 1993;168:756-9.

50. Philipp T, Philipp K, Reiner A, Beer F, Kalousek DK. Embryoscopic and cytogenetic analysis of 233 missed abortions: Factors involved in the pathogenesis of developmental defects of early failed pregnancies. Hum Reprod 2003;8:1724-32.

51. Kurjak A, Pooh RK, Merce LT, Carrera JM, Salihagic-Kadic A, Andonotopo W. Structural and functional early human development assessed by three-dimensional and four-dimensional sonography. Fertil Steril 2005;84(5):1285-99.

52. Dumez Y, Mandelbort L, Dommergues M. Embryoscopy in continuing pregnancies. In proceedings of the annual meeting of the international fetal medicine society. Evian (Eds): France;1992.

53. Buttram Jr VC, Reiter RC. Uterine leiomyomata: Aetiology, symptomatology and management. Fertil Steril 1981;36:433-45.

54. Pritts EA. Fibroids and infertility: A systematic review of the evidence. Obstet Gynecol Surv 2001;56(8):483-91.

55. Donnez J. What are the implications of myomas on fertility? A need of debate? Hum Reprod 2002;17(6):1424-30.

56. Shokeir TA. Hysteroscopic management in submucous fibroids to improve fertility. Arch Gynecol Obstet 2005;273(1):50-4.

57. Bernard G, Darai E, Poncelet C, Benifla JL, Madelenat P. Fertility after hysteroscopic myomectomy: Effect of intramural myomas associated. Eur J Obstet Gynecol Reprod Biol 2000;88(1):85-90.

58. Valle RF. Clinical management of uterine factors in infertile patients. In, Seminars in Reproductive Endocrinology. Sperof L (Ed.) Thieme-Stratton, Inc. Georg Thieme Verlag. New York, NY. 1985;3:149-67.

59. Doridot V, Gervaise A, Taylor S, Frydman R, Fernandez H. Obstetric outcome after endoscopic transection of the uterine septum. J Am Assoc Gynecol Laparosc 2003;10(2):271-5.

60. Buttram VC, Gibbons WE. Mullerian anomalies: A proposed classification (an analysis of 144 cases). Fertil Steril 1979;32:40-6.

61. Valle RF, Sciarra JJ. Hysteroscopic treatment of the septated uterus. Obstet Gynecol 1986;676:253-7.

62. Pabuccu R, Gomel V. Reproductive outcome after hysteroscopic metroplasty in women with septate uterus and otherwise unexplained infertility. Fertil Steril 2004;81(6):1675-8.

6

Endometrial Hyperplasia and Hysteroscopical Diagnosis

Jesus S Jimenez, Carmen Alvarez
Cristina Gonzalez Macho
Gregorio Lopez Gonzalez
Carmen Guillen Gamez

INTRODUCTION

At present, hysteroscopy (endoscopic visualization of the endometrial cavity) is the procedure used in the evaluation of the gynecological pathology like menorrhagia and postmenopausal bleeding. Hysteroscopy provides direct visualization of the lesion, thereby allowing targeted biopsy. Less invasive techniques like Cornier biopsy cannula, and more recently transvaginal ultrasound and hysterosonography have helped to upgrade the sensibility in diagnosis of the endometrial pathology, but no one of them offers the advantages of hysteroscopic study.

The debate on the value of the hysteroscopy in the diagnosis of premalignant and malignant injuries of the endometrium like hyperplasia and cancer continues to be opened. The imprecise and heterogeneous outcomes of limited available studies, make histopathologic validation of the visual endoscopic interpretation continue being controversial. Even though the elevated capacity in diagnosis of endometrial cancer has been demonstrated, it does not occur in endometrial hyperplasia whose sensibility in the diagnosis is between 56 and 82%. The expectations of this procedure for diagnosis of premalignant lesions have not been confirmed. Hysteroscopic images not always present a perfect correlation with the histological study. For this reason targeted biopsy proves to be essential.[1,2]

ENDOMETRIAL HYPERPLASIA

Endometrial hyperplasia is characterized by proliferation of endometrial glands resulting in a greater gland-to-stroma ratio than observed in normal endometrium.[3] The proliferating glands vary in size and shape, and may show cytological atypia, which may progress to or coexist with endometrial cancer. Endometrial hyperplasia virtually always results from chronic estrogen stimulation unopposed by the counterbalancing effects of progesterone. Although this process is often diffuse and not always the whole cavity is affected.

The classification of endometrial hyperplasia is based upon two factors:

1. The glandular/stromal architectural pattern, which is either simple or complex
2. The presence or absence of nuclear atypia.

Already from 1990, Cullen[5] aimed at possibility of progression to carcinoma. This progression is correlated with presence and gravity of nuclear atypia. According to Kurman and Norris[6] this progression is between 1% in case of endometrial hyperplasia without atypia to 29% when nuclear atypias are present.

CLINIC

Abnormal uterine bleeding is the most common clinical symptom, although it can be, at times asymptomatic. Endometrial hyperplasia is common among perimenopausal women or younger women with risk factors causing an hyperestrogenic status, such as obesity, infertility, polycystic ovary syndrome (chronic anovulation) or unopposed estrogen therapy.

DIAGNOSTIC IMAGING

Vaginal ultrasound and saline infusion sonohysterography have improved sensibility in endometrial pathology diagnosis. Recently, Doppler ultrasound and Echo 3D have improved the sensibility even more,[7] but no one of them offers the advantages of the hysteroscopy, than in addition to the direct vision of the lesion, allows to carry out a directed biopsy.

Diffuse endometrial thickening, typical of endometrial hyperplasia may be evaluated by ultrasound (FIGURES 6.1A and B). The sonographic aspects that should make suspect endometrial hyperplasia are the following:
- *Endometrial thickness:* The cut-off point of normality in premenopausal women at the end of the secretory phase, in postmenopausal women with THS and in postmenopausal women in the absence of hormone replacement therapy are 18-20 mm, 8 mm and 5 mm respectively. Endometrial thickening especially in women with abnormal bleeding should be studied (FIGURE 6.1A).
- *Endometrial morphology:* Endometrium presents a increased density, but homogeneous, compared

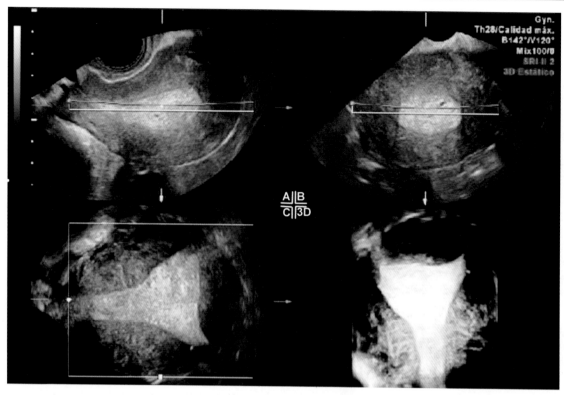

Figure 6.1A: Ecographical aspects: Endometrial thickness

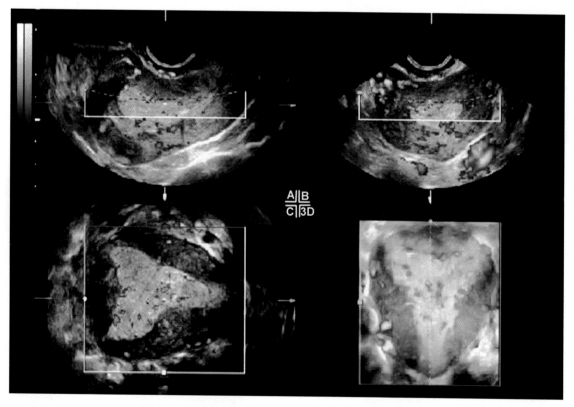

Figure 6.1B: Ecographical aspects: Endometrial vascularization

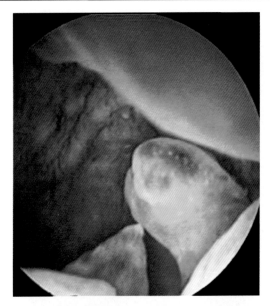

Figure 6.2: Endometrial thickness

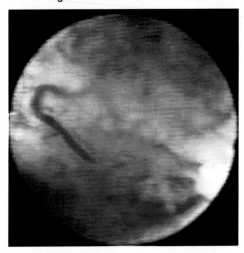

Figure 6.3: Endometrial vascularization

with myometrium. Occasionally, it presents anechoic areas suggesting cystic glandular dilatations.

- *Endometrium-myometrium junction:* It presents a regular and clearly defined contour. Endometrial midline is continuous and uniform with a clear hyperecogenic central line.
- *Endometrial vascularization:* The color Doppler imaging presents regular vascularization coming from myometrium (FIGURE 6.1B).

HYSTEROSCOPICAL DIAGNOSIS OF HYPERPLASIA

A specific pattern does not exist for each kind of hyperplasia. The macroscopic visualization of one or more of the following findings is indicative of its existence:

- Focal or diffuse endometrial thickness with irregular and unequal surface and polypoidal or papillary pattern (FIGURE 6.2).
- Increase in superficial vascularization, with disordered endometrial vessels regarding the normal endometrium's delicate net. Very vascularized mucosa that bleeds easily (FIGURE 6.3).
- Increase of endometrial glandular orifices density, spaced and irregulars, with or without enlargement of the glands' openings (FIGURE 6.4).
- Dilatation of the endometrial glands, cystic glandular changes on a thick endometrium. (FIGURE 6.5).

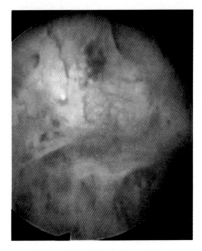

Figure 6.4: Glandular orifices

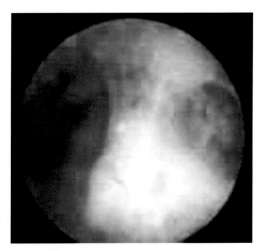

Figure 6.5: Endometrial glands

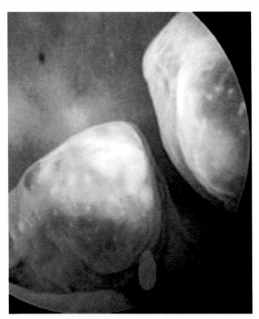

Figure 6.6: Polypoidal mass

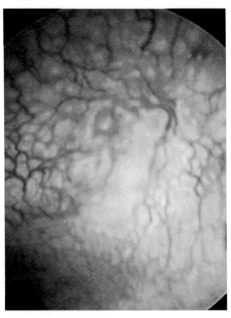

Figure 6.7: Abnormal vascularization

Hysteroscopical diagnosis at the end of prolife-rative phase, when mucosa is in highest thickness might be difficult because of similar appearance with hyperplasia. Likewise the difficulty in uterine cavity distension might interfere in right endometrial thickness and superficial vascularization inter-pretation.[1] In spite of macroscopic criteria are clearly defined, its interpretation is not easy.

Efficacy and histopathologic correlation of hysteroscopy in this entity is between 56% and 83%, showing a 63.5% PPV and 79.4% PNV.[3,8-11] A review of 65 studies with 26346 patients, who underwent hysteroscopical study for diagnosis of endometrial hyperplasia or carcinoma, showed limitations for endometrial hyperplasia diagnosis (78% sensitivity and 95.8% specificity).[12] Better data were found in endometrial cancer diagnosis where hysteroscopy showed 86.4% of sensitivity and 99.2% of specificity.[10]

In an attempt of improving diagnostic capacity of hysteroscopy in diagnosis of hyperplasia, some authors[13] have defined macroscopic criteria that present a better histopathologic correlation like:

*   Diffuse and polypoid endometrial growth
*   Whitish glandular orifices with elevated borders, unequal size and irregular distribution with zones of group.

The diagnosis becomes more difficult if we have in account that hysteroscopical vision does not allow differentiation between a high-risk hyperplasia (complex with atypia) and a diffuse highly differen-tiated adenocarcinoma, finding both even in 29% cases of hyperplasia.[14,15]

In addition to hysteroscopic criteria of endo-metrial hyperplasia, exists several discoveries that raise the probability of finding graver endometrial pathology (RR 51.1).[14-17]

*   Increase of the endometrial thickness
*   Polypoidal formations, cerebroids and irregular mass (FIGURE 6.6)
*   Abnormal vascularization (FIGURE 6.7)
*   Friable excrescences
*   Necrosis
*   Spontaneous and to the contact bleeding.

REFERENCES

1. Mencaglia L, Valle RF, Perino A, Gilardi G. Endometrial carcinoma and its precursors: early detection and treatment. Int J Gynecol Obstet 1990;31:107-16.
2. Hamou JE. Microhysteroscopy. A new procedure and its original applications in Gynecology. J Repro Med 1981;26:375-9.
3. Uno LH, Sugimoto O, Carvalho FM, Bagnoli VR, Fonseca AM, Pinotti JA. Morphologic hysteroscopic criteria suggestive of endometrial hyperplasia. Int J Gynecol Obstet 1995;49:35-40.

4. Loverro G, Bettochi S, Cormio G et al. Diagnostic accuracy of hysteroscopy in endometrial hyperplasia. Maturitas 1996;25:187-91.

5. Cullen TS. Cancer of the uterus. Saunders: Philadelphia, 1990.

6. Kurman RJ, Norris HJ. Evaluation of criteria for distinguishing endometrial atypical hyperplasia from well differential carcinoma. Cancer 1982;49:2547-59.

7. Odeh M, Vainerovsky I, Grinin V, Kais M, Ophir E, Bornstein J. Three-dimensional endometrial volume and three-dimensional power Doppler analysis in predicting endometrial carcinoma and hyperplasia. Gynecol Oncol 2007;106:348-53.

8. Mencaglia L, Perino A. Hysteroscopy and micro-colpohysteroscopy in gynecologic. In Baggish MS, Barbot J, Valle RF (Eds): Diagnostic and operative hysteroscopy. A text and atlas. Saunders (edition): Philadelphia, 1988.

9. Garuti G, Cellani F, Garzia D, Colonnelli M, Luerti M. Accuracy of hysteroscopic diagnosis of endometrial hyperplasia: A retrospective study of 323 patients. J Min Inv Gynecol 2005;12:247-53.

10. Bassil R, Barrozo PR, Pinho de Oliveira MA, Silva E, Dias R. Validation of hysteroscopic view in cases of endometrial hyperplasia and cancer in patients with abnormal uterine bleeding. J Minimally Invasive Gynecol 2006;13:409-12.

11. Garuti G, Sambruni I, Colonnelli M, Luerti M. Accuracy of hysteroscopy in predicting histopathology of endometrium in 1500 women. J Am Assoc Gynecol Laparos 2001;8:207-13.

12. Clark TJ, Voit D, Gupta JK. Accuracy of hysteroscopy in the diagnosis of endometrial cancer and hyperplasia: A systematic quantitative review JAMA 2002;288:1610-21.

13. Inafuku K, Nakayama M. Hysteroscopic diagnosis of adenomatous hyperplasia according to the type of endometrial glandular opening. Act Obstet Gynecol 1987;39:2069-74.

14. Trimble et al. Concurrent endometrial carcinoma in women a biopsy diagnosis of atypical endometrial hyperplasia. A Gynecologic Oncology Group Study. Cancer 2006;106: 812-9.

15. Bakur H, Dwaraskanat S, Khan S, Newton J. The diagnosis accuracy of outpatient miniature hysteroscopy in predicting premalignant and malignant endometrial lesions. Gynecol Endoscopy1999;8:143-8.

16. Lo KW, Yuen PM. The role of outpatient hysteroscopy in identifying anatomic pathology and histopathology in the endometrial cavity. J Am Gynecol Laparosc 2000;7:380-5.

17. Butureanu SA, Socolov RM, Pricop F, Gafitanu DM. Diagnostic hysteroscopy in endometrial hyperplasia. Gynecologic and Obstetric Investigation 2005;59:59-61.

7

Hysteroscopy and Endometrial Carcinoma

Enrique Cayuela Font
Juncal Pineros Manzano
Purificación Regueiró Espin
Alberto Puig Menem

INTRODUCTION

Endometrial cancer continues to be the most frequent female genital tract malignancy. In Western countries, endometrial cancer has an incidence of 17/100,000 per year and a mortality of approximately 7/100,000 per year. In the United States, the number of new cases is 40,100 per year, with 7470 deaths annually.[1] Ninety-percent of cases are diagnosed in women older than 50 years, with a peak incidence between 70 and 74 years. Only 25% of endometrial carcinomas occur in premenopausal women, with 3-4% of cases diagnosed in women younger than 40 years of age.[2]

Approximately 80% of endometrial cancers share the following characteristics: Endometrioid histological features, well-differentiated tumors and lesion confined to the uterine fundus at the time of diagnosis. The most important prognostic factors include FIGO stage, histologic grade and depth of myometrial invasion. Other factors that should be considered are the age of the patient, histologic type, positive peritoneal cytology, invasion of the lymphovascular space, activity of progesterone receptors, hormonal status, and tumor size.

Postmenopausal women with uterine bleeding have a probability of endometrial cancer ranging between 3.7 and 19.9%.[2]

Risk Factors

Risk factors for endometrial cancer[1] are shown in TABLE 7.1.

Types of Endometrial Cancer

Three types of endometrial cancer have been described.[3]

- Type I is estrogen dependent (exogenous and endogenous estrogens) and is known to arise from atypical hyperplasia. It is considered that endometrial hyperplasia has a high malignant potential. Bergeron et al[4] have proposed a simplification of the WHO classification of endometrial hyperplasia into the three categories of simple, complex, and complex with atypia. The primary differentiating factor is the presence of cytologic atypia, which significantly increases the likelihood of

Table 7.1: Risk factors for endometrial carcinoma

Major risk factors	Menarche before 12 years of age Late menopause (after 50 years old) Never having children Infertility Tamoxifen therapy Use of hormone replacement therapy (HRT)
Minor risk factors	Hereditary nonpolyposis colorectal cancer Diabetes Polycystic ovarian disease Obesity High animal fat diet Family history of endometrial cancer History of breast or ovarian cancer Prior pelvic radiation therapy

progression to cancer.[5] The risk of progression to endometrial cancer has been reported as low as 1.1% for simple hyperplasia, between 2 and 36.7% for complex hyperplasia, and between 52 and 88.9% for atypical hyperplasia.[5] Estrogen-dependent endometrial cancer accounts for 80-85% of cases of malignancy of the endometrium, and most tumors are well or moderately differentiated endometrioid adenocarcinomas. Risk factors for endometrial cancer shown in TABLE 7.1, are usually present in patients with this type of endometrial carcinoma. Obesity is an independent risk factor and in Western Europe, overweight is associated with endometrial cancer in about 40% of cases.

- Type II endometrial cancer is not estrogen dependent and appears unrelated to endometrial hyperplasia. This pathogenetic variant is more aggressive and affects older postmenopausal women. Poorly differentiated tumors usually arise, predominantly with papillary serous and clear cell adenocarcinomas as well as other types with high nuclear grade.[3]

- Type III endometrial cancer or Lynch syndrome II, often called hereditary nonpolyposis colorectal cancer, is a type of autosomal inherited cancer of the digestive tract and accounts for 10% of cases of endometrial carcinoma.[4] Women with this disorder have an increased risk of cancers of the gastrointestinal tract (colon, rectum, stomach, small intestine, liver, biliary tree), and also a high-risk of cancer of the endometrium. Individuals with this disorder are more likely to have a genetic predisposition to obesity.

Survival

Mortality has been estimated to be 3% of all female cancers. The 5-year survival depends on the stage of the disease at the time of diagnosis. In the United States, survival at 5 years for stage I endometrial cancer is about 90%.[1] Survival rates for the different stages[5] are shown in TABLE 7.2.

Clinical Manifestations

Metrorrhagia is the cardinal symptom of endometrial carcinoma. Bleeding from the uterus in a post-menopausal woman is suggestive of endometrial cancer. Persistent bleeding, unresponsive to standard treatment measures, in a premenopausal woman older than 35 years is also suggestive of endometrial hyperplasia or endometrial cancer.

In a clinical series of 4200 diagnostic hysteroscopies, endometrial cancer was identified in 156 cases (Cayuela E, unpublished data). The most common indications for hysteroscopy are shown in TABLE 7.3. Abnormal uterine bleeding in the postmenopausal woman was the most frequent indication of hysteroscopy followed by metrorrhagia in women over 40 years of age. Other indications included abnormal endometrial findings in asymptomatic women undergoing transvaginal ultrasonography or abnormal cervical cytology (Pap smear) or nuclear atypia or the endometrial gland cells found on biopsy.

DIAGNOSIS OF ENDOMETRIAL CANCER

Endometrial biopsy together with transvaginal ultrasound and hysteroscopy are the main diagnostic methods for benign and malignant lesions of the endometrium.

Histopathological examination is the gold standard for the diagnosis of cancer of the endometrium.

Fractional dilatation and curettage under general anesthesia, which has been a common diagnostic method in the past cannot be currently recommended. Limitations of this procedure include inadequate amount of tissue (in many cases less than 50% of endometrial thickness is obtained), 10% of endometrial conditions are undiagnosed, polyps and, myomas and in some cases, endometrial hyperplasia

Table 7.2: Survival at 5 years for the different stages of endometrial cancer

Stage	Survival rate
I	81 to 89%
II	72 to 80%
III	51 to 63%
IV	17 to 20%

Table 7.3: Indications of hysteroscopy in 156 women

Indication	Percentage
Postmenopausal metrorrhagia patients	83
Premenopausal metrorrhagia patients	8
Abnormal endometrial findings on transvaginal ultrasound (asymptomatic woman)	3
Abnormal Pap smear or endometrial biopsy	3
Tamoxifen treatment	1
Endocervical polyp	1
Control of treatment of endometrial hyperplasia	1

and focal endometrial carcinomas are not diagnosed. Curettage has a sensitivity of 20% and a positive predictive value of 50%. Moreover, hospitalization, general anesthesia and dilatation of the cervix are necessary, with the risk of complications, such as uterine perforation or infection.[8,9] For these reasons, blind curettage was abandoned and substituted by hysteroscopy.[10]

However, when a diagnostic hysteroscopy should be performed is still controversial. In the presence of postmenopausal metrorrhagia, which is (are) the diagnostic method(s) of choice: Ultrasonography, endometrial biopsy, hysteroscopy, or a combination of them? Under a cost-effectiveness perspective, transvaginal ultrasonography should be performed firstly. Numerous studies measuring endometrial thickness with the use of transvaginal ultrasonography have indicated that an endometrial thickness of less than 5 mm is rarely associated with carcinoma. The combination of transvaginal ultrasonography and endometrial biopsy improves the negative predictive value.

In office, endometrial biopsy is performed with 2.3 to 3 mm cannules. One of the disadvantages of biopsy is that solid tumors (polyps and myomas) are not always diagnosed but in remaining intrauterine conditions, the diagnostic accuracy is very high, ranging between 87 and 100%.[11]

Endometrial sampling using the Pipelle device has a low probability of getting an adequate endometrial sample, when the endometrial thickness is < 5 mm. Therefore, in the investigation of postmenopausal bleeding, it seems reasonable to avoid endometrial sampling when the endometrial thickness is < 4 mm.[12]

In a meta-analysis of 39 studies that included 7914 women undergoing endometrial sampling by means of dilatation and curettage or hysteroscopy for the detection of endometrial carcinoma, the detection rate was higher in postmenopausal women compared with premenopausal women. In both postmenopausal and premenopausal women, the Pipelle was the best device, with detection rates of 99.6 and 91%, respectively.[13] Pipelle biopsy yields an insufficient amount of material for analysis in 16 to 25% of cases.[14] In a multicenter study of 1168 women, with postmenopausal bleeding scheduled for curettage, risk of finding pathologic endometrium at curettage when the endometrium was < 5 mm, as measured by transvaginal ultrasonography was 5.5%. Thus in women with postmenopausal bleeding and an endometrium < 5 mm it would seem justified to refrain from curettage.[15]

A definite diagnosis of endometrial cancer cannot be made by transvaginal ultrasonography but this procedure allows to suspect the presence of an endometrial malignancy. Numerous studies have assessed the efficacy of transvaginal ultrasonography in the diagnosis and/or screening of endometrial cancer in postmenopausal women. The negative predictive value for an endometrial thickness < 5 mm is 99 to 100%,[16-18] and in these cases, diagnostic studies should include hysteroscopy and/or endometrial biopsy.

Although transvaginal ultrasonography is a cost-effective procedure as an initial diagnostic technique in women with postmenopausal bleeding, hysteroscopy is also considered a first choice procedure.[19-21]

Hysteroscopic Images of Malignant Tumors of the Uterus

A morphologic classification of hysteroscopic images of neoplasms of the uterus is difficult to establish. After a review of the literature, the only morphologic

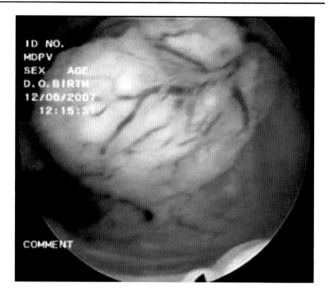

Figure 7.1: Polypoid neoplasm. Atypical vascularization

Table 7.4: Morphologic classification of hysteroscopic images adapted from Sugimoto et al.[22]

Involvement	Gross appearance	Origin
Circumscribed	Polypoid	Primary
Diffuse	Nodular	Metastatic
	Papillary	
	Ulcerated	

classification of hysteroscopic images is that described by Sugimoto et al[22] and depicted in TABLE 7.4.

Polypoid type endometrial carcinoma is the most frequent, and consists of polypoid, cerebroid projections with irregular excrescences (FIGURE 7.1). The tissue has cotton-like aspect and is usually thin, fragile, and bleeds spontaneously in contact with the hysteroscopy biopsy forceps. Abnormal vascularization with sinuous and tortuous atypical vessels is clearly visible. A thick and translucent secretion blurring the image is usually present. Dark brown necrotic areas with whitish, yellowish, fine points are occasionally observed (FIGURE 7.2).

Papillary serous tumor is frequently found in a small atrophic uterus. The tumor is composed by numerous papillae of dendritic type, with a vessel in each one. The tissue is also extremely friable and bleeds easily when comes into contact with the biopsy forceps.

Neoplasms appearing as tumor masses are tumors of mesenchymal origin, adenosarcoma, leiomyosarcoma, stromal sarcoma, mixed mesodermic

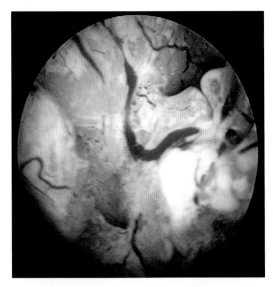

Figure 7.2: Whitish spots and atypical vessels

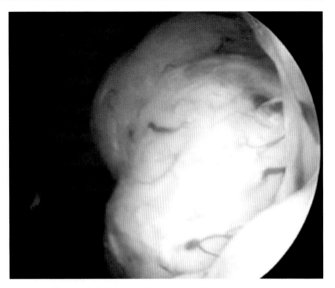

Figure 7.4: Intrauterine metastatic ovarian tumor

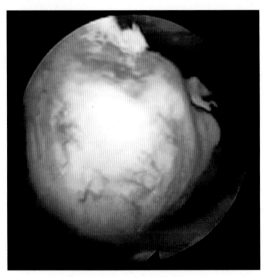

Figure 7.3: Mixed Müllerian tumor

Table 7.5: Gross assessment of invasion in endometrial cancer

Focal or circumscribed	A very small area of the uterine cavity is involved. Anatomy of the uterus is preserved
Less than one-third of the cavity	Affects a larger area but the anatomy of the uterus is still visible
Between one- and two-thirds of the cavity	Affects a larger area and there are difficulties to recognize the remaining of the uterus
More than two-thirds of the cavity	The entire cavity is involved. The ostiums and the remaining anatomy are unrecognizable
Cervical involvement	Endocervical spread

tumors, etc., which resemble a myoma because of its gross appearance and tissue hardness, which makes difficult to obtain adequate samples for histologic examination. In many cases, these tumors may easily be misdiagnosed as uterine myomas (FIGURE 7.3). The remaining endometrium is frequently atrophic.

Intrauterine metastatic tumors of primary carcinomas of the ovary (FIGURE 7.4), breast, etc. can also be occasionally found.

Tumor Invasion

Invasion of the uterine cavity can be easily assessed following the scheme depicted in TABLE 7.5.

Different studies have assessed the accuracy of hysteroscopy in the diagnosis of endometrial cancer (TABLE 7.6). In most series, hysteroscopy revealed sensitivity between 80 and 93%, and specificity 100%.

Hysteroscopy has some limitations in the differentiation between endometrial hyperplasia and endometrial cancer. In fact, pathologists who carried out histological examination of tissue specimens under microscope with × 400 magnification and with specific stains, sometimes have problems for diagnosing not only atypical hyperplasia, but also to differentiate atypical hyperplasia from grade 1 endometrial cancer.[4,26-28] There are various different histological classifications for the differentiation between complex hyperplasia with atypia and grade 1 endometrial

Table 7.6: Sensitivity and specificity of hysteroscopy in comparison with biopsy for diagnosing endometrial cancer

Author, year	Sensitivity (%)	Specificity (%)	Positive predictive value (%)	Negative predictive value (%)
Labastida, 1990[22]	91.1	99.6	78.8	99.8
Pérez-Medina et al, 1994[25]	88.9	100	100	99.2
Haller et al, 1996[18]	93	93.9	95	93.9
Clark et al, 2002[23]	86.4	99.2		
Lasmar et al, 2006[24]	80	99.5	81.6	99.5
Cayuela (Personal data)	92.3	99.7	92.3	99.6

carcinoma. The possibility of misdiagnosis of hyperplasia is inherent in the technique, given the morphological *in vivo* study and without staining methods that is carried out by means of hysteroscopy. This would account for the risk of detecting adenocarcinomas in surgical resected specimens in cases previously diagnosed of atypical hyperplasia by hysteroscopy. The percentage of endometrial carcinomas that remain undiagnosed ranges between 21 and 50%.[29-31] Diagnosis of malignancy in endometrial polyps is another limitation of hysteroscopy. The malignant potential of endometrial polyps varies between 0.5 and 4.8% (see Chapter of Endometrial Polyps).

Possibility of Diagnosing Cervical Invasion

Invasion of the cervix occurs in 10-20% of endometrial cancers through direct extension and invasion (FIGURE 7.5), or by lymph node metastasis affecting the cervical stroma.

Invasion of the cervical stroma increases the rate of spread of the disease and involvement of the parametria. In these cases, the survival at 5 years decreases to 60-70%. For this reason, it is very important to determine the extension of cervical invasion to decide the most appropriate treatment.

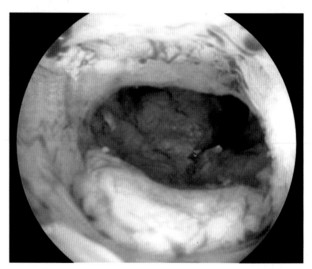

Figure 7.5: Direct invasion of the endocervix

Hysteroscopy is partially effective in the diagnosis of cervical involvement (TABLE 7.7). The positive predictive value is low, whereas the negative predictive value is notably better. Diagnostic accuracy of hysteroscopy is limited for several reasons, including atypical vessels bleeding on touch and directed biopsies which bleed easily leading to blurred vision, as well as difficulties in maintaining adequate distention to visualize clearly the endocervix. Moreover, metastases in the cervical stroma are not visible by hysteroscopy giving rise to false negative cases.

Table 7.7: Diagnostic accuracy of hysteroscopy in the diagnosis of cervical invasion

Author, year	Sensitivity (%)	Specificity (%)	Positive predictive value (%)	Negative predictive value (%)
Toki et al, 1998[32]	82	90	64	96
Lo et al, 2001[33]	68	99	93	92
Avila et al, 2008[34]	87	47	66	75
Cicinelli et al, 2008[35]	93	88	58	98
Cayuela (Personal data)	62	92	57	93

Hysteroscopy and Positive Peritoneal Cytology

Distension of the uterine cavity during hysteroscopy has been suspected to cause tumor cell dissemination into the abdominal cavity in patients with endometrial carcinoma. Disseminating endometrial carcinoma cells into the peritoneal cavity during hysteroscopy is therefore a matter of concern. In 1989, the International Federation of Gynecology and Obstetrics (FIGO) included peritoneal cytology in the staging of endometrial carcinoma (stage IIIA, tumor invades serosa or adnexa, or malignant peritoneal cytology).[36] The clinical and prognostic significance of malignant peritoneal cells in the absence of extrauterine disease is unclear.[37]

Does Hysteroscopy Facilitate Tumor Cell Dissemination into the Peritoneal Cavity?

Many controversial results have been reported in the literature. Different authors[38-42] have shown dissemination of tumor cells into the abdominal cavity during diagnostic hysteroscopy (FIGURE 7.6), whereas others indicated that hysteroscopy does not produce spread of endometrial cancer cells.[43-48]

A systematic review of five studies with 756 patients, 79 of which presented a positive peritoneal cytology demonstrated that diagnostic hysteroscopy did not increase significantly the risk of abdominal dissemination of tumor cells.[49] In addition, it has been shown that hysteroscopy does not increase the risk of penetration of tumour cells into the peritoneal cavity more than estimates in dilatation and curettage[44] or endometrial biopsy.[46] Other studies confirmed that the diagnostic method, dilatation and curettage, hysteroscopy, or pipelle endometrial biopsy, does not influence upon the percentage of positive peritoneal cytology.[45,48]

On the other hand, spreading of endometrial cells at diagnostic hysteroscopy comparing the two distension media, carbon dioxide and normal saline, was found to be more likely after the use of normal saline in one study,[50] whereas in a prospective, randomized, cross-over comparison, transtubal dissemination occurred irrespectively whether

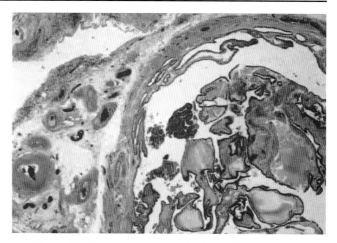

Figure 7.6: Tumor cells floating in the pelvicl cavity after diagnostic hysteroscopy

normal saline or carbon dioxide is used for gaseous distension.[51] On the other hand, threshold intrauterine perfusion pressures for intraperitoneal leakage of dye from the fallopian tube have been reported to exceed either 70 mm Hg[52] or 40 mm Hg.[53]

Are Endometrial Carcinoma Cells Disseminated into the Peritoneal Cavity Functionally Viable?

In a study of 24 uteri obtained at total abdominal hysterectomy/bilateral salpingo-oophorectomy in patients with endometrial carcinoma, in vitro fluid hysteroscopy was performed and fluid running off through the tubes was collected and, viable cells, cultured. The endpoint of the analysis was the adherence of culture tumor cells to the polyvinyl chloride well plate, which was taken as a proxy for functional cell viability. Tumor cells were found in 17 specimens (71%), and in 10 (42%) specimens the disseminated tumor cells were functionally viable. This model suggests that hysteroscopy can cause dissemination of malignant cells into the abdominal cavity from uteri containing endometrial carcinoma, and that these cells can be functionally viable and adhere to a matrix.[54] These data, however, have not yet been demonstrated in vivo.

A prospective study in which sonohysterography was performed on 16 patients with endometrial adenocarcinoma at laparotomy, the median volume that was required for adequate sonohysterography was 8.5 ml, no critical spill volume was identified, and only disseminated benign cells demonstrate viability.[55]

Malignant cells in the peritoneal washing are found in about 12% (5-20%) of patients with stage I endometrial cancer. In our experience, 3.3% of stage I endometrial cancer patients had positive peritoneal cytology at the time of surgery. Positive peritoneal cytology rates of 10.4% have been reported in the series of Yazbeck et al.[49] and 12.5% in the study of Takac et al.[56] In contrast, in the study of Grimshaw et al.[57], in which diagnostic hysterectomy was not performed, extrauterine disease at surgery was documented in 2.3% of the patients. The frequency of positive peritoneal cytology in stage I endometrial cancer in different studies independently of previous diagnostic hysterectomy is shown in TABLE 7.8.

How Positive Peritoneal Cytology Affects 5-year Prognosis?

Different studies have shown that although there is an increased risk of peritoneal dissemination of malignant cells at diagnostic hysterectomy, which is similar to that associated with any intrauterine manipulation procedure, there is no evidence suggesting a poor prognosis for these patients.[47,58-60] In a clinicocytopathological study of 250 patients with stage I endometrial cancer carried out to assess the prognostic value of positive peritoneal cytology, the 5-year disease-free survival of patients positive or negative for malignant cells was 98.1% and 100%, respectively.[61] In a retrospective cohort study of 43 consecutive patients with endometrial carcinoma FIGO stage I, diagnosed with hysteroscopy and tissue sampling and treated by abdominal hysterectomy with bilateral salpingo-oophorectomy, the 5-year disease-specific survival rate was 91.8%.[62] This data indicate that diagnostic hysteroscopy has no adverse effect on prognosis in stage I endometrial cancer patients.

CONCLUSION

Despite limitations of the studies published in the literature related to the retrospective design, small sample size and methodological drawbacks,

Table 7.8: Positive peritoneal cytology in stage I endometrial carcinoma

Author	Hysteroscopy	Year	Cases	Positive cytology
Grimshaw et al.[57]	No	1990	305	2.3%
Cayuela (personal data)	Yes	2001	123	3.3%
Yazbeck et al.[49]	Yes	2005	756	10.4%
Takac et al.[56]	Yes	2007	146	12.5%

hysteroscopy has an important role in the work-up studies of patients with endometrial cancer, which can be summarized as follows.

- Hysteroscopy with an endometrial biopsy is an adequate procedure for the diagnosis of endometrial cancer.
- In the presence of a qualified hysteroscopist, adequate equipment and facilities, hysteroscopy with an endometrial biopsy is the procedure of choice in women with postmenopausal bleeding
- Hysteroscopic assessment of endocervical invasion of endometrial cancer is difficult.
- Distension of the uterine cavity during hysteroscopy may cause tumor cell dissemination into the abdominal cavity, which may be related to the pressure of the distension media. Therefore, the minimal pressure allowing visualization of the uterus should be used. If the diagnosis of endometrial cancer has been already obtained by an endometrial biopsy, the practice of hysterectomy is not necessary.
- It seems that malignant cells disseminated into the peritoneum cavity are rarely viable.
- Diagnostic hysteroscopy has no adverse effect on 5-year survival in endometrial cancer patients.

REFERENCES

1. American Cancer Society database. Cancer statistics 2006. Available at: www.cancer.org/downloads/PRO/EndometrialCancer.pdf
2. Gallup DG, Stock RJ. Adenocarcinoma of the endometrium in women 40 years of age or younger. Obstet Gynecol 1984;64:417-20.
3. Bokhman JV. Two pathologic types of endometrial carcinoma. Gynecol Oncol 1983;15:10-7.
4. Bergeron C, Nogales FF, Masseroli M, Abeler V, Duvillard P, Müller-Holzner E, Pickartz H, Wells M. A multicentric European study testing the reproducibility of the WHO classification of endometrial hyperplasia with a proposal of

a simplified working classification for biopsy and curettage specimens. Am J Surg Pathol 1999;23:1102-8.

5. Marsden J, Sturdee D. Cancer issues. Best Pract Res Clin Obstet Gynaecol. 2009;23:87-107.

6. Sorosky JI. Endometrial cancer. Obstet Gynecol 2008;111:436-47.

7. Creasman WT, Odicino F, Maisonneuve P, Beller U, Benedet JL, Heintz AP, Ngan HY, Sideri M, Pecorelli S. Carcinoma of de corpus uteri. J. Epidemiol Biostat 2001;6:47-86.

8. Mencaglia L, Valle RF, Tonellotto D, Tiso E. Early diagnosis of endometrial carcinoma and precursors and mass screening for endometrial cancer. In: Mencaglia L, Valle RF, Lurain J (eds). Endometrial carcinoma and precursors. Diagnosis and treatment. Herndon, VA: Books International, 1999, pp 13-43.

9. Valle RF. Office hysteroscopy. In: Baggish MS, Barbot J, Valle RF (Eds). Diagnostic and operative hysteroscopy. 2nd edition. St. Louis: Mosby Inc., 1999;171-83.

10. Siegler AM. Office hysteroscopy. Obstet Gynecol Clin North Am 1995;22:457-71.

11. Svirsky R, Smorgick N, Rozowski U, Sagiv R, Feingold M, Halperin R, Pansky M. Can we rely on blind endometrial biopsy for detection of focal intrauterine pathology? Am J Obstet Gynecol 2008;199:115.e1-e3.

12. Elsandabesee D, Greenwood P. The performance of Pipelle endometrial sampling in a dedicated postmenopausal bleeding clinic. J Obstet Gynaecol 2005;25:32-4.

13. Dijkhuizen FP, Mol BW, Brölmann HA, Heintz AP. The accuracy of endometrial sampling in the diagnosis of patients with endometrial carcinoma and hyperplasia: A meta-analysis. Cancer 2000;89:1765-72.

14. Machado F, Moreno J, Carazo M, León J, Fiol G, Serna R. Accuracy of endometrial biopsy with the Cornier pipelle for diagnosis of endometrial cancer and atypical hyperplasia. Eur J Gynaecol Oncol 2003;24:279-81.

15. Karlsson B, Granberg S, Wikland M, Ylöstalo P, Torvid K, Marsal K, Valentin L. Transvaginal ultrasonography of the endometrium in women with postmenopausal bleeding: A Nordic multicenter study. Am J Obstet Gynecol 1995;173:1637-8.

16. Gull B, Carlsson S, Karlsson B, Ylöstalo P, Milsom I, Granberg S. Transvaginal ultrasonography of the endometrium in women with postmenopausal bleeding: Is it always necessary to perform an endometrial biopsy? Am J Obstet Gynecol 2000;182:509-15.

17. Bakour SH, Dwarakanath LS, Khan KS, Newton JR, Gupta JK. The diagnostic accuracy of ultrasound scan in predicting endometrial hyperplasia and cancer in postmenopausal bleeding. Acta Obstet Gynecol Scand 1999;78:447-51.

18. Haller H, Matecjciæ N, Rukavina B, Kraseviæ M, Rupciæ S, Mozetic D. Transvaginal sonography and hysteroscopy in women with postmenopausal bleeding. Int J Gynaecol Obstet 1996;54:155-9.

19. Cayuela E. Grupo Histeroscopia. Documentos de Consenso Sociedad Española de Ostetricia y Ginecología (SEGO). Meditex Madrid 1996;11-45.

20. Valle RF. Manual of clinical hysteroscopy. New Cork: Taylor and Francis 2005;25-37.

21. Van Herendael BJ, Valle R, Bettocchi S. Ambulatory hysteroscopy. Diagnosis and treatment. Oxfordshire, UK: Blandon Medical Publishing, 2004;7-11.

22. Labastida R. Tratado y atlas de histeroscopia. Barcelona, Spain: Editorial Salvat 1990;167-90.

23. Clark TJ, Voit D, Gupta JK, Hyde C, Song F, Khan KS. Accuracy of hysteroscopy in the diagnosis of endometrial cancer and hyperplasia: A systematic quantitative review. JAMA 2002;288:1610-21.

24. Lasmar RB, Barrozo PR, de Oliveira MA, Coutinho ES, Dias R. Validation of hysteroscopic view in cases of endometrial hyperplasia and cancer in patients with abnormal uterine bleeding. J Minim Invasive Gynecol 2006;13:409-12.

25. Pérez-Medina T, López-Mora P, Rojo J, Martínez-Cortes L, Huertas MA, Haya J, Bajo J. Comparación de la histeroscopia-biopsia con el legrado en el diagnostico de la hemorragia uterina anormal. Prog Obst Gin 1994;37:479-86.

26. Zaino RJ, Kauderer J, Trimble CL, Silverberg SG, Curtin JP, Lim PC, Gallup DG. Reproducibility of the diagnosis of atypical endometrial hyperplasia: A Gynecologic Oncology Group study. Cancer 2006;106:804-11.

27. Kendall BS, Ronnett BM, Isacson C, Cho KR, Hedrick L, Diener-West M, Kurman RJ. Reproducibility of the diagnosis of endometrial hyperplasia, atypical hyperplasia, and well-differentiated carcinoma. Am J Surg Pathol 1998;22:1012-9.

28. Ronnett BM, Kurman RJ. Precursor lesions of endometrial carcinoma. In Kurman R (Ed): Blaustein's Pathology of the Female Genital Tract, 5th edn. Springer-Verlag: New York, 2002.

29. Trimble CL, Kauderer J, Zaino R, Silverberg S, Lim PC, Burke JJ 2nd, Alberts D, Curtin J. Concurrent endometrial carcinoma in women with a biopsy diagnosis of atypical endometrial hyperplasia: A Gynecologic Oncology Group study. Cancer 2006;106:812-9.

30. Edris F, Vilos GA, Al-Mubarak A, Ettler HC, Hollett-Caines J, Abu-Rafea B. Resectoscopic surgery may be an alternative to hysterectomy in high-risk women with atypical endometrial hyperplasia. J Minim Invasive Gynecol 2007; 14:68-73.

31. Shutter J, Wright TC Jr. Prevalence of underlying adenocarcinoma in women with atypical endometrial hyperplasia. Int Gynecol Pathol 2005;24:313-8.

32. Toki T, Oka K, Nakayama K, Oguchi O, Fujii S. A comparative study of preoperative procedures to assess cervical invasion by endometrial carcinoma. Br J Obstet Gynaecol 1998;105:512-6.

33. Lo KW, Cheung TH, Yim SF, Chung TK. Preoperative hysteroscopic assessment of cervical invasion by endometrial carcinoma: A retrospective study. Gynecol Oncol 2001;82:279-82.

34. Avila ML, Ruiz R, Cortaberria JR, Rivero B, Ugalde FJ. Assessment of cervical involvement in endometrial carcinoma by hysteroscopy and directed biopsy. Int J Gynecol Cancer 2008;18:128-31.

35. Cicinelli E, Marinaccio M, Barba B, Tinelli R, Colafiglio G, Pedote P, Rossi C, Pinto V. Reliability of diagnostic fluid hysteroscopy in the assessment of cervical invasion by endometrial carcinoma: A comparative study with transvaginal sonography and MRI. Gynecol Oncol 2008;111:55-61.

36. International Federation of Gynecology and Obstetrics. Corpus cancer staging. Int J Gynecol Obstet 1989;28:190-7.

37. Balagueró L, Comino. R, Jurado M, Petschen I, Sainz de la Cuesta R, Xercavins J. Endometrial Carcinoma. Consensus Documents. Spanish Society Gynecology and Obstetrics 1999;89-137.

38. Romano S, Shimoni Y, Muralee D, Shalev E. Retrograde seeding of endometrial carcinoma during hysteroscopy. Gynecol Oncol 1992;44:116-8.

39. Schmitz MJ, Nahhas WA. Hysteroscopy may transport malignant cells into the peritoneal cavity. Case report. Eur J Gynaecol Oncol 1994;15:121-4.

40. Egarter C, Krestan C, Kurz C. Abdominal dissemination of malignant cells with hysteroscopy. Gynecol Oncol 1996;63:143-4.

41. Rose PG, Mendelsohn G, Kornbluth I. Hysteroscopic dissemination of endometrial carcinoma. Gynecol Oncol 1998;71:145-6.

42. Benifla JL, Darai E, Filippini F, Walker-Combrouze F, Crequat J, Madelenat. Operative hysteroscopy may transport endometrial cells into the peritoneal cavity: Report of a prospective longitudinal study. Gynaecol Endosc 1997;6:151-3.

43. Zerbe MJ, Zhang J, Bristow RE, Grumbine FC, Abularach S, Montz FJ. Retrograde seeding of malignant cells during hysteroscopy in presumed early endometrial cancer. Gynecol Oncol 2000;79:55-8.

44. Kudela M, Pilka R. Is there a real risk in patients with endometrial carcinoma undergoing diagnostic hysteroscopy (HSC)? Eur J Gynaecol Oncol 2002;22:342-4.

45. Gutman G, Almog B, Lessing J, Bar-Am A, Grisaru D. Diagnosis of endometrial cancer by hysteroscopy does not increase the risk for microscopic extrauterine spread in early stage disease. Obstet Gynecol Surv 2005;60:579-80.

46. Gu M, Shi W, Huang J, Barakat RR, Thaler HT, Saigo PE. Association between initial diagnostic procedure and hysteroscopy and abnormal peritoneal washings in patients with endometrial carcinoma. Cancer 2000;90:143-7.

47. Revel A, Tsafrir A, Anteby SO, Shushan A. Does hysteroscopy produce intraperitoneal spread of endometrial cancer cells? Obstet Gynecol Surv 2004;59:280-4.

48. Ferrero A, Obispo C, Bravo G, Lamas MJ. Citología peritoneal en pacientes con carcinoma de endometrio según la realización previa de histeroscopia diagnóstica y biopsia dirigida frente al legrado fraccionado. Clin Invest Gin Obst 2004;31:353-8.

49. Yazbeck C, Dhainaut C, Batallan A, Benifla JL, Thoury A, Madelenat P. Diagnostic hysteroscopy and risk of peritoneal dissemination of tumor cells. Gynecol Obstet Fertil 2005;33:247-52.

50. Lo KW, Cheung TH, Yim SF, Chung TK. Hysteroscopic dissemination of endometrial carcinoma using carbon dioxide and normal saline: A retrospective study. Gynecol Oncol 2002;84:394-8.

51. Nagele F, Wieser F, Deery A, Hart R, Magos A. Endometrial cell dissemination at diagnostic hysteroscopy: A prospective randomized cross-over comparison of normal saline and carbon dioxide uterine distension. Hum Reprod 1999;14:2739-42.

52. Baker VL, Adamson GD. Threshold intrauterine perfusion pressures for intraperitoneal spill during hydrotubation and correlation with tubal adhesive disease. Fertil Steril 1995;64:1066-9.

53. Solima E, Brusati V, Ditto A, Kusamura S, Martinelli F, Hanozet F, Carcangiu ML, Maccauro M, Raspagliesi F. Hysteroscopy in endometrial cancer: New methods to evaluate transtubal leakage of saline distension medium. Am J Obstet Gynecol 2008;198:214.e1-4.

54. Arikan G, Reich O, Weiss U, Hahn T, Reinisch S, Tamussino K, Pickel H, Desoye G. Are endometrial carcinoma cells disseminated at hysteroscopy functionally viable? Gynecol Oncol 2001;83:221-6.

55. Berry E, Lindheim SR, Connor JP, Hartenbach EM, Schink JC, Harter J, Eickhoff JC, Kushner DM. Sonohysterography and endometrial cancer: Incidence and functional viability of disseminated malignant cells. Am J Obstet Gynecol 2008;199:240.e1-8.

56. Takac I, Zegura B. Office hysteroscopy and the risk of microscopic extrauterine spread in endometrial cancer. Gynecol Oncol 2007;107:94-8.

57. Grimshaw RN, Tupper WC, Fraser RC, Tompkins MG, Jeffrey JF. Prognostic value of peritoneal cytology in endometrial carcinoma. Gynecol Oncol 1990;36:97-100.

58. Obermair A, Geramou M, Gücer F, Denison U, Graf AH, Kapshammer E, Medl M, Rosen A, Wierrani W, Frech I, Preyer O, Speiser P, Kainz C. Impact of hysteroscopy on disease-free survival in clinically stage I endometrial cancer patients. Int J Gynecol Oncol 2001;10:275-9.

59. Vilos GA, Edris F, Al-Mubarak A, Ettler HC, Hollett-Caines J, Abu-Rafea B. Hysteroscopic surgery does not adversely affect the long-term prognosis of women with endometrial adenocarcinoma. J Minim Invasive Gynecol 2007;14:205-10.

60. Sáinz de la Cuesta R, Espinosa JA, Crespo E, Granizo JJ, Rivas F. Does fluid hysteroscopy increase the stage or worsen the prognosis in patients with endometrial cancer? A randomized controlled trial. Obstet Gynecol Reprod Biol 2004;115:211-5.

61. Takeshima N, Nishida H, Tabata T, Hirai Y, Hasumi K. Positive peritoneal cytology in endometrial cancer: Enhancement of other prognostic indicators. Gynecol Oncol 2001;82:470-3.

62. Biewenga P, DeBlock S, Birnie E. Does diagnostic hysteroscopy in patients with stage I endometrial carcinoma cause positive peritoneal washing? Gynecol Oncol 2004;93:194-8.

8

Instrumentation and Distension Media in Diagnostic and Surgical Hysteroscopy

Enrique Cayuela Font
Sonia Moros
Josep Grau Galtes

INSTRUMENTATION

The first documented endoscopy, which was a cystoscopy, was performed by Bozzini in 1807. It was not until 1970 that hysteroscopy began to develop. The design of the optical system by Hopkins (FIGURE 8.1A) entailed a significant technological change, with the introduction of thinner, brighter lenses with excellent image clarity. Development of hysteroscopy and all other endoscopic techniques began at this time.

Hysteroscopes

Of the different options, two main types of hysteroscopes can be distinguished depending on the flexibility of the body of the hysteroscope: Rigid and flexible.

Rigid Hysteroscopes

They are characterized by having a rigid lens and sheath. It is important to be familiar with the foroblique system (FIGURE 8.1A) that determines the visual field that can be viewed by the observer, depending on the angle at the distal end of the lens. There are three types of lenses (0°, 12° and 30°), each of which has different applications. The diameter of the lens and sheath vary depending on the manufacturer. Therefore, the maximum and minimum diameters have been indicated, and we have attempted to include as many models available on the market as possible. The most well known manufacturers are Olympus, Storz, Wolf, Circon-Acmi and Gynecaretic.

Rigid Diagnostic Hysteroscopes

Single flow distension
Conventional: This is an exclusively diagnostic single flow hysteroscope. It has a 30° foroblique lens with a diameter of 2.9 to 3 mm and a 4 to 4.5 mm detachable external sheath. The distension medium, which may be CO_2 or liquid media, passes through the inside of the sheath. At present hysteroscopy with CO_2 distension is used less than continuous flow hysteroscopy with liquid distension media (TABLE 8.1).

Table 8.1: Classification of endoscopes

Outer sheath diameter	Classification
> 5 mm	Conventional
2 to 5 mm	Minihysteroscopes
< 2 mm	Microhysteroscopes

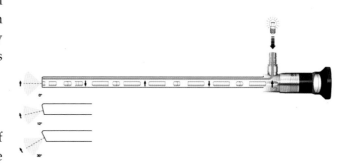

Figure 8.1A: Hopkins lens system.
Field of view: Lens 0°, 12°, 30°

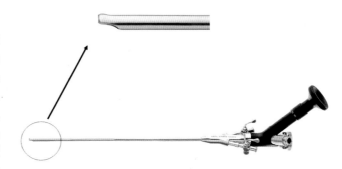

Figure 8.1B: Distal view of the Storz minihysteroscope

Minihysteroscopes: Introduced recently. They have a 30° lens with a diameter of 1.2 to 1.9 mm and a 2.5 to 3 mm external sheath. Image quality is similar to conventional hysteroscopes (FIGURE 8.1B).

Microhysteroscopes: They have a diameter of less than 2 mm and they are made of fiber optics. They are very fragile and image quality is not very good.

Continuous flow distension: One characteristic of continuous flow hysteroscopes is that they are equipped with two separate canals: One for inserting the liquid distension medium and another for discharge (FIGURE 8.2). One advantage of the use of liquid media for distension of the uterus is that the cavity undergoes continuous lavage. This eliminates blood, mucus, detritus and bubbles, and a good

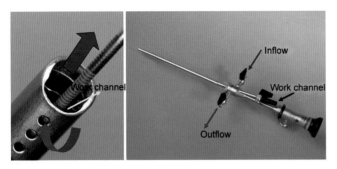

Figure 8.2: Olympus continuous flow hysteroscope, Arrow blue: Inflow, Arrow red: Outflow

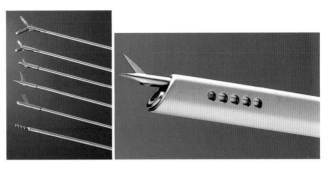

Figure 8.3: Storz types of ancillary instruments

image is obtained even in patients with not very intense mehrorrhagia.

There are two types:

Exclusively diagnostic hysteroscope: External diameter of 4 to 4.5 mm and 30° foroblique lens with a diameter of 2 to 3 mm.

Diagnostic and therapeutic hysteroscope I: External diameter of 5 to 5.5 mm, 30° foroblique lens with diameter of 2 to 3 mm. It has an accessory working canal of 5 Fr. where scissors, capture forceps, biopsy forceps, scalpel electrode and coagulation electrode can be inserted (FIGURE 8.3). With these instruments guided biopsies; minor interventions such as removal of polyps, intrauterine devices and small pedunculated myomas; as well as dissection of mucous or fibrous adherences that are not very complex and thin septa can be performed. Tubal sterilization is also performed with the Essure method.

Diagnostic and therapeutic hysteroscope II: External diameter of 7 to 8.3 mm with a 30° lens with a diameter of 4 mm and a working canal of 7 Fr. Due to the external diameter, local anesthesia and dilatation with Hegar's rods are required.

(*Note:* 1 Fr. French = 1.3 mm)

Flexible Hysteroscopes

These are fiber optic hysteroscopes: Those with a diameter of 3.1 to 3.7 mm are used for diagnosis, whereas 4.9 to 5.3 mm diameters with a working canal are used for surgery (Olympus, Fujinon, Storz, Circon Acmi, Mochida). They are equipped with a mechanism that allows 100° guidance of the tip of the hysteroscope so that areas which are not visible with the rigid hysteroscope can be seen (e.g. forced

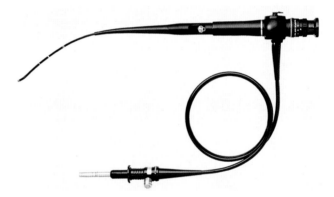

Figure 8.4: Olympus diagnostic flexible hysteroscope

uterine retroflexion or uterine horns with very sharp angles). Since it is optical fiber, the image shown is a cell similar to the honeycomb of bees, and quality is lower. They are not continuous flow, with the exception of the hysteroscope manufactured by Olympus, which can be equipped with a rigid external sheath. The price is high (FIGURE 8.4).

Monopolar surgery: It uses the same generator as that used daily in operating theatres. Since current is monopolar, the return plate for the generator must be used. The distension medium must be ion-free.

Types: Diagnostic-therapeutic hysteroscope equipped with button-shaped 5 Fr. monopolar electrodes for coagulation and a cutting needle (FIGURE 8.3). Use of this hysteroscope is reserved for very specific cases of small polyps and thin septa.

Monopolar resectoscope: It is formed basically by an external sheath, internal sheath, working element, lens, seal and electrodes (FIGURES 8.5 and 8.6). The working element has been designed so that it adapts to the surgeon's hand (FIGURE 8.7). It is equipped with a connection for the electrical cable from the

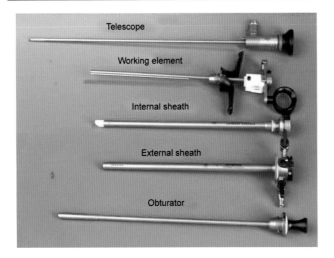

Figure 8.5: Resectoscope elements

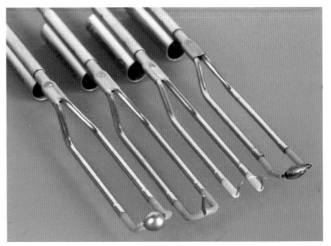

Figure 8.8: Olympus resectoscope electrodes

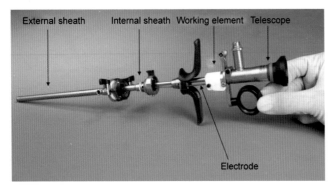

Figure 8.6: Resectoscope

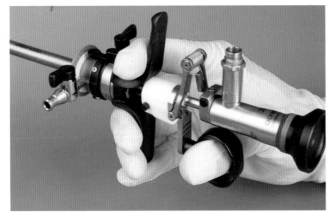

Figure 8.7: Hand position in the working element

electrode comes out from inside of the sheath, and cutting or coagulation can be performed. There are three types of resectoscopes, depending on the external diameter: 7, 8 and 9 mm. The 7 mm resectoscope is equipped with a 0° or 12° lens with a diameter of 3 mm and loop electrodes, ball and needle. Use is limited to minor interventions in patients who are sterile or have a stenotic cervix. It has the disadvantage that the electrodes are very small and fragile. The 8 mm resectoscope is equipped with the same 0° and 12° lens with a diameter of 3 mm and the same electrodes. Interventions of greater breadth can be performed in all types of patients. It is equipped with a seal so that the cervix will not be injured. The 9 mm hysteroscope is the one that is used most frequently. It has a 12° or 30° foroblique lens with a diameter of 4 mm; however, use of the 12° lens is usually the most appropriate. There are also rolling ball electrodes, cylinder, handle, needle or scalpel (FIGURES 8.8 and 8.9). The cylinder is also available with tips that are used to vaporize myomas and for endometrial ablations. All of them operate with the continuous flow system (FIGURE 8.10) and with ion-free distension media.

Bipolar surgery: Electrodes for bipolar use are currently available. The advantages over monopolar energy are: The return plate is not needed, and physiological saline is used as distension medium. They require a specific current generator.

current generator. The thumb is placed on the back handle, and the next three fingers are placed on the front handle. It has a spring that keeps the electrode inside of the sheath when it is at rest. When the thumb is pressed against the other three fingers, the

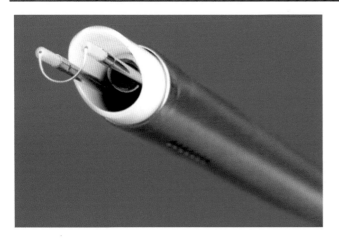

Figure 8.9: Detail of resectoscope

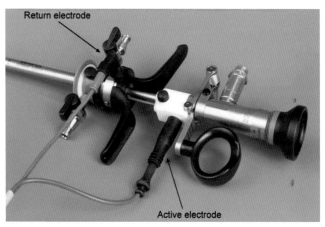

Figure 8.11: Olympus bipolar resectoscope

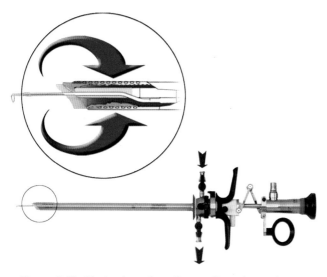

Figure 8.10: Mechanism of continuous flow of resectoscope

The Versapoint™ system: This consists of a specific bipolar current generator that is connected to some electrodes. The diameter is 5 Fr. and it is compatible with the working canal of continuous flow hysteroscopes. Minor surgery such as removal of polyps, small type 0 myomas, and septa can be performed in the consulting room.

Bipolar resectoscope: The main characteristics is that both electrodes are in the working element (FIGURE 8.11). There are three differences compared to the monopolar resectoscope. First of all, the size of the loop and ball electrodes is very small. Therefore, surgery takes a bit longer since a smaller amount of

tissue is obtained at each cut. Secondly, electrical power (watts) greater than that used in monopolar surgery is needed. Thirdly, as mentioned, since the distension medium is physiological saline, it is considered to be safer. This is the future of surgical hysteroscopy once the drawbacks have been resolved.

Laser surgery: For this type of surgery there must be a 75 W source of Neodymium: Yttrium-aluminium-garnet (Nd: YAG). Energy is transmitted through a 0.4-0.8 mm teflon-coated quartz fiber. These therapeutic hysteroscopes are used for conventional surgery. They are equipped with a 5 Fr. working canal. All hysteroscopic surgery can be performed with Nd: YAG laser. It has the drawback of the high purchase price and maintenance. In recent years, use in hysteroscopy has decreased significantly.

Light Sources

There are several commercial brands on the market with applications in all fields of endoscopy. In diagnostic hysteroscopy with CO_2, a 250 W 24 V tungsten halogen light source is sufficient. Although it is also more expensive, the ideal light source is equipped with a 300 W 50-60 Hz xenon lamp that gives off light similar to natural light (FIGURE 8.12). Most light sources have a 150 W auxiliary halogen emergency lamp. When the light source and the tele-

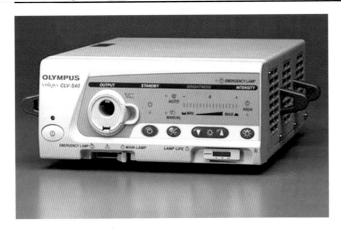

Figure 8.12: Xenon light source

vision camera are made by the same manufacturer, there is automatic self-regulation of light: When the television camera detects excess or defective light, it sends a signal to the light source to adapt to the new light status without losing image quality due to conditions that are too bright or too dark. The fiber optic cable has the function of taking the light from the source to the hysteroscope; some cables are equipped with a condenser on the end. They have the drawback of being extremely fragile. It is easy for the fibers inside to break when it is bent or receives blows. Therefore, as all endoscopic material, it should be handled with great care.

Camera

The same cameras used in laparoscopy are also used in hysteroscopy. The cameras used most frequently have a "chip" with resolution of 470,000 pixels and 1 lux sensitivity. Cameras with 3 chips have not been demonstrated to be more effective in hysteroscopy. The system must be compatible with NTSC and PAL formats. The outgoing connections for the video signal are important for recording surgery or examinations. Most cameras have several different BNC connectors (less quality); Y/C connectors, which use a S-VHS signal; RGB connectors; and DV connectors (firewire) which use a digital signal, and provide high quality images for recording. It can be connected to a video recorder or a PC with the appro-

priate software. In view of the future, some of these cameras already have fiber optic connections.

TV Monitor

Until commercialization of high definition, televisions and monitors are introduced, three types of monitors are presently available.

Conventional cathode ray monitors: At present the 14 or 20 inch Trinitron tube still offers the highest quality image. Although the technology is old, at this time it is still the best image available.

Plasma: This type of screen is made of two glass panels separated by a very small space (0.1 mm). Between the panels, gas is stored in the form of plasma. This gas is activated by electrical impulses and converted into red, green and blue pixels (RGB). These thousands of light points generate images with good stability, high fidelity in reproduction and good quality in terms of color and contrast. They are used on large screens. Image quality is not as good as the conventional Trinitron monitor.

Liquid crystal display or thin film transistor (LCD-TFT): This is a liquid crystal screen that contains one transistor for each pixel. The set of transistors regulates the light coming from the back of the monitor. With this technology, image quality is hardly affected if the viewing angle is not located in front of the screen. Image quality is similar to that of the Trinitron tube.

Recording Images

Recording images is very important. It can be used for several purposes. First of all, and most important, for teaching purposes. It can be used for resident gynecologists who want to learn the technique. Moreover, one can recover the recording and compare it with the histological diagnosis. Secondly, it may be useful for legal purposes, although this is a controversial subject.

There are many image recording media, including the nearly obsolete VHS and S-VHS video as well as the more recent DVD, and the mini-DV or DVCAM, which are digital formats.

Auxiliary Material

This is the material required on the work table:
- Collins speculum
- Forceps
- Tenaculum (Pozzi)
- Half size Hegar tents 3 to 7 (3 to 10 for resectoscopic procedures)
- Tweezers
- Hysterometer
- Aqueous iodine
- 10 ml syringe and long needle (0.9 × 70 mm)
- Local anesthetics
- Sterile swabs (10 × 10)

DISTENSION MEDIA

The endometrial cavity is a virtual space which is only distended in pathological situations (polyps, myomas). Except in these cases, the uterine walls are joined, and together with the endometrium they form something similar to a sandwich. In order to achieve good visualization the cavity must be distended. Since 1914, when Heineberg was able to distend the uterus with water, several different elements were used to do so, with poor results. This continued until 1970, when Edstrom and Fernstrom were able to achieve good distension with an excellent image using dextran-70, a high viscosity fluid. In 1981, Goldrath used a low viscosity fluid to perform an endometrial ablation for the first time. At present many different distension media are available, which we will describe below.

High Viscosity Fluids

Hyskon is a distension medium that is used for diagnostic and surgical hysteroscopy. It was used frequently in the 1980's in Anglo-Saxon countries, but it is difficult to find in Spain. At present it has been replaced by other media.

Low Viscosity Fluids with Electrolytes

These fluids are introduced regularly in daily clinical practice as intravenous infusions, since they have an expansive effect and can be used as a vehicle for drugs. An important characteristic associated with these fluids is the fact that they conduct electricity. Therefore, in surgical procedures with a monopolar current generator they are clearly contraindicated due to the risk of causing lesions.

These distension media are suitable for continuous flow diagnostic and surgical hysteroscopy. The advantages are as follows:
- Greater margin in fluid intravasation (to patient bloodstream). Nevertheless, pulmonary or cerebral edema can not be ruled out if too much fluid is lost, particularly in patients with heart failure or renal failure
- Easy to obtain
- Low cost.

Interventions such as guided biopsies, polypectomies, septostomy, myomectomies, synechotomy, removal of foreign bodies, etc. can be performed using scissors, biopsy forceps and forceps for removal of remains with diagnostic-therapeutic hysteroscopes. They are also appropriate for bipolar resectoscope, Versapoint and laser surgery. The most frequently used are:

Physiological saline: Solution composed of 0.9% isotonic sodium chloride that contains 154 mEq/l of NaCl and has an osmolarity of 310 mOsm/l. Na^+ is the principal cation in this solution. It is also the principal cation of the extracellular space, where it has important functions in controlling fluids and in acid-base metabolism.

Lactated Ringer's solution: Solution formed by sodium chloride, sodium lactate, potassium chloride and calcium chloride. Contains 130 mEq/l of sodium, 4 mEq/l of potassium, 3 mEq/l of calcium and 110 mEq/ l of chloride. Osmolarity is 275 mOsm/l. It is used less than physiological saline.

Low Viscosity Fluids without Electrolytes

In order to practice electrosurgery, particularly in hysteroscopic surgery with monopolar current, distension media without electrolytes should be used.

Types
- *5% glucose:* Osmolarity of 256 mOsm/l. This media has the drawback of presentation in 1 liter containers. It is used in short interventions.

Excess intravasation causes hyperglycemia and aqueous intoxication (described below).

- *1.5% glycine:* This is the medium used most frequently. It is also the medium with which there is most experience, since it has been used in urology in transurethral resections since 1948. Glycine is an amino acid that is metabolized in the form of ammonium, serine and glyoxylic acid. It is a hypotonic solution with an osmolarity of 200 mOsm/l. If the patient absorbs more than 1000.
- 1500 cc, serious complications may arise, including aqueous intoxication. Pathophysiology and treatment of this condition are described in the chapter on complications.

  - In order to prevent complications we should: Maintain strict control of the balance of distension medium inflow and outflow.
  - Respect infusion pressures and flows.
  - Not exceed 60 minutes of intervention.
  - Use infusion pumps that provide immediate information on the balance of the distension medium, and stop the intervention if there is intravasation or loss of over 1,000 ml of distention medium.

- *Sorbitol/mannitol:* Referred to as Cytal or Mein's solution. It is a solution with 2.7% sorbitol and 0.54% mannitol. Mannitol is an osmotic diuretic. Nevertheless, in spite of the preventive effect of diuresis, aqueous intoxication may occur. The mechanisms that cause aqueous intoxication after massive absorption are similar to those described in glycine. The clinical consequences of intravasation are the same, but hyperglycemia is also associated. For treatment, the regimen used is the same as for glycine intoxication.

DISTENSION SYSTEMS

Diagnostic Hysteroscopy

If CO_2 is used as distension medium, use of a specific hystero-insufflator is essential.

If fluid media are used, there are several options:

- *Gravity infusion:* Consists of placing a 3 liter bag of physiological saline at a height of 1 to 1.5 meters from the hysteroscope. At this height there will

be an infusion pressure of 85-105 mm Hg. Good distension is achieved and the flow rate is usually 300 to 500 ml. Complications are exceptional.

- *Pressure sleeve infusion:* There are several devices on the market that have a pressure sleeve around the bag of serum. Manual insufflation may be used, with a ball similar to that used in sphygmomanometers, presetting pressure to 100-150 mm Hg, or electrical insufflation by a compressor that inflates a sleeve bag automatically at the same pressure.
- Pump infusion.

Surgical Hysteroscopes

Surgery with resectoscope requires use of distension media. In this situation there are several options:

- *Gravity infusion:* The technique is the same as that described previously, but the difference is that a 3 liter bag of 1.5% glycine is used instead of physiological saline (height and pressure are the same). Since these procedures take longer, one must be especially careful in balancing glycine inflow and outflow in order to prevent aqueous intoxication. Therefore, the fluid remaining in the bags and the fluid collected in the suction device must be measured. In order to measure vaginal fluid loss, a bag must be adhered to the buttocks of the patient. In some circumstances, surgery can be performed with this system (e.g. in minor surgery of short duration). However, it is not advisable due to the risk of intravasation of distension medium and the severe consequences the patient may suffer.
- *Pump infusion:* With this type of pump, the inflow pressure can be preset. The usual working pressure ranges between 80 and 100 mm Hg with flow from 100 to 400 ml/min. The pump regulates pressure and flow depending on the resistance of the uterine walls, and it calculates the actual intrauterine pressure (FIGURE 8.13). In order to calculate electronically the amount of distension medium that has been absorbed by the patient, a weighing machine is used. A system of tubes collects the distension medium discharged through the hysteroscope evacuation canal, and

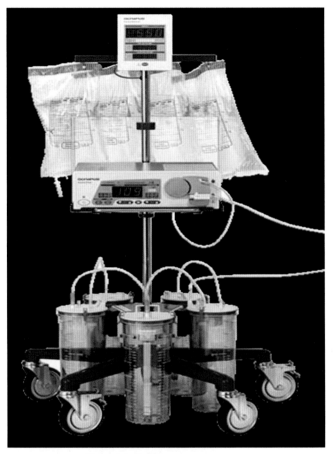

Figure 8.13: Hysteroscopy pump

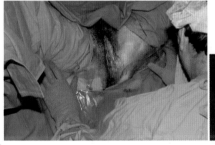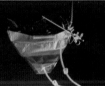

Figure 8.14: Liquid retriever bag

vaginal loss is collected in a bag (FIGURE 8.14). The main advantage of this type of pump is that the intervention can be stopped when the glycine balance indicator indicates that there is 1000 ml of intravasation. The American Association of Gynecologic Laparoscopists recommends use of the infusion pump in hysteroscopic surgery in order to prevent human failure in fluid calculation.

BIBLIOGRAPHY

1. Brooks PG. Distension media in hysteroscopy. In Pasic RP, Levine RL (Eds): A practical manual of hysteroscopy and endometrial ablation techniques. London: Taylor & Francis 2004;25-33.
2. Cayuela E, Cararach M, Gilabert J, Perez Medina T, Rivero B, Torrejón R. Histeroscopia. In Documentos de consenso de la SEGO (Eds): Sociedad Española de Ginecología y Obstetricia, Ed Madrid: Meditex 1996;11-45.
3. Cayuela E. Instrumentación en histeroscopia. Medios de distension. In Comino R, Balagueró L (Eds): Cirugía endoscópica en Ginecología. Prous Science. Barcelona 1998:261-73.
4. Cicinelli E. Diagnostic minihysteroscopy with vaginoscopic approach: Rationale and advantages. J Minim Invasive Gynecol 2005;12:396-400.
5. Hitta P, Bertaud N. Troubles neurologiques graves après hystéroscopie opératoire sous irrigation de glycocolle. Ann Fr Anesth Réanim 1993;12:604-12.
6. Hopkins H. Optical principles of endoscope. In Endoscopy. Berci G (Ed): New York: Appleton, Century, Crofts Publish 1976;3-26.
7. Levine RL. Hysteroscopic instruments. In Pasic RP, Levine RL (Eds): A practical manual of hysteroscopy and endometrial ablation techniques. London: Taylor & Francis 2004;13-24.
8. Lin BL, Iwata Y, Liu KH, Valle RF. The Fujinon diagnostic fiber optic hysteroscopy. J Reprod Med 1990;35:685-9.
9. Lin BL. Comparison of flexible hysteroscopes: theoretical and practical considerations. In Van Herendael B, Valle R (Eds): Ambulatory Hysteroscopy. Oxford (edn): Bladon Medical Publishing. 2004:19-24.
10. Munro MG. Electrosurgery in the uterus. In Pasic RP, Levine RL (Eds): A practical manual of hysteroscopy and endometrial ablation techniques. London (edn): Taylor & Francis 2004;49-65.
11. O'Donovan PJ, Nakade K. Diagnostic outpatient hysteroscopy service: Semi-rigid hysteroscopy. In Van Herendael B, Valle R (Eds): Ambulatory Hysteroscopy. Oxford (edn): Bladon Medical Publishing 2004;7-11.
12. Ruiz JM, Neuwirth RS. The incidence of complications associated with the use of Hyskon during hysteroscopy: Experience in 1793 consecutive patients. J Gynecol Surg 1992;8:219-24.
13. Rullo S, Sorrenti G, Marziali M, Ermini B, Sesti F, Piccione E. Office hysteroscopy: Comparison of 2.7 mm and 4 mm hysteroscopes for acceptability, feasibility and diagnostic accuracy. J Reprod Med 2005;50:45-8.
14. Valle RF. Operative hysteroscopy. In Sciarra JJ (Ed): Gynecology and obstetrics. Lippincott: Philadelphia 1995;35:1-28.
15. Valle RF, Baggish MS. Instrumentation for hysteroscopy. In Baggish MS, Barbot J, Valle RF (Eds): Diagnostic and operative hysteroscopy. Text and atlas (2nd edn). St Louis: Mosby 1999:97-126.

16. Valle RF, Baggish MS. Accessory instruments for operative hysteroscopy. In Baggish MS, Barbot J, Valle RF (Eds): Diagnostic and operative hysteroscopy. Text and atlas (2nd edn) Mosby St Louis 1999:127-38.

17. Valle RF. Manual of clinical hysteroscopy. Oxon (Ed): Taylor & Francis, 2005.

18. Van Herendael BJ. Instrumentation in hysteroscopy. In Siegler AM (Ed): Obstetrics and Gynecology Clinics of North America. Philadelphia: WB Saunders Co. 1995;22:391-408.

19. Wamsteker K, Block S, Emanuel MH. Instrumentation for transcervical hysteroscopic endosurgery. Gynecol Endoscopy 1992;2:59-67.

20. Witz CA, Silverberg KM, Burns WN, Schenken RS, Olive DL. Complications associated with the absorption of hysteroscopic fluid media. Fertil Steril 1993;60:745-56.

9

Basic Principles of Electrosurgery

Tirso Pérez-Medina

INTRODUCTION

In spite of the fact that use of electricity in medicine began long ago, the myths regarding, discharges and burns it causes discouraged many physicians. Therefore, for many years there was little academic interest in studying the principles of electrosurgery.

The current generators are much better than those of ten or twenty years ago. The digital panels can better adjust the desired cutting power and coagulation power at a given time. New electrodes have been designed for specific surgical procedures. All of this has contributed to the renewed use of electricity in medicine. Therefore, it is very important to have some knowledge of basic electrosurgical physics, that allows us to effectively use the apparatus we manage with the least possible number of accidents.

BASIC ELECTRICITY

Electricity is a flow of electrons. When energy particles with negative load are driven through a conductor by a generator, this leads to caloric energy that is used in medicine to destroy, coagulate or cut tissues. The power required to drive these electrons is the voltage (V). This power is measured in volts and is related to the difference between the positive and the negative pole. When these electrons are set in motion in the same direction, an electric current (I) is produced that is measured in Amperes. The difficulty in driving the electrons through tissue or other materials is defined as resistance (R), and is measured in Ohms.

These three parameters are dependent each other (Ohm´s law):

$$V = I \times R$$

The power is measured in Watts is the work produced or consumed by electrons. It depends on the amount of electrons (current) and the power required to drive them (voltage). Applying the Ohm´s law

$$W = I \times V$$

Therefore, power transmitted to tissue increases as a function of both the square of the current and the square of the voltage.

$$W = I^2 \times V \text{ and } W = V^2 / R$$

If an analogy is made between electricity and water, an electron would be equivalent to a water molecule and the voltage would be analogous to the water pressure. If a volume of water is driven through a tube at a constant pressure, after a certain time, a current or flow is created. As the resistance increases (with constant voltage or pressure), the current flow decreases.

There are basically three types of electric current, depending on the oscillographic path of the electrons: Continuous, alternating and pulsating.

The continuous and unidirectional interchange of electrons between opposite poles is called continuous current.

Pulsating current is a large electrical discharge in a short period of time.

Alternating current is a bidirectional interchange of electrons which change polarity rhythmically in a sinusoidal pattern. This is the type of current used most frequently. On the oscillometer this current produces a sinusoidal wave that, starting at zero or neutral polarity, advances first in one direction and then travels back in the opposite direction. Initially, a maximum level or peak is created in the positive direction, and then another maximum level or peak in the negative direction. This sinusoidal path of the electrons or cycle is measured in Hertz. Each cycle is a hertz. The electrical frequency is measured in cycles or hertz per second (FIGURE 9.1).

Electrical generators are apparatuses that produce alternating electrical current with a specific frequency

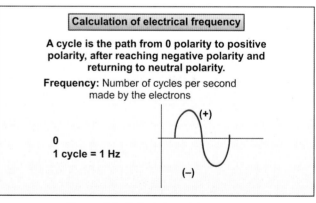

Figure 9.1: Calculation of frequency

that can vary according to the type of generator. Today most generators produce electrical current that is called high frequency since the current emitted is over 10.000 cycles per second (10 KHz/s). These are the currents that, since they go through the body so quickly, do not change the potential of the muscle fiber membrane. Therefore, they do not produce the painful muscle contractions associated with Faradic current, which has a lower wavelength. These currents are also called radiofrequency, since they are the frequencies used by radio waves. They may be found between 350,000 and 5 million cycles per second, or equivalent to between 350 kHz/s and 5 MHz/s.

The measurement from zero polarity to positive or negative polarity is called maximum voltage. By changing the maximum voltage, the same generator can produce cutting currents or coagulation currents.

It has been verified experimentally that in order to obtain a cutting effect in the tissue, the maximum voltage of the electrical wave must reach a peak of 200 volts (FIGURE 9.2). However, in order to obtain a coagulation effect, the peak must be 500 volts (FIGURE 9.3).

Moreover, modern generators can combine wavelengths of cutting and coagulation. This is known as mixed current (FIGURE 9.4). This mixed current can be formed by a variable proportion of cutting waves and coagulation waves that is selected previously according to one's needs.

The electrons driven with a certain voltage concentrate in a specific location, produce a rapid increase in heat at that point in the tissue. This phenomenon of concentration of electrons is known as current density.

When a monopolar electrode is used, the electrons driven by the generator are emitted by the active pole. They enter the body at the point where the electrode is applied, and reach the maximum current density at this point. Then, they are scattered through the tissues or regions where there is least resistance until they reach the passive electrode or return pole that leads them back to the generator, thus closing the circuit.

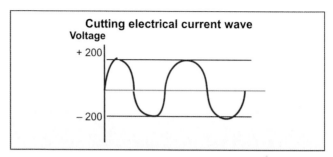
Figure 9.2: Cutting waveform. Low voltage. High current

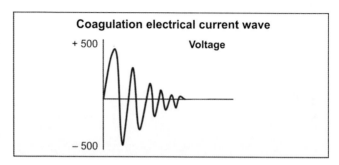
Figure 9.3: Coagulation waveform. High voltage. Low current

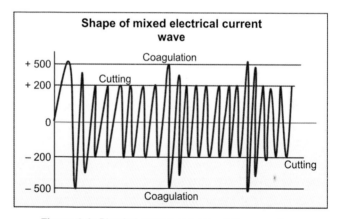
Figure 9.4: Blended cutting and coagulation waveform

One-terminal or monopolar electrodes can lead to more complications than two-terminal or bipolar electrodes. The further apart the poles are located, the greater the possibility of dispersion of the electrodes in the body, with the subsequent danger of current leaks and greater risk of burns.

The smaller the size of the active electrode, the greater the current density at the point of application and, consequently, the heat accumulated at this point. Therefore, the smaller the surface of the active electrode, the deeper the burn produced, and vice versa. Likewise, when the electrons leave the body by the return electrode or passive electrode, if this is very small, they can also cause a burn. Therefore, large return plates are recommended in order to prevent excessive current accumulation at a small point.

BIPOLAR ELECTROSURGERY

In order to avoid the drawback associated with absorption of glycine in hysteroscopic surgery, a coaxial bipolar electrode has been developed that can cut and coagulate in a liquid medium with ions (physiological saline), by cutting the electrical arc generated between the active pole and the passive pole. Both poles are only separated by a small insulating plate that prevents dispersion of the electrons by the distension fluid. In **bipolar mode**, the electron flow passes through the first pole (loop, twizzle, etc.), crosses the tissue interposed between and returns to the electrogenerator through the second pole (external sheath) (FIGURES 9.5 to 9.7).

Bipolar electrodes carry an active electrode and a return electrode into an electrosurgical instrument with two poles (e.g. hysteroscopic loop and external sheath). The flow of alternating current is symmetrically distributed through the tissue between the poles, reversing direction of every semicycle and eliminating the risk of capacitive coupling and aberrant alternate current pathways.

Power requirements are significantly lower than in monopolar surgery due to the current concentration between the poles. Therefore, an unmodulated cutting waveform with low peak-to-peak voltage is used during bipolar electrosurgery. These factors intrinsically limit the thermal effects to desiccation and coagulation of tissue.

The power output from a bipolar circuit is normally calibrated to smaller internal generator impedance than the one used in monopolar surgery. Therefore, thorough desiccation of tissue is better ensured by higher current flow at higher tissue impedances.

Although the flow of current and the correspondent thermal effects are restricted to the tissue located between both poles, the risk of undesired

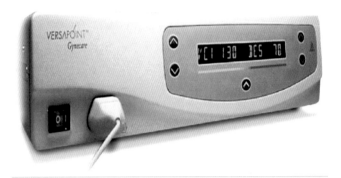

Figure 9.5: Bipolar generator (gynecare)

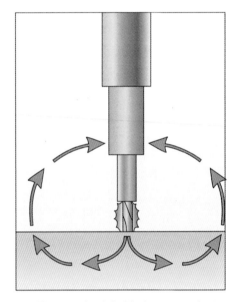

Figure 9.6: Electron circuit in bipolar current hysteroscopy

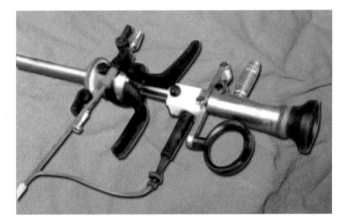

Figure 9.7: Bipolar resectoscope (olympus™)

thermal effects to organs distant from the operative site are not eliminated. The use of bipolar current leads to gradual desiccation of the intervening tissue.

The tissue coagulation is dependent on the applied surface area between the poles, the formation of a vapor layer between the poles and tissue, and the degree of tissue hydration. Impedance is maximal when the vapor phase is ended and the tissue is completely desiccated. If the current is further applied, a second thermal attack passes to surrounding tissues from a correspondingly rapid rise in tissue temperature. Thus, tissues at some distance from the operative site may suffer thermal damage.

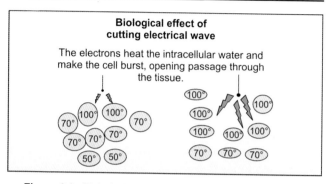

Figure 9.8: Biological effect of cutting current. Vaporization

CLINICAL CORRELATION

By varying the rate and extent of the thermodynamic effects of electric current in biological tissue, high frequency electrosurgery is used to cut and/or coagulate. Although the efficiency of hemostasis is related to the depth of coagulation, it is of paramount importance that no more tissue suffers thermal damage than is absolutely needed. The art of electrosurgery is balancing between the need for absolute hemostasis and the least amount of deep coagulative necrosis.

Operation of the emitting electrode depends on the size and shape, frequency and modulation of the electrical wave emitted by the generator, the maximum voltage, and the current connected against the output resistance. Therefore, the tissue can be cut gently and without resistance or it can burn and carbonize. The success of surgery depends to a great extent on proper use of these different parameters.

Modern digital generators provide pure cutting waves or pure coagulation waves, as well as waves that are a mixture of them. The lower the proportion of coagulation waves, the lower the amount of caloric energy that builds up in the tissue. Therefore, the tissue will be better conserved for subsequent histological study.

In these generators, the power of these waves can be preset, to overcome the resistance of the tissue to be treated in each case.

The biological effect of cutting is achieved when the intracellular water reaches boiling temperature and the cell vaporizes due to energy released by passage of electrons through the cell (FIGURE 9.8). The extremely high current density delivered by the arc heats the intracellular water to temperatures above 600°C. Explosive cellular vaporization ensues secondary to the production of highly disruptive pressure (steam occupies 6 times the volume of liquid water) and acoustic forces. Arcing is then enhanced by an envelope of steam vapor that becomes instantly ionized. The use of the unmodulated cutting waveform helps sustain this envelope by producing an uninterrupted current that continuously maintains the same pathways for arc formation.

The depth of coagulation along the edges increases with increasing voltage and length or intensity of the arcs. Therefore, an unmodulated cutting waveform produces a cut with the least amount of coagulative necrosis, while waveforms with greater modulation and higher voltages result in larger zones of coagulation. Tissue contact eliminates the steam envelope and abolishes the cutting arc.

When the power selected in the generator is higher than needed, heat accumulation is excessive and the cell carbonizes. Tissue resistance increases and the desired cutting effect is not achieved, since the electrode can not travel through the tissue properly. When power is lower than needed, the intracellular water does not reach the temperature required for boiling and the cell does not vaporize. In this case, since it can not advance easily across the tissue, the electrode comes into contact with the cell for longer than necessary, and desiccates due to the excessive heat accumulation. Therefore, electrode travel is hindered by the increased resistance. The power of the cutting current produced by the generator must be selected properly beforehand in each case in order to be able to achieve the desired effect.

The biological effect of coagulation is achieved by the denaturalization of tissue proteins caused by heat. Contact of tissue with the surface of an active electrode leads to conduction of current with a low current density. Resistive heating is produced by the high frequency agitation of intracellular ionic polarities. As the tissue is gradually heated to temperatures above 50°C and maintained, irreversible cellular damage is initiated by the denaturation of cellular proteins (white coagulation). Reaching the 100°C leads to complete evaporation of intracellular water (desiccation), hemostasis because of the contraction of vessels and the surrounding tissues, and conversion of collagen to glucose that has an adhesion effect between the tissue and the electrode. Temperatures above 200°C cause carbonization and charring.

This coagulation effect can be produced by desiccation as well as fulguration of the tissue (FIGURE 9.9). When fulguration occurs, the sparks jump from the electrode to the tissue, maintaining a separation of approximately 1 mm between them. This separation causes greater dispersion of the electrons through the tissue. A positive effect is achieved in terms of surface coagulation, but less effect in terms of depth. When desiccation occurs, the electrode is placed in contact with the tissue and achieves a coagulation effect due to the higher concentration of caloric energy at this point of contact. With this process, larger and deeper vessels can be coagulated, but with greater damage to the surrounding healthy tissue. In general, in order to coagulate in fulguration mode, less power is required than this needed for coagulation in desiccation mode.

In each case, the type of current to be produced by the generator and the power of this current must be selected appropriately in order to obtain the desired effect and prevent undesired effects to the greatest possible extent.

Until the tissue reaches a temperature of 100°C and is completely desiccated, the rise in tissue temperature is directly proportional to the tissue resistance (degree of desiccation), time of current flow, and the square of the current density. Therefore, temperature change is faster at superficial depths, and evolves more gradually with larger surface electrodes.

For instance, if a rolling ball electrode is used for endometrial ablation (FIGURE 9.10), it will cause desiccation of the surface of the endometrium, regardless of the type of current wave emitted by the generator. At any rate, if a cutting wave is used at the same power, since the voltage of this wave is lower than that of the coagulation wave, the caloric energy that accumulates at the point of application and the depth of destruction will also be less. At the same power, the greater the surface of the electrode used, the less the depth, since there is greater dispersion of energy on the surface. In other words, in order to achieve the same effects, greater power must be applied to a cylinder than to a ball.

If the endometrium is to be resected with the loop, the power selected in the generator will depend on the size of the loop, its thickness, and the depth of the cut (FIGURE 9.11). The greater the size, thickness, and depth, the higher the power required. In order to resect a leiomyoma, since it is harder than the endometrium and offers greater resistance, even higher power must be applied.

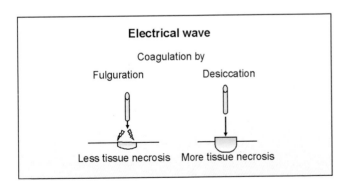

Figure 9.9: Biological effect of coagulation

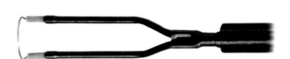

Figure 9.10: Close view of the roller ball electrode

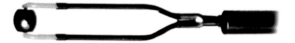

Figure 9.11: Close view of the cutting loop electrode

In all cases, if there are bleeding vessels at the time of resection, instead of a pure cutting current, a mixed current or balanced current is used. The larger the calibre of the vessels to be coagulated, the greater the proportion of coagulation waves needed.

When the cutting process begins, tissue resistance is low since there is intracellular water. However, when this dries due to the effect of the heat, resistance increases and the electrical contact is broken. Since the electrode is no longer in contact with the wet tissue, whenever the voltage is high enough the sparks will jump to the nearby tissue that is wet, vaporizing the cells and opening passage through the cell, producing the cutting effect. After this, the electrode should not be in further contact with the tissue since a safety zone is created between them.

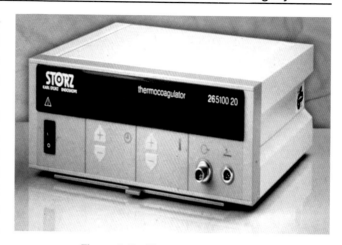

Figure 9.12: Electrosurgical generator

RISKS OF ELECTROSURGERY

Sixty-six percent of the electrical accidents during surgical endoscopy occur at the site of the return electrode. Therefore, operating theater personnel must have the technical knowledge required so that they can resolve the problems that may arise at any time. The return electrode should be large. It should not be obligated to come into direct contact with the patient, although it should be as close as possible to the emitting pole in order to prevent possible electrical leaks. It is better for this plate to be disposable, since lack of coating in a small area of the plate can cause burns.

The generator and the patient form a closed circuit which the electrical current circulates through (FIGURE 9.12). Any small deficiency in the cutting or coagulation indicates that there is a minor failure in the system, either due to lack of cable coating or lack of conductivity at a point on the circuit. In this case, before increasing the generator power, the entire electrical circuit should be checked. Moreover, it is important to ensure that the distension fluid used does not contain electrolytes.

At any rate, today most of the generators have alarm and safety systems that issue a warning when the return current flow is lower than the output current flow, and block the apparatus.

Patient contact with small metal objects that are insufficiently insulated should be avoided (i.e., electrocardiographic monitoring electrodes or metal bolts on the operating table, if the table is not sufficiently insulated from the floor by rubber plugs). Generators can also interfere with heart pacemakers. Appropriate precautions should be taken.

Finally, it must be borne in mind that on very rare occasions the sparks caused by cutting or coagulation can cause small fires of different inflammable substances in the operating theater like some anesthetic gases, alcoholic skin disinfectants, or intestinal methane gas.

BIBLIOGRAPHY

1. Advincula A, Wang K. The evolutionary state of electrosurgery: Where are we now? Curr Opin Obstet Gynecol 2008;20:353-8.
2. Brill AI. Bipolar electrosurgery: Convention and innovation. Clin Obstet Gynecol 2008;51:153-8.
3. Massarweh NN, Cosgriff N, Slakey DP. Electrosurgery: History, principles, and current and future uses. J Am Coll Surg 2006;202:520-30.
4. Veck S. An introduction to the principles and safety of electrosurgery. Br J Hosp Med 1996;55:27-30.
5. Vilos G, Latendresse K, Gan BS. Electrophysical properties of electrosurgery and capacitive induced current. Am J Surg 2001;182:222-5.

10

Hysteroscopic Myomectomy

Ramón Cos Plans
Enrique Cayuela Font
Federico Heredia Prim

INTRODUCTION

Uterine myomas are benign encapsulated solid tumors that originate in the muscle tissue of the uterus. They are formed by connective tissue and smooth muscle fiber. They are surrounded by a thin pseudocapsule of areolar tissue and compressed muscle fiber.

They represent 20% of all benign tumors in women and risk of malignancy is less than 0.2-0.5%. These myomas appear more frequently in young women. It is estimated that they affect one out of every four women in reproductive age. Nevertheless, actual incidence is unknown since in half of the cases they are asymptomatic.

Depending on their location in the uterus, they can be classified as subserous, intramural and submucous. Submucous myomas represent 5-10% of all myomas. However, some authors cite higher figures, between 16.6 and 55%.[1] They originate in the myometrial wall and extend towards the endometrial cavity. They may become completely pedunculated and even protrude through the cervical orifice (spontaneous expulsion of the myoma). These types of myomas are important because they are the most symptomatic. They are the most frequent organic cause of heavy menstrual bleeding in women of reproductive age.

Since Neuwirth[2] performed the first hysteroscopic myomectomy in 1978, this technique has become the treatment of choice for resection of submucous myomas. The advantages of this technique compared to abdominal myomectomy are unquestionable (less morbidity, rapid recovery and decreased cost).

Moreover, with this technique the patient can have vaginal childbirth in future pregnancies. This differs from abdominal myomectomies in which, although controversial, cesarean childbirth is considered advisable due to the risk of subsequent uterine rupture.

CLINICAL SIGNS OF SUBMUCOUS MYOMA

Submucous myomas are the myomas that produce the most of the symptoms. They can cause the following problems.

Irregular Menstrual Bleeding

They cause hypermenorrhea, menorrhagia or metrorrhagia that can lead to severe iron-deficient anemic states in women.

Bleeding intensity is related to the amount of myoma that emerges in the endometrial cavity. There are large, tortuous, highly fragile vessels of thick calibre on the surface of submucous myomas that bleed easily. Moreover, the presence of these myomas cause irregularities in uterine contractility and inflammatory abnormalities in the surrounding endometrium that lead to disorders in local hemostasis.

Sterility-infertility

The actual involvement of myomas in sterility-infertility problems is not known. In 1-4% of the cases, incidence of myomas are the only cause of sterility.[3]

Different mechanisms have been postulated to explain the negative effect on fertility associated with myomas. These include irregularities in spermatic and embryonic transport, endometrial abnormalities that interfere with implantation, irregularities in uterine contractility, and interference with expansion and growth during pregnancy.

There are no well performed studies comparing women with or without myomas and desire for offspring. At present, based on indirect studies in patients who underwent in-vitro fertilization (IVF), we can state that only submucous or intramural myomas that affect the uterine cavity decrease or worsen the implantation and pregnancy rates, whereas their removal improves fertility. Therefore, these types of myomas should only be treated in young asymptomatic women with reproductive desire.[4,5]

Pelvic Pain and/or Dysmenorrhea

In cases with pedunculated submucous myomas that the uterus attempts to eject through the endocervical channel, there may be colic episodes of hypogastric pain accompanied by genital bleeding (spontaneous expulsion of the myoma). There may also be pain due to torsion of pedunculated submucous myomas or degeneration of large submucous myomas.

Metrorrhagia in Postmenopause

During treatment with hormone replacement therapy (HRT) the presence of a submucous myoma can cause the onset of abnormal bleeding.

TREATMENT OF SUBMUCOUS MYOMA

Indications

Submucous myomas can be resected by hysteroscopy through the uterine cervix. Hysteroscopic myomectomy is the best conservative surgical option for women with symptomatic intracavitary myomas.[6]

The advantages of hysteroscopic myomectomy compared to laparotomic myomectomy are: Lower economic cost, less operative time, decreased hospital stay, less convalescence and rapid reintegration in normal life, lower complication rate, elimination of risk of adherences and possibility of subsequent vaginal childbirth. Of the disadvantages, it should be mentioned that in some cases it may be necessary to repeat the intervention, if complete resection is not achieved.

Submucous myomas that should be resected by hysteroscopy[3,4] (TABLE 10.1). include symptomatic myomas that cause irregular menstrual bleeding or pain as well as asymptomatic myomas in women with sterility problems (especially if they must undergo IVF) and repeated abortions. This improves the implantation and pregnancy rates.

Submucous myomas should also be resected in postmenopausal patients with abnormal bleeding and no other endocavitary cause.

Even if there is no change in symptoms, resection with biopsy should be performed in myomas that begin rapid growth.

PREOPERATIVE EVALUATION

The success of the surgical intervention depends on optimal selection of patients. It is essential to perform proper evaluation of the uterine cavity (TABLE 10.2). The characteristics of the myoma that is going to be

Table 10.1: Indications for hysteroscopic myomectomy

- Abnormal uterine bleeding
- Infertility
- Abnormal growth

Table 10.2: Preoperative evaluation

- Preoperative evaluation
- Size/volume
- Localization
- Number
- Degree of intramural affectation
- Classification
- Endometrial and myoma biopsy

resected should be known precisely: The number of myomas, size, location, and the degree of intramural affectation of each myoma.

These factors, along with the surgeon's experience, will determine the success of total resection of the myoma.

The most important factor is the degree of intramural affectation: Complete resection of myomas with over 50% volume inside the uterine cavity is easier. In order to examine all of these characteristics, the following diagnostic tests are available:

Diagnostic Hysteroscopy

This is considered to be the diagnostic method of choice for preoperative evaluation of possible hysteroscopic resection of the myoma.[7] It facilitates precise examination of the uterine cavity. A biopsy is performed to rule out the presence of other disease and confirm that the process is benign.

The degree of intramural extension of the myoma can be studied by observing the angle between the fibroma and the endometrium in the region of the uterine wall. If it is an acute angle this means that the myoma is primarily intracavitary and, therefore, resectable. Otherwise, if the angle is obtuse, this indicates that over 50% of the myoma is intramural, and it would not be resectable. The hysteroscopic classification proposed by Wamsteker and De Blok[36] and adopted by the European Society of Hysteroscopy,

Table 10.3: Classification of submucous myomas

Type 0	Myoma with development limited to the uterine cavity, pedunculated or with limited implant base
Type I	Myoma with partial intramural development. Endocavitary component > 50%. Angle of protrusion between the myoma and uterine wall < 90°
Type II	Myoma with predominantly intramural development. Endocavitary component < 50%. Angle of protrusion between the myoma and uterine wall > 90°

differentiates between three types of myomas (TABLE 10.3). This is a classification that is easy to use and helps catalogue the surgical difficulty (FIGURES 10.1 and 10.2).

The uterine cavity should be inspected carefully with different degrees of distension, reducing the inflow pressure of the distension medium since the endometrium can level the actual angle (FIGURES 10.3 to 10.5).

Nevertheless, diagnostic hysteroscopy provides subjective information on the size of the myoma and indirect information on the actual depth of the myoma in the myometrium. One must bear in mind that only the intracavitary part of the myoma is visible. If the true extent of the myoma (size, volume, depth) is unknown, complete resection may be a failure or there may be complications such as uterine perforation and bleeding.

Therefore, preoperative examination of submucous myomas should not be limited to hysteroscopic diagnosis.[8] Vercellini reports that complete resection of the myoma is only achieved in 69% of women selected using the hysteroscopic criterion.[9]

A prospective study[10] performed by the author of the hysteroscopic classification showed that the degree of intramural affectation had little influence on the success of hysteroscopic resection of submucous myomas. In women with type I myomas (< 50% myometrial extension), complete resection was achieved in 60% of the procedures (12/20) compared to 50% (10/20) in type II myomas (>50% myometrial extension). After repeating the procedure, complete resection was achieved in 85.7% (12/14) of type I myomas with identical results, and in 83.3% (10/12) of type II myomas.

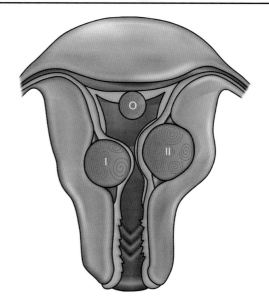

Figure 10.1: Wamsteker and de Blok classification: Types of submocous myoma

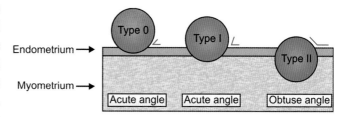

Figure 10.2: Angle myoma/endometrial surface

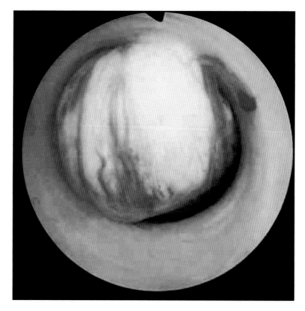

Figure 10.3: Hysteroscopy. Myoma type 0

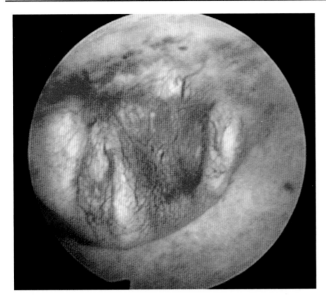

Figure 10.4: Hysteroscopy. Myoma type I

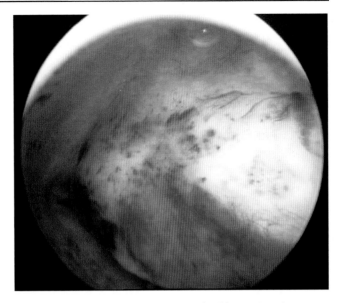

Figure 10.6: Hysterosonography. Myoma type I

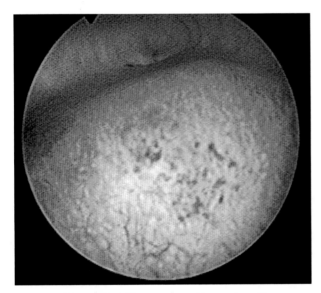

Figure 10.5: Hysteroscopy. Myoma type II

Ultrasound

The sensitivity and specificity of the diagnosis of submucous myomas by vaginal ultrasonography is 90%.

Transvaginal ultrasound is better than abdominal ultrasound to determine the size of the myoma, specify its location, and assess the degree of intramural extension. However, for preoperative assessment of submucous myoma (size, location and degree of intracavitary growth), sonohysterography appears to be the most valid technique, superior to diagnostic hysteroscopy.[11]

There is a good correlation between ultrasound sonohysterography and diagnostic hysteroscopy for diagnosis of submucous myomas (FIGURE 10.6). In classification of submucous myomas, the correlation is very good for myomas that are completely intracavitary or type 0. This correlation decreases as the degree of myometrial affectation of type I and II myomas increases. Ultrasound sonohysterography provides us with more precise information on the part of the myoma embedded in the myometrial wall.[12]

Another very important fact that can be determined from the ultrasound examination is measurement of the distance between the edge of the myoma and the serosal layer. In submucous myomas with significant intramural affectation (type I or II), resection can be performed, if this distance is greater than or equal to 5 mm (safety margin).

Magnetic Resonance

This diagnostic tool is more sensitive than transvaginal ultrasound or sonohysterography for topographic study and preoperative localization (FIGURES 10.7 and 10.8) of uterine myomas.[13,14] The images obtained are very clear. They can even be used to examine lesion volume and the existence of degeneration within the tumor.

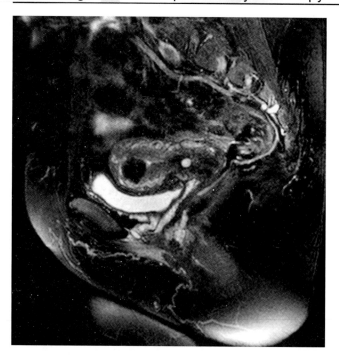

Figure 10.7: MRI myoma type II

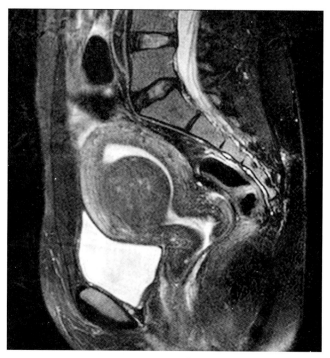

Figure 10.8: MRI myoma type I

The disadvantage is high cost and limited availability. Therefore, it cannot be used in the initial examination of all patients with suspected myoma. MRI is indicated in those cases in which ultrasound or sonohysterographic findings are either inconclusive or technically limited, in order to be able to make a decision on the type of surgery to be performed.

In summary, preoperative assessment of the resectability of submucous myomas should not be performed only by hysteroscopic examination. This examination must be complemented by techniques such as sonohysterography or MRI that provide more precise assessment of the size and intramural extension of the submucous myoma.[10]

PREOPERATIVE PREPARATION

In order to facilitate hysteroscopic resection it is important that the endometrium have limited thickness and vascularization in order to have a clear, unobstructed view of the entire cavity throughout surgery.

There are several options:

Initial Phase of Menstrual Cycle

Perform intervention during the initial proliferative phase, when there will be a thin, slightly vascularized endometrium. This is ideal in patients with small, completely intracavitary submucous myomas.

Pharmacological Treatment

Administer drugs that cause thinning or atrophy of the endometrium. Progestogens, oral contraceptives, danazol and GnRH analogs have been used. Most authors use the latter, most frequently since they offer a series of advantages, although their cost is higher.

GnRH analogs: They cause a state of transitory hypestrogenism. Preoperative administration of this drug for 2-3 months may entail a series of advantages (TABLE 10.4).[15,16,34]

Table 10.4: Advantages of preoperative administration of GnRH analogs

- Reduction of tumor size and volume
- Recovery from anemia
- Decrease in intraoperative bleeding
- Decreased surgical time

- *Substantial reduction of tumor size and volume:* Although the decrease is not constant, it occurs in most cases. It facilitates resection of the myoma. In some cases, myomas that were initially rejected for surgical hysteroscopy may even become accessible.
- *Recovery from anemia:* Endometrial atrophy with elimination of menstruation helps control symptoms such as bleeding disorders and facilitates correction of patient anemia.
- *Decrease in intraoperative bleeding:* By causing atrophy of the endometrium and decreased vascularization, women who receive three doses prior to the intervention have less bleeding during resection that can obstruct intraoperative vision.
- *Decreased surgical time:* The reduction in size, absence of endometrium, and less bleeding during surgical hysteroscopy facilitate resection and reduce resection time.

All of these advantages are more evident in resection of large myomas. In completely intracavitary solitary myomas less than 3 cm use of analogs is not required.[17]

The disadvantages of treatment with GnRH analogs are the appearance of side effects such as hypestrogenism (e.g. hot flushes, sweating) and its high economic cost. Some authors also cite the increase in intraoperative absorption of glycine due to the endometrial atrophy they cause. Cases of necrobiosis of submucous myomas with preoperative administration of GnRH analogs have been described, causing uncontrolled bleeding during treatment. Moreover, some authors find it more difficult to perform cervical dilation after administration of this drug.

Progestogens, Danazol and Oral Contraceptives

Used infrequently. These treatments can not produce endometrial atrophy equivalent to that associated with GnRH analogs. Neither do they have an effect on the volume and vascularization of the myoma. Although the side effects are more tolerable than GnRH analogs, they are much less effective due to the pseudodecidualization of the endometrium.

Contraindications

The situations with greatest risk of failure of hysteroscopic resection of submucous myomas are:[18,34]

- Multiple uterine myomas (> 3 intracavitary myomas) that affect 50% of the endometrial cavity (FIGURES 10.9A and B)
- Submucous myoma >5 cm diameter (FIGURE 10.10A)
- Intramural extension >50% or type II (FIGURE 10.10B)
- Size of uterus (hysterometry > 12 cm)

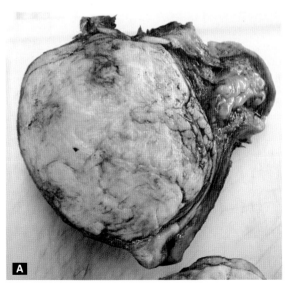
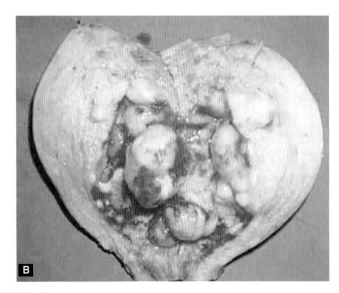

Figures 10.9A and B: Multiple submucous myomas

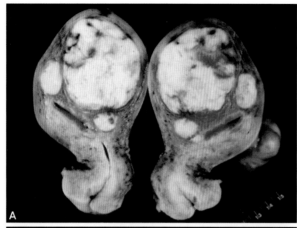

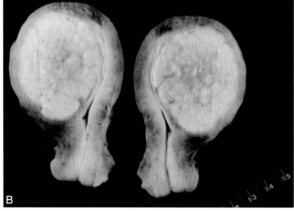

Figures 10.10A and B: Giant myoma

The size and type of myoma are not absolute contraindications, but rather depend on the experience of the surgeon.

ANESTHESIA

The most advisable types of anesthesia are that in which the patient remains conscious. In interventions that are expected to last a long time, such as myomectomies, risk of intravasation is greater. The initial clinical manifestations of aqueous intoxication are disorientation, nausea, vomiting, and cephalea. These may encourage the anesthetist to begin early treatment. If the patient is under general anesthesia, these symptoms do not appear. Therefore, regional anesthesia or conscious sedation is the most advisable in this type of surgery (This topic can be found in Chapter 18).

Myoma Resection Surgical Technique

There are different instruments for performance of a hysteroscopic myomectomy: Scissors, monopolar or bipolar resectoscopy, VersaPoint™ system, intra-uterine morcellator and laser.

The myomectomy technique will vary depending on the size, type, and location of the myoma.

Monopolar Resectoscopy

Use glycine as distension medium. Before beginning resection, coagulate the large vessels located on the surface of the myoma with the electrode handle in order to prevent bleeding that obstructs vision. After activation, the electrode handle should always be under visual control. The handle is placed in the back part of the tumor and the electrical current is activated. The handle is always moved forwards from behind the myoma rather than in the opposite direction, ensuring that it is removed from the anterior part of the tumor and that lesions to the healthy myometrium and endometrium in this region are prevented.

Resection begins from the surface of the free intracavitary portion to the border between the intramural portion of the myoma and the endometrium. This border is identified by having the pinkest color, the least firm consistency, and bleeding easily. Resection is performed homogeneously by layers, attempting to ensure that none of the edges of the myoma remain after resection (FIGURES 10.11 and 10.12). The fragments or sheets of myoma produced should be removed when they obstruct vision. A fenestrated curette or a hysteroscope can be used for this, through the internal sheath or removing the entire hysteroscope as a single unit through the cervical channel, placing it between the deactivated handle and the optical tip.

After resecting the entire intracavitary portion of the myoma one must wait a few seconds, allowing time so that the uterine contractions cause the intramural portion of the myoma to protrude towards the cavity. Expulsion of this portion can also be favored by administering intravenous

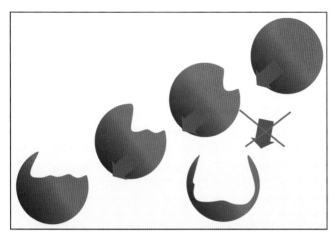

Figure 10.11: Resection technique I

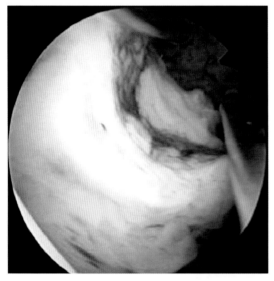

Figure 10.12: Resection technique II

oxytocin (10-20 IU) or pushing the edge of the myoma with the handle.

If the intervention takes longer than 60 minute or intravasation of the distension medium is greater than 1000 cc, completion of surgery should be assessed at that time. Surgery may be prolonged slightly only if it is nearly complete, ensuring that intravasation is less than 1500 cc. If the remaining myoma is large, a second surgical intervention can be scheduled in 2 or 3 weeks, taking advantage of the effect of the GnRH analogs. In the cases in which the remaining portion of myoma is small, a second resection is not required. The remaining myoma will undergo a process of hyalinization and remain asymptomatic, or even be eliminated.

Bipolar Resectoscopy

This is the same technique. However, since saline solution is used as distension medium rather than glycine, it is safer than monopolar resectoscopy. Even though aqueous intoxication due to excess absorption is less frequent, it is not completely ruled out. The inflow and outflow of distension medium should be monitored.

VersaPoint™ System

The VersaPoint system uses a 200 W bipolar current to vaporize the myomas. A 5 or 5.5 mm continuous flow hysteroscope is used with a 5 Fr. working channel. A specific, single-use 1.6 mm electrode passes through the working channel. Myomas less than 2 cm and type 0 and type I myomas can be treated with this system. The advantage is that it can be used as an outpatient and with no need for dilatation. Saline solution is used as distension medium.

Disadvantages: It can not be used in myomas over 2 cm and type II myomas. During vaporization, bubbles appear that can reduce visibility. No material is obtained for histological analysis.

Nd:YAG Laser

In pedunculated myomas, it can be used with a cutting technique. In myomas with intramural component, the laser facilitates vaporization of the myoma with no need for cutting. This eliminates the need to remove the fragments of resected tissue that obstruct or prevent a good visual field.[19] The major disadvantage is its high cost and the lack of material for histological analysis.

Intrauterine Morcellator (IUM)

This is a new hysteroscopic method that consists of inserting a double tube formed by an internal rotator tube within an external tube into the working channel of a 9 mm, rigid, continuous flow, and hysteroscope. Both tubes have an open window with sharp teeth on the distal end. The internal tube rotates at a velocity of 750 rotations per minute. By means of a suction system, the tissue is drawn into the windows, and cut like shaving by the rotation of the internal tube. At the same time, the cut fragments are sucked in. The mechanism is similar to that used by traumatologists to perform arthroscopic surgery. The advantages of this new technique include the possibility of using saline solution as distension medium, which prevents the complications caused by glycine absorption. Moreover, suction of the fragments of cut tissue through this internal tube eliminates the need to remove the fragments with the hysteroscope, and implies a decrease in operative time. The only disadvantage is that, bleeding vessels can not be coagulated if necessary.[20] This is a method that is being studied, and when this chapter was written it was available commercially.

Immediate Postoperative Control

If there have not been any other complications, the only item that should be controlled is vaginal blood loss. Depending on the type of anesthesia, the blood pressure and pulse should be monitored. When regional anesthesia is used, recovery of limb mobility should also be considered. Pain can be controlled with a NSAID. Discharge can be prescribed 4 hours after the intervention, recommending relative rest of 24-48 hours. If there is pain, patients can take a NSAID. The patient should be informed of the possible complications.

Subsequent Postoperative Control

In women who are sterile-infertile or desire offspring in the future, it is advisable to perform hysteroscopic control after 2 months in order to rule out the formation of intrauterine adherences. Postoperative synechia have been detected after hysteroscopic myomectomies in 10-13% of the cases.[21,22] If they are detected within a short time they can be easily eliminated, even with the tip of the hysteroscope, since they will be fine, mucous, slightly rigid and non-fibrous.

In cases in which it is not clear that complete resection has been achieved, a subsequent hysteroscopic examination will indicate whether or not another intervention is needed.

RESULTS

Bleeding Disorders

In resolution of bleeding symptoms, patients with short-term follow-up have a success rate of over 90%. With longer follow-up periods, the results are less favourable.[21] Derman[23] reported that, after a 9 year follow-up, 84% of the patients who underwent hysteroscopic myomectomy did not require additional surgery. Overall, in patients with long-term follow-up of 5 years or more, success rates range between 70-85%.[24]

In myomas over 5 cm and in myomas with a greater intramural component, the results are worse. In type 0 myomas, failure occurs in 13.5%. In type I and type II myomas, this figure is slightly higher, approximately 17%.[22]

In patients with multiple submucous myomas, bleeding disorders recur in nearly one-third of the patients (27%).[19] Nevertheless, other authors[22] have not detected a significant relationship between failure and the number of myomas (17% with multiple myomas vs 12.4% with solitary myoma).

Fertility

In terms of reproductive results, according to the literature, between approximately 30 and 77% of the patients became pregnant after hysteroscopic myomectomy (TABLE 10.5). The average is approximately 55%, although lower results have been recorded in some studies. The abortion rate decreased by 15%. In the largest study[18] with 134 sterile patients, 79 patients became pregnant after hysteroscopic myomectomy (58.9%).

These rates are influenced by patient's age, presence or absence of other factors that affect sterility, and myoma size. Therefore, the best results are achieved in patients less than 35 years with no other sterility factors and with myomas over 5 cm.[26, 27]

Regarding the type of submucous myoma, the best pregnancy rates (49%) are achieved in resection of type 0 myomas, compared to type I myomas (36%) and type II myomas (33%).[28]

Table 10.5: Reproductive outcome after hysteroscopic myomectomy

	Number of cases	Number of pregnancies	Pregnancy rate (%)	Delivery rate (%)
Donnez et al (1991)	24	16	67	67
Valle (1990)	16	10	62	50
Corson and brooks (1991)	13	10	77	61
Hucke (1992)	14	4	28.7	-
Goldenberg et al (1995)	15	7	47	40
Ubaldi et al (1995)	134	79	58.9	-
Preutthipan et Theppisai (1998)	12	2	16.7	-
Giatras et al (1999)	41	25	60.9	48.7
Varasteh et al (1999)	36	19	52.8	36.1
Vercellini et al (1999)	40	15	37.5	32.5
Fernandez et al (2001)	59	16	27.1	10.0

Incomplete Resection

The need for a second intervention due to the fact that total resection of the submucous myoma has not been achieved is related primarily to intramural extension of the myoma. However, there are also other factors such as size, number and position.[10]

In type II myomas, incomplete resection and the need for a second surgical intervention occurs in 50% of the cases. In pedunculated myomas and type I myomas, the rate is only 26%.[28]

Recurrences

Risk of recurrence and additional surgery is related to the size of the uterus and the number of submucous myomas.[25]

• Normal uterine size and < 2 myomas: 10% recurrence at 5 years.

• Increased uterine size and > 3 myomas: 36% recurrence at 5 years.

Therefore, in patients who do not desire offspring in the future and have large multiple uterine myomas, the best alternative is hysterectomy. Nevertheless, Cravello[22] did not find any statistical differences in therapeutic failure in cases with multiple myomas compared to solitary myoma (17.1 vs 12.4%).

Another important factor in recurrence is the degree of resection completed. When resection of the myoma has been incomplete, half of the patients require additional surgery due to recurrence of the myoma within the next 2 years.[10, 25]

The risk of repetition of hysteroscopic myomectomy due to tumor recurrence is also related to the degree of intramural extension of the submucous myoma. Therefore, risk is greater in type II myomas in which it is more difficult to achieve complete resection.[28]

COMPLICATIONS

Myomectomy is the hysteroscopic procedure with the greatest number of complications.[29] Although next chapter is fully devoted to general hysteroscopic complications, the specific complications of myomectomy will be now discussed. The overall surgical risk of hysteroscopic myomectomy is approximately 3%.[18] The most common complications are uterine perforation, bleeding, infection, and the risks associated with the distension medium.

Bleeding

Hysteroscopic myomectomy is the technique with the greatest risk of causing bleeding, with rates of 2-3%.[30] Bleeding is more frequent in myomectomy due to lesions of the intratumoral vessels and intramyometrial vessels, especially in myomas with large intramural extension with affectation of the deepest network of myometrial blood vessels.

Treatment consists of performing uterine compression by inserting a Foley catheter in the cervix. Thirty cc of saline solution are instilled. After 6 hours, the balloon is deflated and patient bleeding is verified in semi-Fowler's position without removing the catheter. If blood loss is limited, the catheter is removed completely. If bleeding continues, the balloon should be inflated again and maintained for 24 hours. After this period of time, it is very rare for bleeding to continue.

Infection

The risk of infectious complication is also the highest in myoma resection: Rates of 2% or even 3.5% have been cited.[31] This may be related to the fact that multiple fragments of myoma have to be removed with several maneuvers of inserting and withdrawing the resector, and due to the longer surgical time required for resection. Treatment with wide spectrum antibiotics or selective antibiotics should be administered if culture results are available.

Aqueous Intoxication

The greatest absorption of distension fluid occurs in myomectomy. Therefore, there is greater risk of aqueous intoxication with hyponatremia. This occurs in 2.1 to 3% of myomectomies.[21,32] it is estimated that the patient absorbs 20 ml/min of glycine during myoma resection. Therefore, resection should not be prolonged for over 60 minutes to prevent excessive glycine absorption. In resection of large myomas with significant myometrial extension, absorption is greater.[33] Treatment depends on the result of the monogram. It is based on endovenous infusions of sodium and diuretics under strict control in an intensive care unit. Pulmonary and cerebral edema should be avoided, as this could lead to death of the patient.

Uterine Perforation

There is greater risk of uterine perforation in resection of type II myomas, and myomas located in the fundal and the cornual region. In the event of detection, surgery should be discontinued. If perforation has been performed by hysterometer or resectoscopy without electricity, a channel can be established to monitor blood pressure, pulse, and hematocrit/hemoglobin with wide spectrum antibiotic coverage. If perforation has been performed with electrical instruments or cutting instruments, a laparoscopy should be performed to evaluate damage on the level of the blood vessels, intestine or urinary tract.

Uterine Synechia

When submucous myomas located on opposite sides are resected, especially the anterior and posterior sides, there is risk of formation of postoperative synechia. In these cases, in women who desire offspring, administration of estrogens is recommended in order to enhance rapid endometrial regeneration and prevent appearance of uterine synechiae.[18] Some authors place intrauterine devices for 1 month to prevent contact between the two sides. A control hysteroscopy should be performed after 1-2 months. Administration of antibiotics can also reduce the risk of formation of synechia.

REFERENCES

1. Novak ER, Woodruff JD. Myoma and other benign tumors of the uterus. In Novak ER, Woodruff JD (Eds): Novak's gynecologic and obstetric pathology. Philadelphia: WB Saunders 1979;260-79.
2. Neuwirth RS. A new technique for and additional experience with hysteroscopic resection of submucous fibroids. Am J Obstet Gynecol 1978;131:91-4.
3. Buttram VC (Jr), Reiter RC. Uterine leiomyomata: Aetiology, symptomatology and management. Fertil Steril 1981;36:433-45.
4. Pritts EA. Fibroids and infertility: A systematic review of the evidence. Obstet Gynecol Surv 2001;56(8):483-91.
5. Donnez J. What are the implications of myomas on fertility? A need of debate? Hum Reprod 2002;17(6):1424-30.
6. Lefebvre G, Vilos G, Allaire C, Jeffrey J. The management of uterine leiomyomas. J Obstet Gynaecol Can 2003;128:396-405.
7. Wamsteker K, De Blok S, Gallinat A, Lueken RP. Fibroids. In Lewis BV, Magos AL (Eds): Endometrial Ablation. Churchill Livingstone, Edinburgh 1993;161-81.
8. Fedele L, Bianchi S, Dorta M, Brioschi D, Zanotti F, Vercellini P. Transvaginal ultrasonography versus hysteroscopy in the diagnosis of uterine submucous myomas.Obstet Gynecol 1991;77:745-8.
9. Vercellini P, Cortesi I, Oldani, Moschetta M, De Giorgi O, Crosignani P. The role of transvaginal ultrasonography and outpatient diagnostic hysteroscopy in the evaluation of patients with menorrhagia. Hum. Reprod 1997;12:1768-71.
10. Wamsteker K, Emanuel MH, De Kruif JH. Transcervical hysteroscopic resection of submucous fibroids for abnormal uterine bleeding: Results regarding the degree of intramural extension. Obstet Gynecol 1993;82:736-40.

11. Cicinelli E, Romano F, Silvio Anastasio P, Blasi N, Parisi C, Galantito P. Transabdominal sonohysterography, transvaginal sonography, and hysteroscopy in the evaluation of submucous myomas. Obstet Gynecol 1995;85:42-7.

12. Salim R, Lee C, Davies A, Jolaoso B, Ofuasia E, Jurkovic D. A comparative study of three-dimensional saline infusion sonohysterography and diagnostic hysteroscopy for the classification of submucous fibroids. Hum Reprod 2005;20(1):253-7.

13. Dudiak CM, Turner DA, Patel SK, Archie JT, Silver B, Norusis M. Uterine leiomyomas in the infertile patient: Preoperative localization with MR imaging versus US and hysterosalpingography. Radiology 1988;167:620-30.

14. Dueholm M, Lundorf E, Hansen ES, Ledertoug S, Olesen F. Evaluation of the uterine cavity with magnetic resonance imaging, transvaginal sonography, hysterosonographic examination, and diagnostic hysteroscopy. Fertil Steril 2001;76:350-7.

15. Perino A, Chianchiano N, Petronio M, Cittadini E. Role of leuprolide acetate depot in hysteroscopic surgery: A controlled study. Fertil Steril 1993;59:507-10.

16. Mencaglia L, Tantini C. GnRh agonist analogs and hysteroscopic resection of myomas. Int J Gynecol Obstet 1993;43:285-8.

17. Romer T. Value of premedication with gonadotropin releasing hormone agonists before transcervical resection of solitary submucous myoma. Gynakol Geburtshilfliche Rundsch 1996;36(4):194-6.

18. Ubaldi F, Tournaye H, Camus M, Van Der Pas H, Gepts E, Devroey P. Fertility after hysteroscopic myomectomy. Hum Reprod Update 1995;1:81-90.

19. Smet M, Nisolle M, Bassil S, Donnez J. Expansive benign lesions: Treatment by laser. Eur J Obstet Gynecol Reprod Biol 1996;65:101-5.

20. Emanuel MH, Wamsteker K. The Intrauterine Morcellator: A new hysteroscopic operating technique to remove intrauterine polyps and myomas. Journal of Minimally Invasive Gynecology 2005;12:62-6.

21. Hallez JP. Single-stage total hysteroscopic myomectomies: Indications, techniques and results. Fertil Steril 1995;63:703-8

22. Cravello L, D'Ercole C, Boubli L, Blanc B. Hysteroscopic treatment of uterine fibroids. J Gynecol Surg 1995;11:227-32.

23. Derman SG, Rehnstrom J, Neuwirth RS. The long-term effectiveness of hysteroscopic treatment of menorrhagia and leiomyomas. Obstet Gynecol 1991;77:591-4.

24. Cravello L, Agostini A, Beerli M, Roger V, Bretelle F, Blanc B. Résultats des myomectomies hystéroscopiques. Gynécologie Obstétrique Fertilité 2004;32 :825-8.

25. Emanuel MH, Wamsteker K, Hart AA, Metz G, Lammes F. Long-term results of hysteroscopic myomectomy for abnormal uterine bleeding. Obstet Gynecol 1999;93:743-8.

26. Fernandez H, Kadoch O, Capella-Allouc S, Gervaise A, Taylor S, Frydman R. Résection hystéroscopique des myomes sous-muqueux: Résultats a long terme. Ann Chir 2001;126:58-64.

27. Fernandez H, Sefrioui O, Virelizier C, Gervaise A, Gomel V, Frydman R. Hysteroscopic resection of submucosal myomas in patients with infertility. Hum Reprod 2001;16(7):1489-92.

28. Vercellini P, Zaina B, Yaylayan L, Pisacreta A, De Giorgi O, Crosignani P. Hysteroscopic myomectomy: Long-term effects on menstrual pattern and fertility. Obstet Gynecol 1999;94:341-7.

29. Propst AM, Liberman RF, Harlow BL, Ginsburg ES. Complications of hysteroscopic surgery: Predicting patients at risk. Obstet Gynecol 2000;96:517-20.

30. Cooper JM, Brady RM. Intraoperative and early post-operative complications of operative hysteroscopy. Obstet Gynecol Clin North Am 2000;27:347-66.

31. Neuwirth RS. Hysteroscopic management of symptomatic submucous fibroids. Obstet Gynecol 1983;62:509-11.

32. Phillips DR, Nathanson H, Meltzer SM, Milim SJ, Haselkorn JS, Johnson P. Transcervical electrosurgical resection of submucous leiomyomas for chronic menorrhagia. J Am Assoc Gynecol Laparosc 1995;2:147-53.

33. Emanuel MH, Hart AAM, Wamsteker K, Lammes FB. An analysis of fluid-loss during transcervical resection of submucous myomas. Fertil Steril 1997;68:881-6.

34. Cayuela E, Cararach M, Gilabert J, Pérez Medina T, Rivero B, Torrejón R. Consensus documents. Spanish Society of Gynecologist and Obstetrics: Meditex, Madrid; 1996;11-46.

35. Preutthipan S, Theppisai U. Hysteroscopic resection of submucous myomas: Results of 50 procedures at Ramathibodi hospital. J Med Assoc Thai 1998;81:190-4.

36. Wamsteker K, De Block S. Diagnostic hysteroscopy: Technique and documentation. In Sutton CIG Diamond (Eds): Endoscopic surgery for gynaecologist. London: WB Saunders 1993;263-76.

11

Hysteroscopic Treatment of the Symptomatic Septate Uterus

Rafael F Valle

INTRODUCTION

The septate uterus which represents a congenital uterine anomaly resulting from lack of reabsorption of the original embryonic uterine septum may interfere with normal reproduction in 20-25% of women afflicted with this condition, usually resulting in repetitive abortions and fetal malpresentations, therefore it may require surgical treatment which can be accomplished transcervically via the hysteroscope utilizing different methods such as mechanical scissors, thermal electrical energies via the resectoscope or hysteroscope, laser energy via fiber-optic lasers, and bipolar or vaporizing electrodes.

UTERINE ANOMALIES (SEPTUM)

Uterine anomalies, specifically the uterine septum, may cause repetitive abortions in one out of every five women who achieve pregnancy with this condition. The anomaly is due to a lack of reabsorption of an original septum, which results from a fusion of the two Müllerian ducts in the midportion to form the uterus. Because the remaining septum is usually avascular and composed of fibrotic tissue, when implantation occurs at this site, the blastocyst may not have sufficient nutrients and eventually is aborted. Additionally, the uterine cavity's volume decreased by this septations, may also contribute to repetitive abortions and malpositions, when the pregnancy reaches the third trimester. The diagnosis is best obtained with a hysterosalpingogram and when symptomatic, the uterine septum is best treated by hysteroscopy. The uterine septum may be of different lengths and widths involving only the corporeal portion of the uterus or extending also into the cervix. Occasionally it results in septation of the vagina.[1]

The relationship between the septate uterus and infertility remains controversial; the consensus is that this type of uterine anomaly does not cause infertility. Nonetheless, as the therapeutic approach of this anomaly has evolved, patients with primary infertility requiring assisted reproductive technologies or difficult and expensive treatments for infertility have been considered lately as candidates for treatment of the uterine septation.

Preoperative Evaluation

It is important to evaluate other factors that may cause pregnancy wastage before deciding on surgical treatment of the uterine septum. A karyotype should be performed involving husband and wife, and a normal maturation of the endometrium should be evaluated with a late-luteal phase endometrial biopsy, and mid-luteal phase serum progesterone. Endocrine conditions such as subclinical hypothyroidism should be evaluated with a thyroid stimulating hormone assay (TSH).[1]

Autoimmune and alloimmune conditions must be ruled out with a lupus anticoagulant factor study, partial thromboplastin time (PTT), as well as anticardiolipin antibodies (ACA) and antinuclear antibodies (ANA). Human leukocyte antigen (HLA) testing should only be selectively performed in patients with multiple early abortions who do not show any other reason for the abortions. Chronic endometritis is ruled out with an endometrial biopsy.[2]

Finally, because of the close embryologic relationship of Müllerian structures to the mesonephric ducts, when these uterine anomalies occur, renal anomalies should be ruled out. Although these urinary tract anomalies are not as marked and frequent with a septate uterus, duplication of caliceal systems, renal ptosis, and other such abnormalities have been described. Therefore, it is important to evaluate these patients with a screening intravenous pyelogram (IVP).[3]

Methods of Treatment

While surgical treatment requiring laparotomy and hysterotomy were performed in the past only in women with habitual abortions, women experiencing more than three spontaneous miscarriages in the early or mid second trimester of pregnancy, with new less invasive approaches such as hysteroscopic treatment, the indications for treating the uterine septum have been liberalized to focus the attention on each individual patient and her unique reproductive failure.

Hysteroscopic Metroplasty

Hysteroscopic treatment provides a less invasive approach to divide the uterine septum. The treatment offers minimal discomfort to the patient as well as minimal morbidity, as it is performed on an outpatient basis. Because the uterine wall is not divided, a subsequent cesarean section is required only for obstetrical indications. The healing process with reepithelialization of the uterine cavity takes only 4 to 5 weeks, and patients are allowed to conceive sooner than with abdominal metroplasty. Hospitalization is not required, so expenses are markedly reduced.

Four hysteroscopic methods can be used to divide the uterine septum. The mechanical hysteroscopic (semirigid) scissors, the resectoscope, the fiberoptic lasers, and the bipolar vaporizing electrodes. The most commonly used method for treatment of the uterine septum is with semirigid hysteroscopic scissors. The fibrotic consistency of a septum permits this division without significant bleeding and the procedure is performed by systematically dividing the septum in the middle from its nadir to its base, having as landmarks, both uterotubal junctions and the translucency of the hysteroscopic light as seen by an assistant utilizing a laparoscope with dimmed or no light. While this observation is indirect, it can be most helpful to the physician performing the procedure. Nonetheless, the best landmark to avoid invasion of the uterine wall or even possible perforation, is the knowledge by the practitioner of the anatomic landmarks of the uterus. Systematic, delicate, and shallow cuts should be performed in order to observe at all times the symmetry of the uterine cavity. The use of hysteroscopic scissors permits to distend the uterine cavity with saline solutions[4,5] (FIGURES 11.1 to 11.6).

While sonography can be used also guide the division of the uterine septum, it becomes somewhat more cumbersome to maintain in the same plane the uterus and the hysteroscopic scissors, with the sonographic transducer while the surgeon is operating and moving the organ. Nonetheless, it is another alternative of monitoring the surgery.

Another method of hysteroscopic division of the septum is the utilization of the resectoscope with a thin knife electrode that can divide these anomalies systematically by contact. This method becomes most useful in broad septa that may be more difficult to

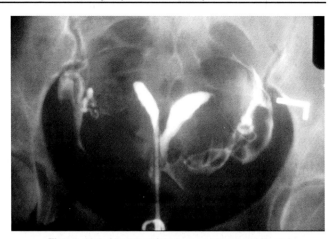

Figure 11.1: Hysterosalpingogram shows a thin and complete uterine septum

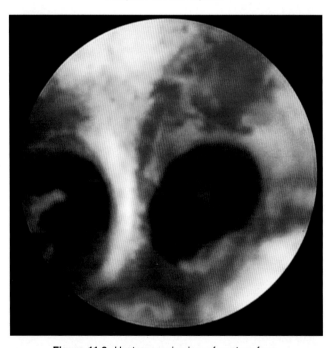

Figure 11.2: Hysteroscopic view of septum from internal cervical os

divide with hysteroscopic scissors. The use of the resectoscope provides continuous washing of the uterine cavity, and avoids any bleeding as minimal as it may be. However, only fluids devoid of electrolytes can be used to avoid conduction and also to permit direct effect of the electrosurgery on tissues.[6] Because this fluid, be it glycine 1.5%, sorbitol 3%, or mannitol 5%, does not contain electrolytes, care should be taken to monitor the deficit of fluid not recovered that may have been absorbed by the patient. A limit of 800-1000 ml of deficit is paramount to assess

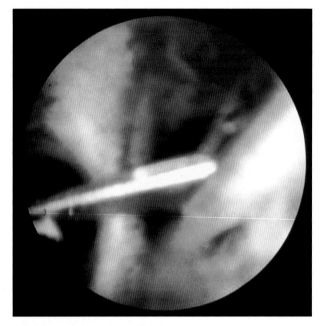

Figure 11.3: Beginning of hysteroscopic division of septum and its medial part

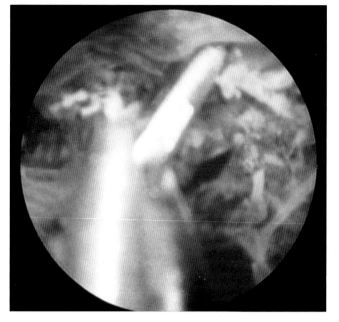

Figure 11.5: Final sculpturing of fundal portion of uterine cavity

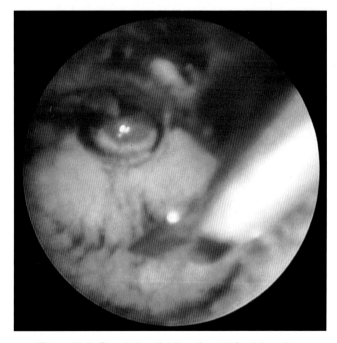

Figure 11.4: Completing division of septal fundal portion.

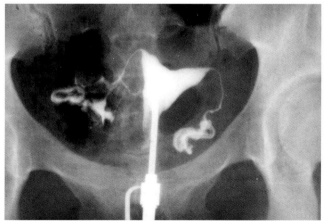

Figure 11.6: One month following treatment, a hysterosalpingogram shows a normal uterine cavity

the condition of the patient and her levels of serum sodium. Should hyponatremia occur, specific measures for treatment should immediately be established (FIGURES 11.7 and 11.8).

Finally, fiberoptic lasers, Neodymium YAG, KTP-532, or argon lasers can be used to divide the uterine.

The precautions to take are similar to those with electrosurgery to avoid invading the fundal myometrial wall, as when using this type of energy, coagulation of the small vessels that cross the septum occur, therefore, obscuring a landmark's junction between septum and myometrium at the uterine wall.

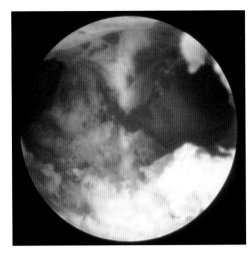

Figure 11.7: Hysteroscopic view of broad uterine septum

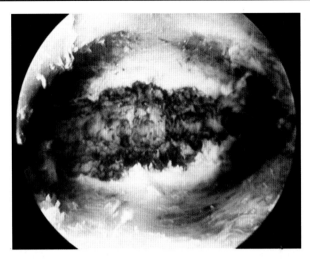

Figure 11.10: Hysteroscopic view of immediate postoperative results following laser division of septum

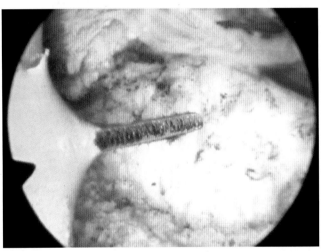

Figure 11.8: Resectoscopic division of the septum

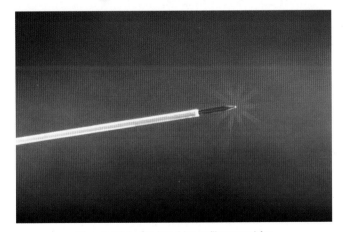

Figure 11.9: Sculpted laser fiber used for septal division (lasersonics)

Fluids with electrolytes can be used, as lasers do not produce conductive energy[7] (FIGURES 11.9 and 11.10).

The newly introduced bipolar vaporizing electrodes also can be used for this purpose, permitting the use of electrolytic fluids, nonetheless, care should be taken to avoid peripheral damage and scattering to the endometrium and impede reepithelialization. Furthermore, the energy should be controlled to avoid excessive bubbling and possible intravasation of the products of combustion.

Adjunctive Intraoperative and Postoperative Management

While prophylactic antibiotics are optional, their use is based on the multiple manipulations and perhaps contaminations that may occur while operating in the uterus. Additionally, being infertile the patients are treated, all measures should be at hand to avoid possible tubal contamination. Perioperative cephalosporins or doxycycline are most useful. While the use of postoperative hormonal therapy is controversial, when used, natural conjugated estrogens are the option, utilizing Premarin 2.5 mg bid orally for 30 days to expedite re-epithelialization with terminal progesterone in the last ten days of the cycle with 10 mg/day to allow withdrawal bleeding. A hysterosalpingogram may be performed after the completion of the hormonal therapy to evaluate uterine symmetry.

Table 11.1: Reproductive performance before and after treatment of septate uterus
(658 patients from 16 reports)

	Pregnancies No.	Abortions (%)	Preterm (%)	Term (%)
Before treatment	1062	933(88)	95(9)	34(3)
After treatment	941	67(14)	29(6)	395(80)

Homer HA. The Septate Uterus: A Review. Fertil Steril 2000;73:1-14.

Comparison of Results

The reproductive outcome following hysteroscopic treatment of the symptomatic septate uterus has not only equaled but has surpassed the results obtained with traditional abdominal metroplasties, with over 85 to 90% viable pregnancies in women with a history of repetitive abortions. Furthermore, the patient is spared a laparotomy and a hysterotomy, eliminating the potential for pelvic adhesions and secondary infertility as well as the associated pain, disability, and expense. Patients treated hysteroscopically need to wait only four weeks to attempt conception and do not require a mandatory cesarean section[8-10] (TABLE 11.1).

While no large, prospective, randomized studies to evaluate the role of the uterine septum in the causation of abortions have been performed, the results obtained using patients as their own controls pre- and postoperatively, strongly suggest a definite role in the ability of carrying pregnancies at term following treatment.[11,12] Fedele et al. performed serial sonographic evaluations in 12 patients who conceived and were known to have a uterine septum, to evaluate the site of implantation. In 4 women where the implantation occurred away from the septum, the pregnancies progressed normally to viability. Six patients whose implantation was septal aborted; in the other two who also aborted, the implantation was mixed in one, and undetermined in the other.[13] These observations strongly support the role of the uterine septum in subsequent abortions.[14,15]

Some infertile patients, particularly those who require expensive and lengthy treatments for ovulations induction, insemination, or in vitro-fertilization and embryo transfer methods, as well as those with unexplained infertility, may benefit from prophylactic removal of the uterine septum. The routine treatment of uterine septum in asymptomatic patients who have not proven fertility, however, does not seem to be warranted.[16]

CONCLUSION

The uterine septum resulting from failure of reabsorption of the embryonic original fusion of the müllerian ducts may impair reproductive function in 20 to 25% of women affected with this anomaly. The modern treatment of this condition is by hysteroscopic transcervical division of this embryonic remnant. Following treatment, the term pregnancy rate reaches 90%. Several hysteroscopic modalities can be used, but the hysteroscopic scissors and resectoscopic methods are by far the most common. Because of the obvious benefits of this approach; rapid recovery, excellent anatomic and reproductive outcome, avoidance of major invasive surgery with a prolonged healing process, and no necessity for mandatory cesarean section for delivery, the hysteroscopic treatment is now established as the treatment of choice for these uterine anomalies.

REFERENCES

1. Valle RF. Clinical management of uterine factors in infertile patients. In Speroff L (Ed): Seminars in Reproductive Endocrinology. Thieme-Stratton, Inc. Georg Thieme Verlag: New York, NY 1985;3:2,149-67.
2. Carp HJA V, Mashiach S, Nebel L, Serri DM. Recurrent miscarriage: A review of current concepts, immune mechanisms, and results of treatment. Obstet Gynecol Survey 1990;45:657-69.
3. Buttram VC, Gibbons WE. Mullerian anomalies: A proposed classification (an analysis of 144 cases). Fertil Steril 1979;32:40-6.
4. Valle RF, Sciarra JJ. Hysteroscopic treatment of the septated uterus. Obstet Gynecol 1986;676:253-7.
5. March CM, Israel R. Hysteroscopic management of recurrent abortion caused by septated uterus. Am J Obstet Gynecol 1987;156:834-42.

6. DeCherney AH, Russell JB, Graebe RA, Polan ML. Resectoscopic management of Mullerian fusion defects. Fertil Steril 1986;45:726-8.
7. Choe JK, Baggish MS. Hysteroscopic treatment of septated uterine with Neodymium-YAG laser. Fertil Steril 1992;57:81-4.
8. Fedele L, Arcaini L, Parazzini F, Vercellini P, Dinola G. Reproductive prognosis after hysteroscopic metroplasty in 102 women: Life-table analysis. Fertil Steril 1993;59:768-72.
9. Valle RF. Hysteroscopic treatment of partial and complete uterine septum. Int J Fertil 1996;41:310-5.
10. Hassiakos DK, Zourlas PA. Transcervical division of the uterine septa. Obstet Gynecol Survey 1990;45:165-73.
11. Lin K, Zhu X, Xu H, Liang Z, Zhang X. Reproductive outcome following resectoscope metroplasty in women having a complete uterine septum with double cervix and vagina. Int J Gynaecol Obstet 2008 (In press).
12. Patton PE, Novy MJ, Lee DM, and Hickok LR. The diagnosis and reproductive outcome after surgical treatment of the complete septate uterus, duplicated cervix and vaginal septum. Am J Obstet Gynecol 2004;190:1669-78.
13. Fedele L, Dorta M, Brioschi D, Giudici MN, Candiani GB. Pregnancies in septate uteri: outcome in relation to site of uterine implantation as determined by sonography. Am J Roentgenol 1989;781-4.
14. Fedele L, Bianchi S. Hysteroscopic metroplasty for septate uterus. In Siegler AM (Ed): Hysteroscopy. Obstetrics and Gynecology Clinics of North America 1995;22:473-89.
15. Zlopasa G, Skrablin S, Kolefatic D, Bonovic V, Lesin J. Uterine anomalies and pregnancy outcome following resectoscope metroplasty. Int J Gynaecol Obstet 2007;98:129-33.
16. Pabuccu R, Gomel V. Reproductive outcome after hysteroscopic metroplasty in women with septate uterus and otherwise unexplained infertility. Fertil Steril 2004;81:1675-8.

12

Endometrial Polyps

Tirso Pérez-Medina

INTRODUCTION

The endometrial polyps (EP) are excretions of the endometrium containing variable amounts of glands, stroma and blood vessels. Polyps are generally solitary, but in 20% of cases are multiple. Polyps vary in size, ranging from microscopic abnormalities that are only a few millimeters, across to huge lesions that can fill the uterine cavity or prolapse through the endocervical canal. They can be sessile or pedunculated, and originate anywhere in the uterine cavity.[1]

Most EPs appear to originate from localized hyperplasia of the basalis, although their pathogenesis is not well understood.[2] Polyps occur over a wide age range, but are most common in women in the fourth and fifth decades, becoming less frequent after age 60. The prevalence of EPs in the general female population is estimated to be approximately 25%.[3] Usually they present with abnormal uterine bleeding. They have been implicated as a cause of abnormal uterine bleeding in between 2 and 23% of patients. They also have been implicated as a possible cause of infertility, either by physically interfering with blastocyst implantation or by altering the development of secretory phase endometrium, making it less receptive to the implanting embryo. EPs have been found in patients receiving tamoxifen therapy for breast carcinoma. Large polyps that extend into the endocervix and dilate the internal os can cause endometritis. In general, polyps are benign growths with no malignant potential. Occasional cases of carcinoma, including serous carcinoma and even mixed mesodermal tumors, can be confined to a polyp.

Furthermore, polyps have been associated with the occurrence of carcinoma in several studies. Nonetheless, polyps are not regarded as a major risk factor for the development of carcinoma and most lesions are successfully treated with hysteroscopic excision.

PATHOGENESIS

EPs are the cause of 15% of the cases of abnormal uterine bleeding in women of reproductive age and of 25% in postmenopausal women. Benign polyps occur in approximately 50% of all patients with

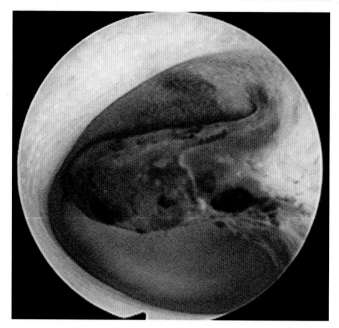

Figure 12.1: Necrotic polyp showing darkened areas corresponding to infarctions inside the polyp

abnormal uterine bleeding[4] and in 25% of women presenting with postmenopausal bleeding.[5] These polyps give rise to abnormal uterine bleeding due to different mechanisms such as continual rubbing against the surrounding normal endometrium, provocation of progressive atrophy in the vicinity, and vascular infarctions in the actual polyp, without overlooking the potential establishment of a malignant degeneration at its core. In addition to these characteristic features, polyps may show evidence of focal glandular and stromal breakdown (FIGURE 12.1), usually due to thrombosis of the dilated superficial veins. Reslova[6] reported that of the 245 having intrauterine polyps, 58% had abnormal uterine bleeding. Preutthipan,[7] comparing premenopausal and postmenopausal women with EP, founds that in the premenopausal group 81% of the patients had abnormal uterine bleeding and 44% in the postmenopausal group.

They also have been found during routine ultrasound or infertility investigations. Although the precise mechanism by which intrauterine polyps cause infertility is unclear, their removal has been reported to increase fertility, and their extraction improves significantly the chance for pregnancy.

We conducted a clinical trial[8] in a series of 204 women with endometrial polyp and scheduled for intrauterine insemination (103 control group no polypectomy and 101 study group hysteroscopic polypectomy), in which a total of 93 pregnancies occurred, 64 in the study group and 29 in the control group. Women on study group have a better possibility to get pregnancy after polypectomy with a relative risk of 2.1 (CI 95% 1.5-2.9). The survival analysis showed that after 4 cycles the pregnancy rate was 51.4% in the study group and 25.4% in the control group ($p < 0.001$). Interestingly, pregnancies in the study group were obtained before the first IUI in 65% of cases. The rest were obtained over the 4 cycles period, without a clear distribution between the cycles (TABLE 12.1).

The cause for this disturbance is unknown. Richlin demonstrated an increase in glycodelin levels in the periovulatory period in women with EP. The glycodelin is a protein that facilitates the implantation by decreasing the NK cell activity. During the normal periovulatory phase during a functional cycle, glycodelin decreases because it inhibits the sperm-oocyte binding. In this situation, the EP produces significant amount of glycodelin thus difficulty in implantation.[9]

Polyps are in general benign growths, although malignancy confined to a polyp has also been identified.[10,11] The incidence of carcinoma confined to EPs varies between 0 and 4.8 % depending on the selection of patients and the methods used in making the diagnosis. Anyway, to consider a polyp to be cancerous, the malignant transformation must be limited to the polyp and the pedicle and the surrounding endometrium must be free of disease.

HISTOPATHOLOGY

Although their etiology is not clear, in general polypoid endometrial structures are considered as local hyperplasia of the endometrium. The pathogenesis of such local overgrowth of tissue is not understood. Possibly they result from local variation in hormone responsiveness, producing the so-called basal hyperplasia, seen in transvaginal

Table 12.1: Number and percentage of pregnancies in both groups (N = 204)

	Polypectomy		Signification
	Study (N = 101)	Control (N = 103)	
Pregnancy (%)			
Yes	64 (63.4)	29 (28.2)	< 0.001
No	37 (36.6)	74 (71.8)	

RR = 2.1 95% CI (1.5-2.9)

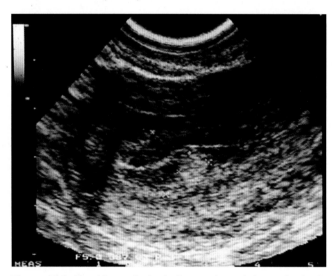

Figure 12.2: Basal hyperplasia. An hyperechogenic image is clearly seen under the surface epithelium. This lesion is not visible hysteroscopically

ultrasonography at first (FIGURE 12.2) and, once becomes manifested as a bulk, in hysteroscopy.

The glands and stroma of EPs can show diverse histologic patterns. Despite their diverse growth patterns, all polyps show several histologic features that facilitate their diagnosis: Polypoid shape, surface epithelium on three sides, dense stroma, thick-walled arteries, glands dilated, and more tortuous than normal glands, glands appear "out of phase" or hyperplastic.

Each type of polyp is identified by the changes that occur in the glands and stroma. Following these changes, 6 different types of EPs have been proposed[3]: hyperplastic, atrophic, functional, mixed endometrial-endocervical, adenomyomatous, and the atypical polypoid adenomyoma. This classification has little clinical significance but is useful for correct identification of these lesions and separation of some polyps from hyperplasia.

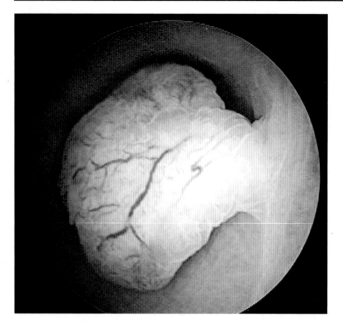

Figure 12.3: Hyperplastic polyp. Note the prominent vascularization in the polyp beneath the polypoid surface endometrium

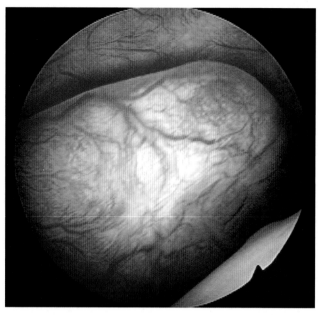

Figure 12.4: Hyperplastic polyp. Hypervascularized surface with irregular vascular network with crowded gland openings

Hyperplastic Polyps

Hyperplastic polyps are most common. They are highly variable in size, measuring up to several centimeters in greatest dimension. Regardless of size, they show irregular, proliferating glands, resembling those in hyperplasia. They have typically clusters of thick-walled arteries in dense stroma (FIGURES 12.3 and 12.4).

The hysteroscopic appearance is a well-defined polyp surrounded by atrophic, hyperplastic or functional endometrium in a postmenopausal patient, with a compact aspect, thick-walled vessels showing an irregular vascular network, and epithelial superficial component with crowded or irregularly spaced glands and no signs of necrosis or suspicious zones. They have a rather fibrous stroma with a leash of thick-walled vessels at the pedicle that, due to the fibrous component, is hard to the touch with the endoscopic scissors.

Atrophic Polyps

Atrophic polyps, or "glandular-cystic polyps" are usually seen in postmenopausal women. These polyps contain scarce atrophic glands lined by low columnar epithelium reflecting no mitotic activity

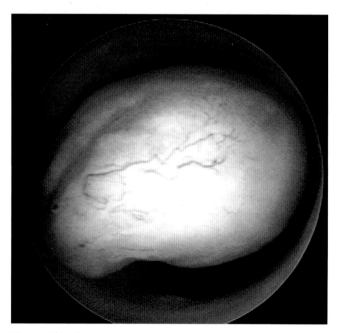

Figure 12.5: Scarce gland openings, atrophic surface epithelium and regular vascular network are the mean characteristics of atrophic polyps

(FIGURES 12.5 and 12.6). Other types of atrophic polyps, the glandularcystic ones, show great dilated glands with round contours that form cysts of retention favored by the fibrotic stroma around them. If biopsied, they extrude a mucous fluid (FIGURE 12.7). Many of these polyps apparently represent

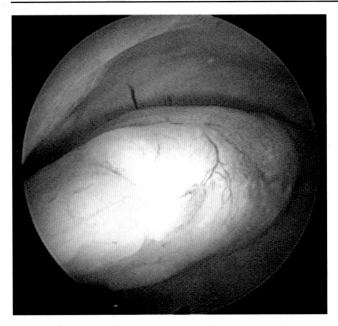

Figure 12.6: Atrophic polyp. The regular trajects of the vessels are clearly appreciated

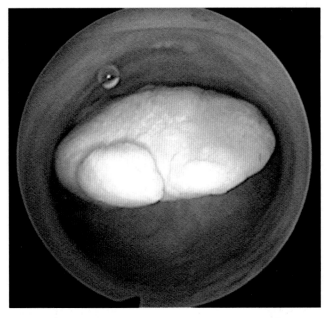

Figure 12.8: Functional polyp showing white spots corresponding to proliferative gland openings in the surface

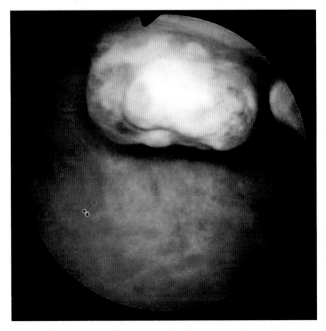

Figure 12.7: Glandulocystic (atrophic) polyp with dark areas of mucus retention

hyperplastic polyps that no longer show proliferative activity. They are inactive and this is clearly seen in their vessels, which are straight and thin.

Functional Polyps

These polyps, like the endometrium around them, are hormonally responsive and show proliferative

or secretory changes. They occur typically in premenopausal patients (FIGURE 12.8).

The most important sign for the hysteroscopic diagnosis is the recognition of multiple gland openings on the surface, reflecting functional activity. The vessels are not apparent, obscured by the surface epithelium. Due to their major epithelial component, they are very soft to the touch and the pedicle is easy to cut, even pushing with the open jaws of the endoscopic graspers.

Mixed Endometrial-Endocervical Polyps

Some polyps originate in the upper endocervix and lower uterine segment and show both endocervical and endometrial type gland development. These polyps tend to have a fibrous stroma resembling the stroma of the lower uterine segment. Hysteroscopically, the most important thing is to identify the attachment area in the isthmus (FIGURE 12.9).

Adenomyomatous Polyps

These polyps have smooth muscle in their stroma, usually as irregular bundles and strands in proximity to thick-walled vessels. Most often these are large hyperplastic polyps in which the stroma has undergone partial smooth muscle change. They are

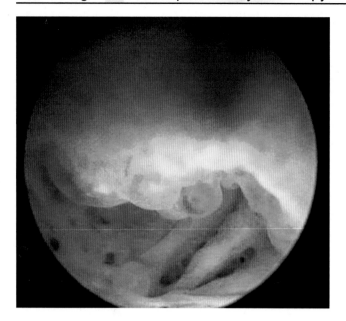

Figure 12.9: Polyp arising from the left tubal ostium

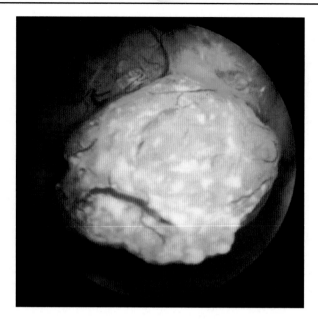

Figure 12.10: Atypical polyp showing atypical vessels. The appearance is of friability

rarely suspected in the hysteroscopy, and the pathologist will make the definitive diagnosis.

Atypical Polypoid Adenomyoma

This is an unusual and distinctive polyp characterized by glands that are lined by atypical epithelium and surrounded by cellular smooth muscle. It typically occurs in premenopausal or perimenopausal women, with a mean age of about 40 years. Often these lesions arise in the lower uterine segment, but they can also arise in the corpus.

There have been a few reports of endometrial adenocarcinoma in association with an atypical polypoid adenomyoma, and we have seen similar cases. Usually this lesion does not show aggressive growth, however, and curettage may be curative.

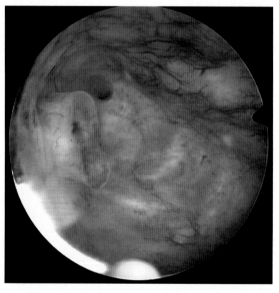

Figure 12.11: Atypical polyp in the right ostium

Atypical Polyps

In some polyps, independent of their histological origin, some atypical characteristics can be seen. Atypical vessels, necrotic areas, and friable touch are observed (FIGURE 12.10). They are often located around the tubal ostia (FIGURE 12.11). In these cases, biopsy is mandatory.

DIAGNOSIS

The large variation in the reported prevalence of polyps reflects the difficulties in establishing the histologic diagnosis. Polyps often are fragmented and removed piecemeal at curettage and therefore they can be difficult to recognize. Hysteroscopy can be useful to confirm the diagnosis of polyp, although in one study as many as 13% of polyp-like structures seen by hysteroscopy were not confirmed histologically.

Diagnosis of EPs is of vital importance because in most cases they are not detected during physical examination or curettage, which explains the persistence or recurrence of symptoms, so we need to find an effective alternative diagnostic method.

Although the presence of EPs is sometimes suspected on account of the patient's case history, these formations are not diagnosable in a standard gynecological examination and require an instrumental technique of some type. Hystero-salpingography was originally considered to be the best diagnostic method, but it gave a high rate of false positives and negatives, as appreciated later in the hysterectomy specimen.[12] Abdominal ultra-sonography then began to be used, although its results left a lot to be desired in terms of efficacy, because the resolution of the instruments was not high. With the improvement of the instruments, and especially with the arrival of the transvaginal probe, more accurate descriptions of this condition have become possible.

Fedele,[13] puts the limitation down to the hypere-choic ultrasound aspect of polyps. Since these are dissimulated by a secretory endometrium, he suggests that they should be explored during the proliferative phase of the cycle, when the endo-metrium in less than 4 mm thick.

Goldstein[14] states that saline infusion sono-hysterography can reliably differentiate between EPs, globally thickened tissue and submucous myomas. To minimize this problem we can use the color Doppler scan all around the suspected EP tracing the pedicle of the polyp in the wall of attachment (FIGURE 12.12). It exhibited a color map image characterized by increased vascularization together with thick low resistance vessels in contrast with color map found in myomata, which show a round, non-pedunculated, peritumoral color Doppler pattern.

Syrop[15] introduced a contrast fluid during the US scan. Thus, Hulka describes the ultrasound appear-ance of polyps as an echogenic endometrium with

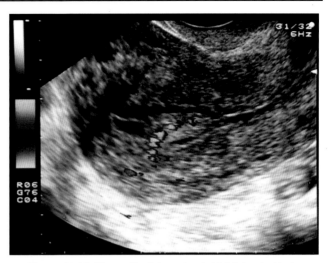

Figure 12.12: The stalk of the polyp is highlighted with the Doppler velocymetry

cystic spaces in its interior.[16] Atri,[17] in turn, describes 3 types of sonographic appearance of the polyp, depending on its hormonal state: Hyperplastic, functional and atrophic (Chapter 4).

At the present time, hysteroscopy is considered the gold standard for the investigation of any intrauterine lesion. Hysteroscopy permits panoramic direct vision and biopsy of lesions, thus increasing precision and accuracy in the diagnosis of intrauterine conditions.[18,19]

MANAGEMENT

As mentioned above, the prevalence of EPs is 24% in the general female population. The prevalence is high and the number of positive diagnoses is increasing, as routine transvaginal ultrasonography in healthy women is becoming mandatory. The clinician has to face the issue of how to treat EPs because they are being diagnosed in growing numbers even in asymptomatic women, and because their malignant potential is not fully understood. The problem will be how to manage so many polyps. We know that all EPs can be resected but hysteroscopic surgery implies some, although minimal, real risk,[20] so removing them all may be too aggressive and leaving them all may be dangerous, but their malignant potential still represents an enigma. Most of the published reports are based on specimens that were obtained by curettage or by other sampling techniques, such as Pipelle.[21] In a consistent proportion of cases, these "blind" methods fail to extract the whole polyp and obtain only a mixed specimen of polyp and endometrial mucosa. In such studies, fragmentation of the polyp, incompleteness of specimen, and the presence of adjacent endometrium hamper the diagnosis, as to whether an endometrial cancer has originated in an antecedent benign polyp or in the surrounding endometrium (FIGURE 12.13). Only hysteroscopy gives the possibility of removing the entire polyp with its stalk, leaving intact the adjacent endometrium, so that the risk of malignancy of EPs can be estimated confidently.[22] Primary malignant degeneration of an EP has been quoted variably in the scientific literature, ranging from 0.5[23] to 4.8%.[24] Savelli[25] demonstrated that in a large unselected population of women with EP, the rate of malignancy is low (0.8%), but the hyperplastic changes are more common (FIGURE 12.14). He described several risk factors (age, menopause status and hypertension) that may increase the risk of premalignant and malignant polyps. They did not find a difference in the prevalence of atypical hyperplasia and endometrial carcinoma between symptomatic and asymptomatic patients and to achieve complete removal of the polyp and a reliable histologic analysis, operative hysteroscopy is the treatment of choice and should be offered to symptomatic patients or to patients with risk factors.[26]

In the other hand, we do not perform surgery on asymptomatic fibroids, being the malignant potential between 0.1 and 0.6%.[27] It is of great concern to know which ones should be resected and which ones can be safety left (as we do with the asymptomatic myomas, with similar malignant potential), thus avoiding the anesthetic and surgical risks (26.8% in our series). Color Doppler map obtained with TVUS color Doppler is an accurate method to diagnose the vascularity of EPs. This vascularity reflects the functionality of the polyps, thus recommending surgery. Contrarily, a negative color Doppler map traduces inactivity and no growth potential inside the polyp, allowing us to follow-up, avoiding hysteroscopic surgery in almost 30% of the patients in our series.

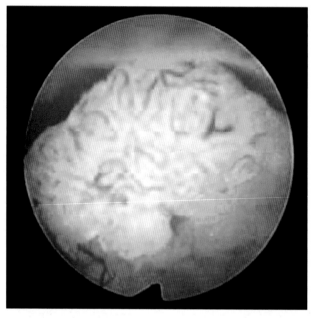

Figure 12.13: Malignant polyp. Necrotic areas in a polypoid mass arising from the upper wall

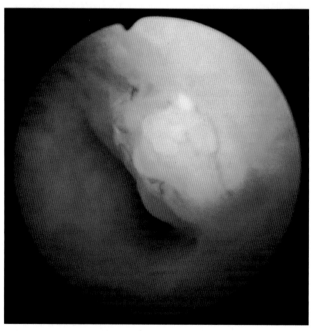

Figure 12.14: Malignant polyp. Suspicious lesion in a polyp located near the left ostium

TREATMENT

Curettage is one of the most frequently performed surgical procedures in gynecology and has long been considered the criterion standard in diagnostic evaluation of abnormal uterine bleeding.[28] Although curettage is used primarily as a diagnostic procedure, the removal of endometrial lesions, especially EPs, should be curative as well.[29] However, correction of bleeding disorders and especially removal of thick endometrium diagnosed by vaginal ultrasonography and curettage is not always successful. Simple curettage, which is a blind procedure, may not be considered as an effective method to treat EPs. Previous study reported that 10 % of intrauterine lesions, mainly polyps, were missed during curettage.[30]

The lack of accuracy in patients with persistently abnormal thick endometrium shown on vaginal ultrasonography after "blind" curettage led to the recommendation that hysteroscopy be included in the management of endometrial lesions.

At the present time hysteroscopy is considered the gold standard for the investigation of any intrauterine lesion. Hysteroscopy has become increasingly common, essential, and popular from the eighties till now in the field of gynecology.[31,32] It is effective and safe to treat submucous myomas, EPs, and other lesions such as septate uterus and intrauterine synechiae. It permits panoramic visualization of the uterine cavity and direct biopsy of lesions, thus increasing precision and accuracy in the diagnosis of intrauterine conditions in contrast to dilatation and curettage, which is a blind technique. It allows the correct diagnosis to be made. The nature of the lesion and its precise localization can be determined. Hysteroscopic surgery reduces the need for major and unnecessary surgery.

Hysteroscopy provides a simple, safe, and effective mean of diagnosing intrauterine abnormality. Hysteroscopic surgery has become a common and important therapeutic procedure in patients with intrauterine lesions. EPs are commonly found during diagnostic hysteroscopy.

Hysteroscopic polypectomy is a minimal invasive operation and it allows the complete removal of the polyps under direct visual control, which prevents the recurrence in situ of these lesions. The type of instruments used depends on the operators experience, and also on the location, and size of the lesion.

Most of the EP can be removed using the diagnostic hysteroscope fitted with an operative sheath and scissors (FIGURE 12.15). The cut must be directed to resect the polyp from its deep origin; this is, from the stroma. Otherwise, as the plants, the polyp will grow back from its germ (FIGURE 12.16).

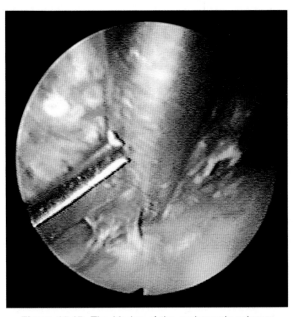

Figure 12.15: The blades of the endoscopic scissors reaching the pedicle

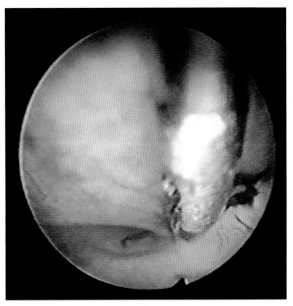

Figure 12.16: The first cut must contain as much pedicle as possible

The extraction should be from outside with the endoscopic graspers and exerting the right pressure to achieve the complete removal. The outside channel should be open to facilitate the drag of the polyp. When this is not possible, it is very helpful to use an endoscopic basket, similar to the one used in gastroenterology, adapted to hysteroscopy (shorter, rigid and lighter) to entrap the polyp (FIGURE 12.17).

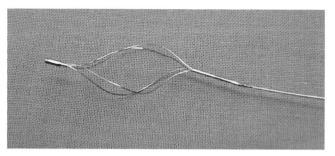

Figure 12.17: Endoscopic polyp basket adapted for hysteroscopy

There are some characteristics that must be kept in mind when planning to resect a polyp in the office with the 5 French endoscopic scissors.

- The stalk of the polyp should be accessible with the scissors.
- Pedicles arising from the fundus are more difficult as the rigid scissors can not easily reach the pedicle in a perpendicular line, thus difficulty in the cuts
- The polyp should not be very large, because it should be difficult to extract it after the resection
- The atrophic and hyperplastic polyps are easier to extract because they are fibrous and hold the pressure exerted by the endoscopic grasper in the narrowest place, as is the os. The functional or glandular cystic polyps break easily when the pressure exerted with the grasper is high.
- The stalk of the polyp should not be too large, as sessile polyps need more cuts to be transected and problems arise when bleeding begins.

With all these characteristics, the surgeon has to be realistic and begin the transection only when complete removal is expected. Each particular surgeon has to know where his own limit is?

Anyway, when once resected the extraction is not possible, there are some clues that are to be followed:

- Always perform biopsy to achieve a throughout diagnosis
- Misoprostol is given the next two following nights trying the expulsion. This is achieved in most of the cases
- Confirmation of the expulsion 3 days later
- No antibiotic is needed meanwhile.

The role of bipolar energy in office hysteroscopy is discussed in Chapter 3.

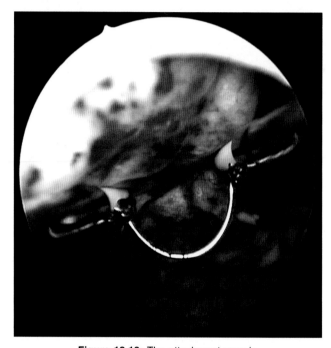

Figure 12.18: The attachment area is identified prior to the resection

Larger polyps may need to be removed using the resectoscope. Larger polyps can be difficult to remove as they may fill the uterine cavity and, because they are vascular, they may bleed if traumatized. The pedicle should always be found (FIGURES 12.18 and 12.19). It is worth to spend some minutes to look for the pedicle as the resection from there should be safer and faster. If the polyp is transected in strips, as is the case for submucous myomas, the soft tissue of the polyp and the strips will surround the resectoscope, difficulting the vision and the risk for complications.

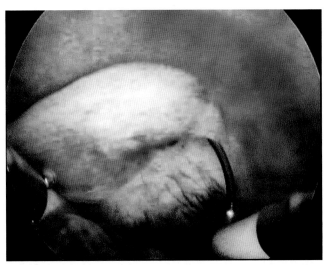

Figure 12.19: The loop in contact with the pedicle. This must be the first step prior to resectoscopic polypectomy

CONCLUSION

The prevalence of EPs in the general female population is estimated to be approximately 25%. Patients having these intrauterine lesions may be totally asymptomatic. When they became symptomatic, the most common cause is abnormal uterine bleeding. EPs may be implicated as possible causes of infertility. Although the precise mechanism by which intrauterine polyps cause infertility is unclear, their removal has been reported to increase fertility.

Simple curettage, which is a blind procedure, may not be considered as an effective method to treat EPs. Previous study reported that 10% of intrauterine lesions, mainly polyps, were missed during curettage. In contrast, hysterectomy is a major procedure at risk of morbidity and mortality for treatment of these isolated benign lesions. Hysteroscopy now plays a major role in the rapidly changing therapeutic approach to both the diagnosis and the treatment of intrauterine lesions. It allows the correct diagnosis to be made. The nature of the lesion and its precise localization can be determined. Hysteroscopic surgery reduces the need for major and unnecessary surgery.

REFERENCES

1. DeWaay DJ, Syrop CH, Nygaard IE, Davis WA, Van Voorhis BJ. Natural history of uterine polyps and leiomyomata. Obstet Gynecol 2002;100:3-7

2. S herman ME, Mazur MT, Kurman RJ. Benign diseases of the endometrium. In: Kurman RJ (Ed): Blaunstein's pathology of the female genital tract. 3rd ed. New York: Springer 2002;421-66.

3. Mazur MT, Kurman RJ. Polyps. In: Mazur MT and Kurman RJ (Eds): Diagnosis of endometrial biopsies and curettings. New York:Springer 1995;146.

4. Nagele F, O'Connor H, Davies A, Badawy A, Mohamed H, Magos A. 2500 outpatient hysteroscopies. Obstet Gynecol 1996;88:87-92.

5. Cronje HS. Diagnostic hysteroscopy after postmenopausal uterine bleeding. S Afr Med J 1984;66:773-4.

6. Reslova T, Tosner J, Resl M, Kugler R, Vavrova I. EPs: A clinical study of 245 cases. Arch Gynecol Obstet 1999;262:133-9.

7. Preutthipan S, Herabutya Yongyoth. Hysteroscopic polypectomy in 240 premenopausal and postmenopausal women. Fertil Steril 2005;83:705-9.

8. Pérez-Medina T, Bajo-Arenas J, Salazar F, Redondo T, SanFrutos L, Alvarez P, Engels V. Endometrial polyps and their implication in the pregnancy rates of patients undergoing intrauterine insemination: A prospective, randomized study. Hum Reprod 2005;20:1632-5.

9. Richlin S, Ramachandran S, Shanti A, Murphy AA, Parthasarathy S. Glycodelin levels in uterine flushings and in plasma of patients with leiomyomas and polyps: Implications and implantation. Hum Rep 2002;17,2742-7.

10. Anastasiadis PG, Koutlaki NG, Skaphida PG, Galazios GC, Tsikouras PN, Liberis VA. EPs: Prevalence, detection, and malignant potential in women with abnormal uterine bleeding. Eur J Gynaecol Oncol 2000;21:180-3.

11. Perez-Medina T, Martinez O, Folgueira G et al: Which EPs should be resected? J Am Assoc Gynecol Laparosc 1999;6:71-4.

12. Preuthippan S, Linasmita V. A prospective comparative study between hysterosalpingography and hysteroscopy in the detection of intrauterine pathology in patients with infertility. J Obstet Gynecol Res 2003;29,33-7.

13. Fedele L, Bianchi S, Dorta M, Brioschi D, Zanotti F, Vercellini P. Transvaginal ultrasonography versus hysteroscopy in the diagnosis of uterine submucous myomas. Obstet Gynecol 1991;77:745-53.

14. Goldstein SR, Monteagudo A, Popiolek D, Mayberry P, Timor-Tritsch I. Evaluation of EPs. Am J Obstet Gynecol 2002;186:669-74.

15. Syrop CH, Sahakian V. Transvaginal sonographic detection of EPs with fluid contrast augmentation. Obstet Gynecol 1992;79:1041.

16. Hulka CA, Hall DA, McCarthy K, Simeone JF. EPs, hyperplasia, and carcinoma in postmenopausal women: Differentiation with endovaginal sonography. Radiology 1994;191:755-8.

17. Atri M, Mazarnia S, Aldis AE, Reinhold C, Bret PM, Kintzen G. Transvaginal US appearance of endometrial abnormalities. Radiographics 1994;14:483.

18. Motashaw ND, Dave S. Diagnostic and therapeutic hysteroscopy in the management of abnormal uterine bleeding. J Reprod Med 1990;35:616-20.

19. Mencaglia L, Perino A, Hamou J. Hysteroscopy in perimenopausal and postmenopausal women with abnormal uterine bleeding. J Reprod Med 1987;32:577-82.

20. Motashaw ND, Dave S. Complications of hysteroscopy. Gynecol Endosc 2001;10:203-10.

21. Armenia CS. Sequential relationship between EPs and carcinoma of the endometrium. Obstet Gynecol 1967;30;524-9, Van Bogaert LJ. Clinicopathologic findings in EPs. Obstet Gynecol 1988;71:771-3.

22. Tjarks M, Van Voorhis BJ. Treatment of EPs. Obstet Gynecol 2000;96:886-9

23. Perez-Medina T, Bajo J, Huertas MA, Rubio A. Predicting atypia inside endometrial polyps. J Ultrasound Med 2002;21:125-8.

24. Wolfe SA, Mackles A. Malignant lesions arising from benign EPs. Obstet Gynecol 1962;20:542-51.

25. Savelli L, De Ianco P, Santini D, Rosati F, Ghi T, Pignotti E, Bovicelli L. Histopathologic features and risk factors for benignity, hyperplasia, and cancer in EPs. Am J Obstet Gynecol 2003;188:927-31.

26. Pérez-Medina T, Bajo JM, Martinez-Cortes L, Castellanos P, Pérez de Avila I. Six thousand office diagnostic-operative hysteroscopies. Int J Gynecol Obstet 2000;71:33-8.

27. Seki K, Hoshihara T, Nagata I. Leiomyosarcoma of the uterus: Ultrasonography and serum lactate dehydrogenase level. Gynecol Obstet Invest 1992;33:114-8.

28. Ben-Yehuda OM, Kim YB, Leuchter RS. Does hysteroscopy improve upon the sensitivity of dilatation and curettage in the diagnosis of endometrial hyperplasia or carcinoma? Gynecol Oncol 1998;68:4-7.

29. Brooks PG, Serden SP. Hysteroscopic findings after unsuccessful dilatation and curettage for abnormal uterine bleeding. Am J Obstet Gynecol 1988;158:1354-7.

30. Word B, Gravlee LC, Widdeman GL. The fallacy of simple uterine curettage. Obstet Gynecol 1958;12:642-8.

31. Gimpelson RJ, Rappold HO. A comparative study between panoramic hysteroscopy with directed biopsies and dilatation and curettage. A review of 276 cases. Am J Obstet Gynecol 1988;158:489-92.

32. Bettocchi S, Ceci O, Nappi L, Di Venere R, Masciopinto V, Pansini V, Pinto L, Santoro A, Cormio G. Operative office hysteroscopy without anesthesia: Analysis of 4863 cases performed with mechanical instruments. J Am Assoc Gynecol Laparosc 2004;11:59-61.

13

Hysteroscopic Techniques for Endometrial Ablation

Tirso Pérez-Medina
Mar Rios Vallejo

INTRODUCTION

Endometrial Ablation (EA) is a surgical technique by which the full extent of the endometrium is eliminated.

EA is considered as an alternative to the hysterectomy for the treatment of the abnormal uterine bleeding (AUB) in women who fail conservative medical treatment.

The endometrium has an extraordinary power of regeneration. To suppress successfully, the menstruation is essential to remove the total thickness of the endometrium along with the superficial myometrium, which includes the deep basal glands that are the primary focus for the uterine re-epithelialization (this include 2.5-3.0 mm of myometrium) (FIGURE 13.1).

Endometrial destruction offers an alternative to hysterectomy as a surgical treatment for heavy menstrual bleeding. Both procedures are effective and satisfaction rates are high. Although hysterectomy is associated with a longer operating time, a longer recovery period and higher rates of postoperative complications, it offers permanent relief from heavy menstrual bleeding. The cost of endometrial destruction is significantly lower than hysterectomy but since re-treatment is often necessary the cost difference narrows overtime.[1]

INDICATIONS

The main indication is the dysfunctional uterine bleeding or menometrorrhagia associated to systemic pathology.

The procedure is designed for patients with:
- Menorrhagia
- Failure of conservative therapy (women have not responded or who have not tolerated)
- Normal uterine cavity
- Normal endometrial histology
- Reproductive desires completed
- Desire of conserving the uterus
- Amenorrhea is not demanded
- No significant dysmenorrhea.

Optionally can be performed in:
- Recurrent postmenopausal metrorrhagia after excluding other pathologies
- Patient on tamoxifen or HRT with persistent metrorrhagia

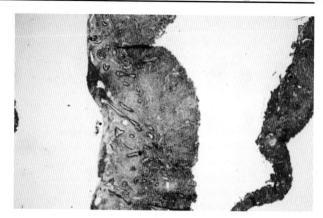

Figure 13.1: Strip of endometrial resection. Endometrium (right) and superficial myometrium (left)

- Associated to endometrial polypectomies or hysteroscopic submucosal myomectomy as prophylactic surgery.

CONTRAINDICATIONS

- *Premalignant or malignant endometrial histology:* The atypical hyperplasia and the endometrial carcinoma are absolute contraindications. The glandular hyperplasia without atypia is a relative contraindication, but compels a more exhaustive surveillance.
- *Intramural or multiple fibroids:* The only presence of fibroids is not a contraindication for the EA. The contraindication will be determined by the size and the localization of the myoma as these problems may not be resolved from the EA. The exception may be the premenopausal women who could really benefit from the EA in spite of having intramural or big fibroids as they are near to the menopause.
- *Adenomyosis:* It is an absolute contraindication as it is strongly associated to a high rate of failures (second surgery or hysterectomy) (FIGURE 13.2).
- *Uterine size longer than 12 cm:* The contraindication for uterine size is explained by the inability of the endoscope to reach the fundus, and tubal ostiums, and the frequent coexistence with other associated pathologies (hypertrophy, fibroids, adenomyosis).

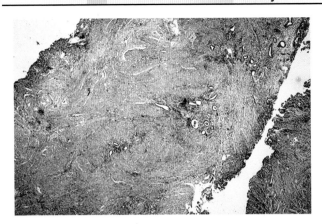

Figure 13.2: Pathological strip of endometrial resection showing adenomyosis when endometrial glands are present in the deep myometrium

- *Pelvic organ prolapse*: For severe prolapse, hysterectomy is the preferred treatment for symptom relief.
- A desire for future fertility.

PATIENTS COUNSELING

The preoperative consultation is essential and every patient should be informed of what can be expected from the offered treatment. Patients should be informed that the usual result after EA is not the amenorrhea but the hypomenorrhea or eumenorrhea. An important reduction in the volume of the menstrual bleeding, however, should be perceived as a satisfactory result by most of the women that consult for menorrhagia. The rates of amenorrhea vary among 25-60%, with significant reduction of bleeding in most of the rest. The satisfaction at five-year follow-up should be more than 75%. Approximately 15-25% of women will require a second surgical procedure such as repeat endometrial ablation and/or hysterectomy (for pain, abnormal bleeding or both). Most common problems or failures are caused by adenomyosis.

Patients should be carefully counseled prior to EA with regard to their contraception following surgery and elective sterilization or an alternative anti-contraceptive method, if desired, should be offered.

PREOPERATIVE ASSESSMENT

Although the EA is a procedure that can be performed inside, the parameters of the day-care surgery, should not be minimized and must be considered as a technique of major surgery. In fact, it is one of the more complex procedures of the hysteroscopic surgery. There are several advantages to a thorough preoperative work-up.

EA has more possibilities of success if the patients are carefully selected. The first thing that must be met for expectations of EA to be realistic is the proper selection of patients.

In the preoperative study the following considerations will be included:
- A complete medical history
- Physical and pelvic examination
- Recent cervical cytology is highly recommended
- Transvaginal ultrasound: It is an indispensable complementary test before the EA, to have precise information about the characteristics of the endometrium, the structure of the myometrium, to exclude ovarian pathology and to rule out other pathologies like fibroids or adenomyosis. Ultrasound will provide data about overall uterine size, endometrial thickness, and the size and location of fibroids. Information concerning fibroids and the ovaries are particularly useful as hysteroscopy only allows the examination of the uterine cavity and gives no details about the rest of the pelvis (FIGURE 13.3).
- Diagnostic hysteroscopy and biopsy (FIGURE 13.4): To evaluate the uterine cavity as well as the endometrium and to perform directed biopsies in any suspicious lesion. The endometrial biopsy is essential before EA. Hysteroscopy will confirm any uterine cavity abnormality. Evenmore, endometrial biopsy will show any premalignant change which would be contraindication for hysteroscopic surgery.
- General analytic examination, electrolyte determinations (in patients with medical disorders), hematocrit, hemoglobin, coagulation, human chorionic gonadotropin (β-hCG) (in any women of reproductive age), and ECG.

ANESTHESIA

The type of anesthesia to perform EA can be:
- General

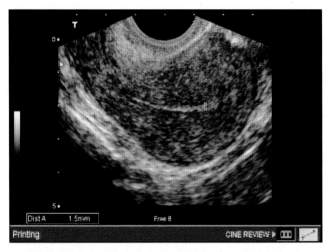

Figure 13.3: Basal transvaginal ultrasound prior to surgery

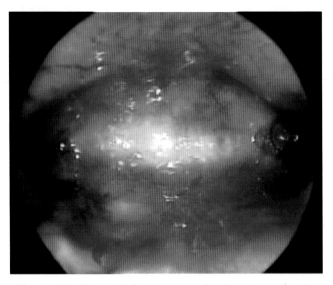

Figure 13.4: Diagnostic hysteroscopy showing a normal cavity

- *Locoregional:* For extensive procedures or for patients with a low pain tolerance, general or regional anesthesia is indicated.
- *Local anesthesia under intravenous sedation:* The uterine innervation is autonomous and this organ is relatively insensitive to the surgical action of section, coagulation, etc. However, the traumatic cervical dilation can cause vagal reactions so patients are to be monitorized. Keeping in mind this exception, EA can be performed with local anesthesia.

    Full patient's recovery is complete in 2-4 hours and she can be safely discharged in 6 hours (Chapter 18).

In the presence of risk factor for thrombosis (hypertension, obesity, metabolic syndrome, etc.) and, especially, if there are thrombophilic antecedents, antithrombotic prevention will be administered by means of low molecular weight heparins 2 hours before the intervention.

The prophylactics antibiotics are not strictly necessary, although in the event of antecedent of previous endometritis, pelvic inflammatory disease, deficient immunologic states, or clinically significant valvular disease, it can be recommended in a similar way to the used in the conventional surgery according to the protocol established in each center.

RECOMMENDATIONS

Cervical Preparation for Hysteroscopic Surgery

It is advisable during the preoperative preparation in every patient previous to hysteroscopic surgery. It is mandatory in nulliparous or postmenopausal women, in patients on tamoxifen and in women with GnRH agonists for endometrial thinning.

Available methods for previous cervical preparation:

- *Synthetic laminaria tents with high hygroscopic power:* Requires previous application
- *Misoprostol 3 hours before surgery:* Very effective in vaginal administration after wetting the capsules. Innocuous and cheap medication. Their action causes softening of the cervical stroma leading to dilation of the canal.[2]

    When cervical preparation has not been performed and the intraoperative dilation is hard.
- *Nitric oxide donors:* Their immediate relaxant conjunctive tissue ability makes it ideal for its use when problems with dilation arise in the theater. The more used is 1% nitroglycerine, diluted in 20 ml of saline, and injecting 1 ml of that solution intravenously. Isosorbide mononitrate also has been used.
- *Half to half progressive:* Hegar tents dilators, to diminish cervical lacerations or perforations.
- It is advisable to introduce the sheath of the hysteroscope with the obturator, before introducing the resector working element.

Endometrial Preparation for Hysteroscopic Surgery

Objectives

- To facilitate the surgical act, by means of thinning the area to resect (endometrium)
- To reduce the surgical bleeding
- To reduce the liquid absorption
- To increase the effectiveness of the procedure (more complete endometrial resection)
- Fewer recurrences.

Available Methods for Endometrial Preparation

- Performing the EA in the early proliferative phase of the cycle. Requires effective surgical programming
- *Progestogens or Danazol:* They are rarely used nowadays because of their limited effectiveness and severe collateral effects. The progestins decidualize the endometrium, resulting in hypervascularity and stromal edema
- GnRH agonists produce slightly more consistent endometrial thinning than danazol, though both agents produce satisfactory results. The effect of these agents on longer term postoperative outcomes such as amenorrhea and the need for further surgical intervention reduces with time.[3]

The advantage of endometrial preparation for EA is immediately apparent when one considers the dimensions of the resectoscope loop; a 27 French resectoscope is equipped with a 4 mm length cutting loop, which means that it will cut to a maximum depth of 4 mm. Ensuring that the endometrial thickness after thinning preparation is about 2 mm, means that the whole endometrium, even the deep basal glands, can be effectively undercut with a single pass of the loop (FIGURE 13.5). To avoid complications, each furrow of the loop should not be repeated, as the 4 mm security margin of the loop will be lost. Surgery is therefore both easier and faster.[4]

On the other hand, some problems may arise with the use of GnRH agonists as cervical atrophy, with the risk of perforation during dilation, the menopausal-like effects, the metrorrhagia after the first dose because of the flare-up, and their cost.

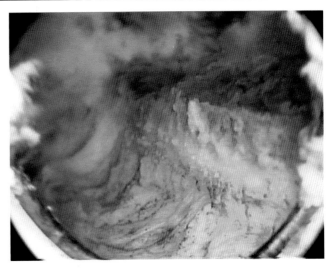

Figure 13.5: Depth of resection with the loop electrode

TECHNIQUE

The patient is placed in the dorsal lithotomy, and draped in the usual fashion as for vaginal surgery. No bladder catheterization is required.

Following bimanual examination of the uterus, the vagina is carefully washed with a disinfectant agent (chlorhexidine, povidone iodine), the cervix is fixed with a tenaculum, the cavity is sounded and the cervix dilated sufficiently to admit the resectoscope comfortably and allow for in and out movements. If a 27 Fr. resectoscope is used, which has an outer diameter of 9 mm, then dilatation to Hegar size 10 is adequate and, while maintaining the intrauterine pressure, the loss of irrigant solution between the sheath and the cervix will be avoided. The sheath is introduced in the endocervical canal with the obturator. The obturator is withdrawn and, after inserting the assembled working element, the irrigation system is turned on. Use of cold distention medium causes vasoconstriction and reduces blood loss and distention fluid deficits.

The uterine pressure is essential to maintain the vision. It is easy to understand that, in one hand, if the pressure is high, the vision is good as there is no bleeding because the endouterine fluid blocks the vessels, but in this case, the water hyperabsorption syndrome is possible, as the endouterine pressure surpasses the blood pressure and the fluid tends to be absorbed. On the other hand, if the pressure is too low, the blood pressure is higher than the endouterine pressure so bleeding occurs, darkening the vision and making the procedure more difficult. The best thing to do is to maintain the pressure below the mean arterial pressure of every patient, without strict rules, and setting up the pressure when the resection is difficult in any area (ostium or fundus). Once inside the uterus, the cavity is inspected, and the resection started. A 12° scope is suggested because it provides a panoramic view of the uterine cavity.

EA can be performed with loop or ball electrode. The loop is a 8 mm diameter metal wire that conducts the current between both poles, cutting the intervening tissue (resection), while the ball is a round electrode that destroys the endometrium under cutting current (ablation). The electric generator is preset to 80 W cut and 40 W coagulation and the blend 1 monopolar current is selected to achieve 20% of coagulation. The full uterine cavity is resected with one type of electrode or combining both, as preferred by the surgeon without a clear benefit by using one instead of the other.

Close monitoring of the patient during surgery is just as mandatory for EA as for the other resectoscopic techniques. EA may seem to be a minor procedure in terms of surgical time, lack of external scars, and hospitalization of the patient, but is still major surgery in terms of potential risks. The safety aspects of EA must always be kept in mind, and careful monitoring of every procedure is a basic component of this.

LOOP ENDOMETRIAL RESECTION

Resection is performed systematically to ensure that all areas are resected, guided by the different color of the brown resected myometrium, and the red areas of resting endometrium. Cutting must only take place when moving the loop towards the resectoscope sheath, as an active loop pushed away from the sheath can easily perforate the uterus.

The uterine cornua and tubal angles are resected first because of their difficulty. The endometrium is undercut between the two cornua in small chips, taking care not to push the loop more deeply into the myometrium than is necessary (FIGURE 13.6). Particular care has to be taken over the two tubal ostia

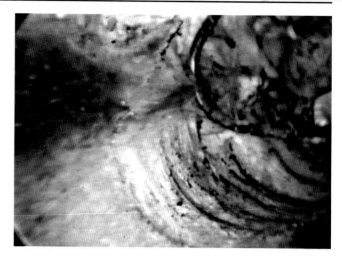

Figure 13.6: Endometrial resection with loop electrode

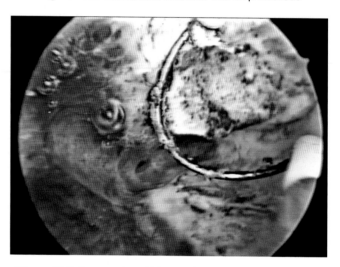

Figure 13.7: Loop endometrial resection in the right tubal ostium

where the myometrium is at its thinnest, and it is best to take a series of shallow shavings until all the endometrium has been resected here rather than make one large cut and risk for perforation (FIGURE 13.7). Although this all sounds somewhat complicated and dangerous, resection of the fundus is not difficult to learn and is also safe.[5] There are surgeons, however, who prefer to coagulate the fundus and cornual regions using a rollerball and then switch to the loop for the rest of the procedure.

Once the fundus has been treated, the standard cutting loop can be used to resect the walls of the uterus. The first furrow is the most important because this will set the depth for the whole of the resection and should stop when the myometrial musculature becomes visible. It is best to treat the posterior wall first, as the endometrial debris collects there and gradually obscures this part of the cavity. The electrode is extended and allowed to passively return towards the sheath at rate of 1.0-1.5 mm/s. It is important to know that each stroke of the loop is just the distance obtained when the loop is totally outside the sheath, so when cutting with the loop, the resectoscope should not be moved, and the loop should be fully brought into the inner sheath before the generator is turned off. Otherwise, a part of the resected tissue will remain attached to the uterus, interfering the vision. Once the posterior side is completed, the lateral and anterior side are tackled. This can be performed in different sequences (clockwise or anticlockwise), and do not resect the same place twice. It is wise to be careful when resecting the anterior wall of the isthmus in presence of previous cesarean scars, as the myometrium in these cases can be thinned and perforation can occur.

Although the chips can be removed from the cavity strip-by-strip, this is slower, there is fluid leakage via the cervix, and, although remote, there is possibility of air embolism. It is too possible to operate without interruption and leave the resected pieces in the uterine cavity until the end of the procedure, keeping them at the fundus.

The endocervical canal has to be shallowly resected, especially in the laterals where the descending branches of the uterine artery are located.

Resecting the endocervix does not seem to cause cervical stenosis, probably because the canal is actually widened previously and the percentage of amenorrhea is higher.

What is removed is sent to the pathologist for histological examination, this being one of the major advantages of endometrial resection compared to the other ablative techniques which destroys the endometrium *in situ*.

ROLLERBALL ENDOMETRIAL ABLATION

The electric generator is preset at a power output of 40-60 W under cutting current. The surgeon holds firmly the electrode against the uterine wall and presses the coagulation pedal. The first thing to learn is the strength required to effectively ablate the endometrium, as this strength is different in each area depending on the anatomical position of the uterus. Obviously, prior to proceeding with electrocoagulation the surgeon explores the uterine cavity for unexpected pathology.

The areas most difficult to reach technically are the areas where complications will arise. It requires quite some maneuvering with the resectoscope to reach areas like the tubal ostia (FIGURE 13.8A). The roller ablation is repeated until the entire fundus and adjacent cornual areas are coagulated. Care is taken not to force the electrode into the tubal ostia.

As in almost all the resectoscopic techniques, the electrode is slowly rolled towards the sheath (FIGURE 13.8B). At all times, coagulation effect has

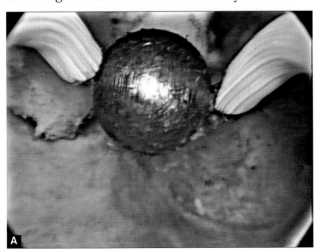
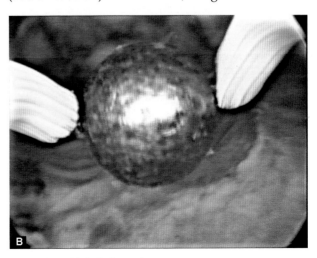

Figures 13.8A and B: Endometrial ablation with ball electrode

to be controlled preceding the electrode. The walls of the uterine cavity are coagulated systematically. Whether one starts on the anterior wall or any other, is of no importance. However, once adopted in every patient, a particular sequence should be religiously adhered to.[6] The internal cervical os represents the limit of coagulation. A last inspection of the uterine cavity is performed. The pressure is reduced, and if bleeding vessels are spotted, these are now coagulated.

EVOLUTION AND NORMAL POSTOPERATIVE FOLLOW-UP

As other minimally invasive surgery techniques, EA is an ideal intervention to be performed under the principles of day-care surgery. The period of admission is from 3 to 6 hours. Postoperatively, the most frequent referred symptoms are nausea and pelvic cramping, never lasting more than 24 hours and easily controlled with antiemetics and NSAIDs. Patient's recovery is fast, returning to the level of habitual activity in 3 to 7 days.

Bleeding is exceptional after the first 12-24 hours, but a serohematic discharge usually happens lasting some more days. Occasionally, a little more intense bleeding happens toward the 10th day, coincident with the detachment of the coagulated endometrium. Cares are limited to avoid vaginal irrigations and coitus while the discharge persists. Habitually the visit is scheduled 30 days postoperatively to evaluate the patient and probe the cervix. Follow-up in 3, 6 months and annually thereafter is recommended.[7]

SPECIFIC COMPLICATION

Related to the moment of appearance, complications can be intra- or postoperative.

Intraoperative Complications

- *Hemorrhage (0.8-1%):* The deep resection in the myometrium with the loop electrode opens vascular vessels that, sometimes, cause hemorrhage. The intrauterine insertion of an inflated balloon of a 15-30 mL Foley catheter for 2-4 hours used to be enough for hemostasis.

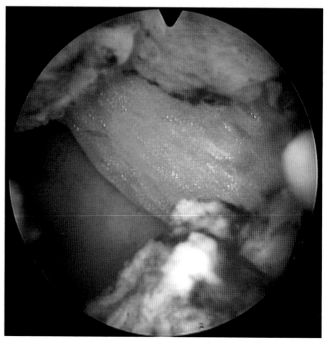

Figure 13.9: Perforation in the uterine fundus—Hysteroscopic view

- *Perforation (1-5%):* They happen during the dilatation in half of the cases. The uterine perforation in the course of the EA with the activated monopolar electrode always obliges to the inspection of the pelvic cavity by means of laparoscopy or laparotomy (FIGURE 13.9). The risks of peritonitis, sepsis, and death are most often associated with unrecognized and untreated thermal injuries to the viscera. If the perforation takes place during the dilation or with the disabled resector, an expectant treatment with admission, antibiotics and observation for 24 hours will be enough (FIGURE 13.10).
- *Cervical tears or lacerations:* In the moment of the cervical dilation or when introducing the resector. Using medical or mechanical preoperative cervical dilators may help to decrease resistance during dilation.
- *False intramyometrial tunnel* (FIGURE 13.11): They are forms of partial perforations. They are important as they may preclude the continuation of surgery by obscuring the endoscopic view.
- Electric burns in the genital tract.
- *Air embolism (3/17000):* It can be provoked by repeated introduction and removal of the hysteroscope,

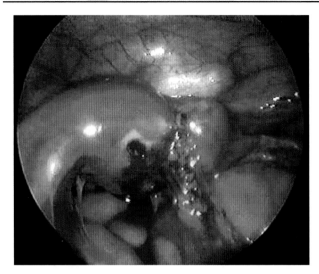

Figure 13.10: Perforation in the uterine fundus. Laparoscopic view

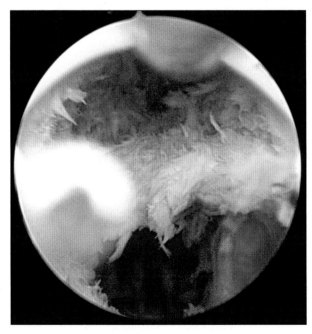

Figure 13.11: Cervical laceration

by the use of pressure pumps without air detectors, and/or by cervical trauma with subsequent dilacerated veins.

* *Transcervical Resection of the Endometrium syndrome (TCRE) (1.8-2%):* The massive pass of the hypo-osmolar distension medium from the uterine cavity to the intravascular space is a relatively frequent fact in the course of a EA and is favored by:
  – Excessive intrauterine pressure of the distension medium (intravasation can occur when

the intrauterine pressure is greater than the patient's mean arterial pressure)[8]
  – Too deep resection in the base of myometrium, where the vessels are bigger
  – Surgical time longer than 60 minutes
  – Uncontrolled liquid balance.

POSTOPERATIVE COMPLICATIONS

Early

Intrauterine infection: If a patient has a preoperative infection (cervical or endometritis) or a significant history of PID, treatment before surgery is recommended, but prophylactic antibiotics do not reduce the risk of infection after surgery.[9] A specific form of infection is the necrotizing endometritis, a severe condition that comports endometritis along with a necrotizing myometritis, with the presence of gram positive as well as anerobic germs. The secondary adnexal, peritoneal, or tubaric infection is exceptional.

* *Thrombosis (0.05%):* In cases associated with risk factors for thrombosis (obesity, diabetes and trombophilic antecedents)
* The embolism is based on the formation of a venous "shunt" with the myometrial vessels, facilitated by an excessive intrauterine pressure and forced Trendelenburg's position
* *Hematometra (0.7%):* Is a consequence of a too deep resection in the isthmus, driving to synechia formation and retention of debrided tissues due to cervical stenosis (FIGURE 13.12). Follow-up in 2-4 weeks is recommended to probe the cervix and break up any scar tissue that may have developed in the isthmus.

Late

* *Gestation:* The reported pregnancy rate after endometrial ablation is quite low, approximately 0.7% (higher in younger patients). These pregnancies were complicated by a high risk of abnormal placentation, spontaneous abortion, preterm delivery, and cesarean hysterectomy.[10] Therefore, the need for contraception after endometrial ablation.

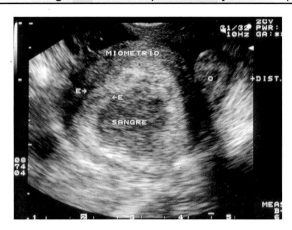

Figure 13.12: Residual hematometra

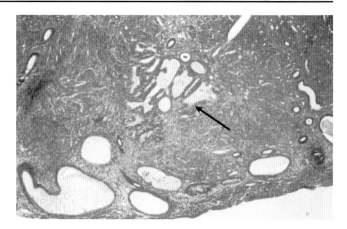

Figure 13.13: Neoplastic endometrial glands in the deep endometrium diagnosed after endometrial resection

- *Atypical hyperplasia and adenocarcinoma (exceptional):* The appearance of a "de novo" most of them are associated with some grade of hyperplasia prior to the EA,[11] although the possibility of finding unexpected pathology after the resection has also been described[12] (FIGURE 13.13).
- *Tubaric postresection syndrome:* Distension fluid accumulate in the tube of a woman with previous tubaric sterilization, causing severe pain, similar to acute hydrosalpinx. The histopathology is that of persistent endometrium in the cornual area. (Further details about Complications are described in Chapter 15).

RESULTS

There are several end points that can be used in describing what can be expected from EA. They are:
- Amenorrhea rate
- Eumenorrhea rate or better
- Patient satisfaction
- Hysterectomy rate
- Cost.

Former studies only informed about short and half term results so their conclusions were little predictive;[13,14] Nowadays, studies on wider populations with long term follow-up have been published.[15,16] EA has better possibilities of success if the patients are carefully selected. It is less effective in women under 35 years because the endometrium

remnants have more time for their regeneration, thus reappearing the hemorrhages, with better results in women older than 40 years. The incidence of recurrence of abnormal uterine bleeding is unknown but it could be around 10% annually. Unger[17] calculates that a third part at five years and the totality of the patients after 13 years of the EA would require hysterectomy.

There are many studies informing on short (follow-up 2 years) and medium term results (2 to 5 years).[18]

The results of the EA to the 2 years reflect an amenorrhea rates that oscillate between 35 and 55%, while the satisfaction of the patients is around 92%.

In the three years follow-up, amenorrhea rate varies equally between the 25 and 45% lowering the index of satisfaction lightly until values around 85%.

In the four years follow-up, the satisfaction is around 80%, while the amenorrhea rates reach just the 30%.

In the long-term results (longer than five years), only 25% of women will remain amenorrheic, but it can be accepted that after 5 years, between 70 and 80% of the patients will be satisfied with their intervention.[19]

Amenorrhea rates generally fall in a range from 25-30% with hysterectomy rates falling between 10 and 15%. The majority of hysterectomies are done for pain rather than heavy bleeding (TABLE 13.1).

The EA long-term result on the menstruation is still not well known.

Vilos,[20] in 800 EA patients, reports on 95% of success (60% amenorrhea, 29% hypomenorrhea and 6% eumenorrhea). In 5% there was not any change. EA was repeated in 4% and hysterectomy in 2%. Garry,[21] with 600 endometrial ablations, reports on 83.4% of success in his series, requiring second surgery in 14.3%. The success increased with the age. The size of the cavity, the length of follow-up and if it was a first or a second procedure did not associate with any difference in the rate of success, although the proportion of hysterectomies tended to ascend as the follow-up increased. In the series of Baggish,[22] on 625 patients, with a mean follow-up of 4.5 years and a minimum of 12 months, amenorrhea was obtained in 58% of the patients and hypomenorrhea in 34%, with the rate of total failure of 8%. Phillips,[23] with a series of 1000 endometrial laser ablations, with follow-up times ranging from 26 to 76 months reports on a projected failure of 21.5% at 6.5 years follow-up. O'Connor,[24] with 525 patients with long-term follow-up (mean 31 months) needed to perform a new surgery in 16%. Again, the failure increased with the length of the follow-up. Finally, the Aberdeen Endometrial Ablation Trials Group, with a minimum of four years follow-up reports on 36% of further surgery.[25] In our series, with 286 patients and a mean follow-up of 47 months, we found that the most dependent significant factor associated with the success of the procedure was the age (than, the time of follow-up), with poor results in the < 35 years old group (TABLE 13.2).

In assessing patient satisfaction with EA, there is evidence to suggest that older patients tend to be more satisfied with the procedure than younger patients, and those with concomitant pain less satisfied than those with a pure menorrhagia. In studies where patients have been randomized to EA and hysterectomy there is a higher percentage of patients who are satisfied with the hysterectomy than with EA, but in most cases there is no statistical difference between the two methods of treatment. In the one study where there was a statistical difference, it would appear that unrealistic patient expectation for EA,

Table 13.1: Clinical outcome directly related to the age of the patient

Age (years)	Amenorrhea (%)	Improved (%)	Failures (%)
< 35	33	33	33
36-40	39	39	22
41-45	42	41	17
> 45	54	41	5

Table 13.2: Clinical outcome directly related to the length of follow-up

Follow-up (years)	Amenorrhea (%)	Improved (%)
3-4	46	89
4-5	49	90
5 or >	55	95

was the reason for the lack of satisfaction. It was clear in these studies that there was a higher rate of complications with hysterectomy, but a lower rate of the need for further surgery.

Although the patient's satisfaction is the best index for success of this technique, the rate of failure increased with the length of follow-up. The proportion of failure reaches a plateau after two years. Turnbull[26] demonstrated by means of magnetic resonance imaging (MRI) that the great majority of the amenorrheic women and the totality of those menstruating after EA have residual endometrium, suggesting that, sooner or later, the endometrium regenerates in almost all of the patients. So, if continued during *enough time*, will all the women recover the menstruation? This takes us to the inverse option. Since that *enough time* finishes sooner or later in every woman, the sooner it finishes, the better the expected results. This is defined in all the series in women that reach the menopause during the follow-up, being the patient's age the major predicting factor for the success of the surgery.

The major negative independent factor is the presence of adenomyosis (TABLE 13.3). The patients with deep penetration in the myometrium (deep adenomyosis) obtain poor results after the EA. The poor outcome of the surgery can be predicted if the classic holes of adenomyosis, mimicking small perforations, are found inside the myometrium during the resection (FIGURE 13.14). The problem

Table 13.3: Cox regression analysis of the relative risk (RR) factors associated with a subsequent hysterectomy after loop endometrial resection

Risk factors	*Univariable regression*		*Multivariable regression**	
	HR (95% CI)	P	RR (95% CI)	P
Adenomyosis	6.96 (2.28-21.26)	0.0007	11.21 (2.70-46.46)	0.0009
Age at surgery (<45 year; >45 year)	0.92 (0.90-0.95)	<0.0001	2.93 (1.59-5.40)	0.002

*Cox multivariate analysis with presence or absence of posterior hysterectomy after loop endometrial resection as the time dependent variable and the presence of adenomyosis and the age at surgery as predictor variables.

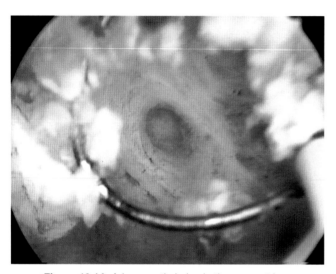

Figure 13.14: Adenomyotic holes in the myometrium during resection

is that adenomyosis is difficult to diagnose preoperatively. McCausland performs a myometrium biopsy in the diagnostic hysteroscopy to look for adenomyosis.[27] The symptomatology, along with the clinical exploration, can rise the suspicion but is the histology the only that warrants an accurate diagnosis. The MRI is being studied as an option but, although initial studies are promising, cannot still be recommended as a reliable method.

The most important thing to obtain a successful procedure is making a good selection of the patients. EA has more possibilities of success if the patients are selected carefully. It is less effective in young women because the remnant endometrium has more time for its regeneration, recurring the metrorrhagia, so the older the patient, the better the results.

Patients will have a hysterectomy after EA for all the same reasons that any patient might undergo a hysterectomy. They include problems involving ovarian tumors, CIN, enlarging uterine fibroids, development of pelvic prolapse, only a very few relate to the previous EA. While there will be some hysterectomies for menorrhagia there would appear to be a disproportionate number of patients who develop pain. The problems of pelvic pain and dysmenorrhea following EA does not appears to be related to the creation of adenomyosis but more probably relates to the creation of small hematometra.

Conditioning Factors of the Results

It is less effective in young women because the remnant endometrium has more time for its regeneration, recurring the metrorrhagia, so the older the patient, the better the results. The first thing that must be met for expectations of EA to be realistic is the proper selection of patients. The frequency of recurrences is not known, but Phillips[23] reports, according to survival curves, an overall hysterectomy rate projected of 21.5% at 6.5 years follow-up. It is influenced by several factors as the characteristics of the patients, the technique elected, the endometrial preparation, the length of follow-up, the correct indication or the presence of concomitant pathology. It is has been exposed previously that the rate of successes lowers as the time of follow-up grows. Nevertheless, in general terms, there are some factors that can affect the outcome of EA:
• Age
• Uterine size
• Preoperative treatment
• Fibroids
• Adenomyosis
• Technique.

Age

The younger the women, the higher the risk for recurrence, because endometrium has more time of hormonal stimulus before menopause.

Uterine Size

It is considered that a uterine size of more than 12 cm increases the rate of failed resections. The high adenomyosis rate, the uterine hypertrophy and the surgical difficulty are possibly the responsible factors for this.

Preoperative Treatment

The endometrial suppression atrophies the endometrium and thus facilitates the surgery.

Fibroids

The uterine fibroids are accompanied of vascular, functional, and morphological anomalies that can hamper the EA results.

Adenomyosis

Preoperative diagnosis of adenomyosis is very difficult. Its eradication during an EA technique is almost impossible, being this disease the more important independent negative factor. Patients with deep penetration in the myometrium (deep adenomyosis) obtain poor results after the EA, so any patient clinical or ultrasonographically suspicious of having adenomyosis should be referred to other technique.[27]

Technique

The experience of the surgeon is very important and is directly related to the depth of penetration of the electrode in the myometrium.

CONCLUSION

In view of these facts, it is difficult to understand why more gynecologists have not adopted EA into their armamentarium of surgical procedures. The answer most likely lies in the fact that it is deceptively skill dependent in order to achieve good results. For that reason, the newer global non hysteroscopic endometrial ablation methods and the use of the progesterone-loaded IUD which require less skill and achieve more uniform and reproducible results may make EA more readily available to patients.

It is very important to make a right indication. It is necessary to remember that EA is an alternative to the hysterectomy, that is why, only patients that otherwise would have had a radical surgery, would really benefit of this technique. They must have tried, and failed, the different medical treatments that exist to indicate an EA. Only in this situation, a reasonable margin of trust in the procedure can be offered to the patient.

EA is undoubtedly a technique which has to be learnt. It is a technique which can be applied to a broad range of menorrhagic women, from those with dysfunctional bleeding and a small uterus, to those with a sizeable uterus enlarged with fibroids. This versatility together with advantages in terms of cost, operative time and histology makes it a skill worth learning.

REFERENCES

1. Lethaby A, Shepperd S, Cooke I, Farquhar C. Endometrial resection and ablation versus hysterectomy for heavy menstrual bleeding. Cochrane Database Syst Rev 2000;CD000329.
2. Preutthipan S, Herabutya Y. Vaginal misoprostol for cervical priming before operative hysteroscopy: A randomized controlled trial. Obstet Gynecol 2000;96:890-4.
3. Sowter MC, Lethaby A, Singla AA. Preoperative endometrial thinning agents before endometrial destruction for heavy menstrual bleeding. Cochrane Database Syst Rev 2002;(3):CD001124.
4. Parazzini F, Vercellini P, De Giorgi O, Pesole A, Ricci E, Crosignani PG. Efficacy of preoperative medical treatment in facilitating hysteroscopic endometrial resection, myomectomy and metroplasty: Literature review. Hum Reprod 1998;13:2592-7.
5. Sutton CJC, Macdonald R, Magos A, Broadbent JAM. Endometrial resection. In Endometrial ablation. Lewis B, Magos A (Eds): Churchill-Livingstone, London 1993;91-32.
6. Vancaillie TG. Electrocoagulation of the endometrium. In: Endometrial ablation. Lewis B, Magos A (Eds): Churchill-Livingstone, London.1993;133-50.
7. The Practice Committee of the American Society for Reproductive Medicine Indications and options for endometrial ablation. Fertil Steril 2008;90:S236-40.
8. Morrison DM. Management of hysteroscopic surgery complications. AORN J 1999;69(1):194-7, 199-209, quiz 210, 213-15, 21.

9. Cooper JM, Brady RM. Intraoperative and early postoperative complications of operative hysteroscopy. Obstet Gynecol Clin North Am 2000;27(2):347-66.

10. Lo JS, Pickersgill A. Pregnancy after endometrial ablation: English literature review and case report. J Minim Invasive Gynecol 2006;13:88-91.

11. Valle RF, Baggish MS. Endometrial carcinoma after endometrial ablation: High-risk factors predicting its occurrence. Am J Obstet Gynecol 1998;179:569-72.

12. Perez-Medina T, Bajo-Arenas J, SanFrutos L, Haya J, Iniesta S, Vargas J. Endometrial intraepithelial neoplasia diagnosed at endometrial resection. J Am Assoc Gynecol Laparosc 2003;10:85-7.

13. O'Connor H, Magos A. Endometrial resection for the treatment of menorrhagia. N Eng J Med 1996;335:151-6.

14. Cravello L, D'Ercole C, Roge P, Boubli L, Blanc B. Hysteroscopic management of menstrual disorders: A review of 395 patients. Eur J Obstet Gynecol Reprod Biol 1996;67:163-7.

15. Seeras RC, Gilliland GB. Resumption of menstruation after amenorrhea in women treated by endometrial ablation and myometrial resection. J Am Assoc Gynecol Laparosc 1997;4:305-9.

16. Pérez-Medina T, Haya J, SanFrutos L, Bajo-Arenas J. Factors influencing long-term outcome of loop endometrial resection. J Am Assoc Gynecol Laparosc 2002;9:73-7.

17. Unger J, Meeks R. Hysterectomy after endometrial ablation. Am J Obstet Gynecol 1996;175:1432-7.

18. Garry R. Endometrial ablation and resection: Validation of a new surgical concept. Br J Obstet Gynaecol 1997;104:1329-31.

19. Saurabh V, Kenneth BC, Sturdee DW. Endometrial resection: Factors affecting long-term success. Gynaecological Endoscopy 1998;8:41-50.

20. Vilos GA, Vilos EC. Experience with 800 hysteroscopic endometrial ablations. J Am Assoc Gynecol Laparosc 1996;4:33-8.

21. Garry R. Good practice with endometrial ablation. Obstet Gynecol 1995;85:144-51.

22. Baggish MS, Sze EH. Endometrial ablation: A series of 568 patients treated over an 11-year period. Am J Obstet Gynecol 1996;174(3):908-13.

23. Phillips G, Chien PFW, Garry R. Risk of hysterectomy after 1000 consecutive endometrial laser ablations. Br J Obstet Gynecol 1998;105:897-903.

24. O'Connor H, Magos A. Endometrial resection for the treatment of menorrhagia. N Eng J Med 1996;335:151-6.

25. Aberdeen Endometrial Ablation Trial Group. A randomized trial of endometrial ablation versus hysterectomy for the treatment of dysfunctional uterine bleeding: Outcome at four years. Br J Obstet Gynaecol 1999;106:360-6.

26. Turnbull LW, Jumaa A, Bowsley SJ, Dhawan S, Horsman A, Killick SR. Magnetic resonance imaging of the uterus after endometrial resection. Br J Obstet Gynaecol 1997;104:934-8.

27. McCausland AM, McCausland VM. Depth of endometrial penetration in adenomyosis helps determine outcome of rollerball ablation. Am J Obstet Gynecol 1996;174:1786-93.

14

Hysteroscopic Tubal Sterilization Essure™ System

Enrique Cayuela Font
Federico Heredia Prim
Ramón Cos Plans
Sonia Moros

INTRODUCTION

Laparoscopic tubal sterilization is the most widely used and undoubtedly the most well-known irreversible contraceptive method, with the exception of sterilization immediately after delivery. In some countries, there is a high rate of use of this method. For example, in the United States, over 2,000,000 tubal sterilizations were practiced from 1994-1996. Incidence was 11.5 per 1,000 or 684,000 per year,[1] and this technique was practiced in nearly 700,000 patients each year.

Nevertheless, laparoscopy is not exempt of risks. Therefore, in the early 1980s, use of hysteroscopy was proposed as an alternative to tubal occlusion. The advantages of this method compared to laparoscopy are rapidity, lack of need for or infrequent use of general anesthesia, as well as the presumably good acceptance by patients. Therefore, the procedure can be performed in an outpatient consulting room suitable for such purposes, and it is not necessary to use the operating theater.

Since, Froriep used silver nitrate to achieve tubal occlusion in 1849, and the first intrauterine exam with hysteroscopy was performed by Pantaleoni[2] in 1869, up until our days, several different methods for tubal sterilization by transcervical route have been tested. The problems and failures of these techniques are described in the literature.

The ideal contraceptive method should have a low failure rate (efficacy), low morbidity (safety), simple application (short intervention time), minimal operative management, no need for general anesthesia, and good acceptance and tolerance by the patient, as well as low cost.

In the early 1970s, with the use of modern hysteroscopy, some of the previous difficulties in tubal sterilization were overcome. Two main types of techniques were introduced: Destructive techniques, in which the intramural segment of the tube is destroyed by electrocoagulation or sclerotic agents, and occlusive techniques that place tampons or devices on the level of the tubal ostium.[3,4]

At present, destructive methods are no longer used due to their limited efficacy and the possibility of severe complications such as uterine perforation or intestinal lesions. In some cases, death in patients who have undergone electrocoagulation has even been reported.[5] Nevertheless, although there is less probability of complications and placement is relatively simple, occlusive devices have not gained acceptance as the ideal method. Some cases of incomplete obstruction and expulsion have been described.[6]

After 20 years of research, seeking to develop a hysteroscopic method of tubal sterilization, this has been achieved.

Since 1998, a phase II, multicentric clinical trial with Essure™ intratubal devices (Conceptus Inc.) is being conducted in five hospitals in the United States, Australia, Belgium and Spain.[7]

In 2000, a multicentric pilot study was begun with a larger number of cases and hospitals to confirm the satisfactory phase II results. According to plans, both trials will be completed in 2010. In July 2001, the EC granted approval for clinical use. In October 2002, the FDA gave its approval in the United States. All authors of this chapter have participated in both of these studies.

DESCRIPTION OF SYSTEM

Essure™ Device

This device (FIGURE 14.1) consists of an expandable spring (outer coil) made of titanium alloy and nickel. The spring is 4 cm long, and has a diameter of 0.8 mm when folded, or 2 mm when unfolded. Its function is

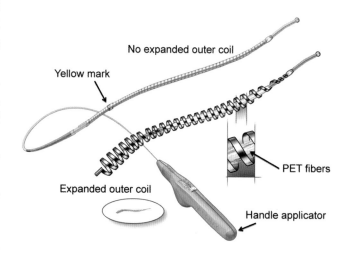

Figure 14.1: Essure (with permission of Conceptus Inc)

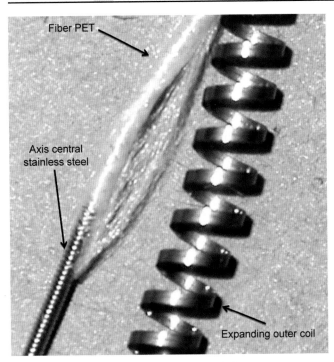

Figure 14.2: Essure description

to anchor itself inside of the tube so that it will be immobilized. Inside the device, there are some terephthalate polyethylene (Dacron) fibers (FIGURE 14.2) that are attached to a central steel shaft (inner coil) made of different metals alloys iron, chromium, nickel. This device is located inside a catheter. For handling, it is equipped with a handle that is connected to the steel shaft of the device by a metal support (FIGURE 14.7).

Mechanism of Action

The objective of the device is to obstruct the channel inside the tube by fibrosis. The dacron fibers induce a benign tissue response characterized by the presence of macrophages, fibroblasts and collagen, which invade the device, creating a second and definitive anchorage. The study by Valle,[8] in which the device was inserted in volunteer patients scheduled for a hysterectomy 3 months before this procedure, offers a histological demonstration of tubal obstruction (FIGURE 14.3). In the phase II and phase III studies, the hysterosalpingography performed 3 months after insertion also showed that tubal obstruction had been achieved.[7,9,10] For this reason we cannot rely on the method only after three months of insertion.

Material

For Application

- A continuous flow hysteroscope with a 5 Fr. working channel (internal diameter 1.7 mm) and biopsy forceps or clamp are needed
- Distension medium: Physiological saline
- Light source: 300 W Xenon
- Pressure bushing/pump: It is important to achieve good distension of the uterine cavity. In order to do so, use of an infusion pump is preferred. With pressures from 80 to 150 mm and flows of 400 ml/L, excellent uterine distension and good image quality are achieved

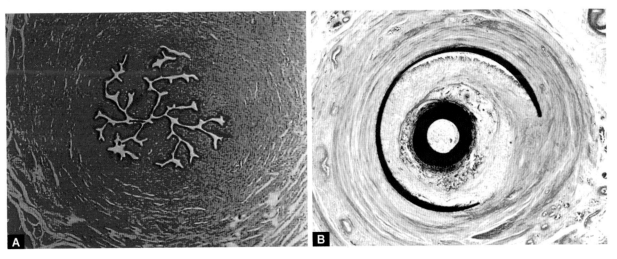

Figures 14.3 A and B: (A) Normal tube, (B) Tubal fibrotic obstruction with Essure (With permission of Conceptus Inc.)

- Camera: A latest generation camera can be used for this purpose
- Television monitor
- Auxiliary material: Aqueous povidone, gauze, clamps for the cervix, speculum with side opening, Hegar's rods (numbers 3-6) increased progressively by ½ mm, material for local cervical/paracervical anesthesia.

APPLICATION

Patient Selection

The procedure is irreversible. Therefore, only patients who have decided not to have any more children should be included as candidates.

Contraindications

Absolute Contraindications

- Patients unsure of decision
- Recent or active inflammatory pelvic disease
- Gynecological cancer
- Currently pregnant.

Relative Contraindications

- Patients with known nickel allergy are included in the contraindications section of the instructions for use of Essure™ because as it has been mentioned before, this device is manufactured from a titanium-nickel alloy. Essure™ has successfully passed all required biocompatibility tests. Moreover, Conceptus has performed bench testing to evaluate the leaching rate of nickel ions from Essure™ in a simulated corrosive environment. Test results show that the amount of nickel ions released from the Essure™ micro-insert is lower than the average daily intake of nickel from food, water, and environmental sources. Furthermore, no adverse event indicative of allergy to nickel has been reported to date in phase II and pivotal clinical trials.[7,10] Although allergy to nickel has not been documented in any clinical trial patient using the Essure™ system to date, conceptus is suggesting the following to

physicians in order to distinguish between contact dermatitis and a severe hypersensitivity reaction that could possibly result in patient injury:

  - If a potential Essure™ patient expresses concern about nickel allergy due to a previous skin reaction (contact dermatitis) to jewellery or endodontic appliance, etc., they recommend that she has a skin patch test performed by a dermatologist or allergist
  - Based on the results of the skin patch test, the dermatologist can recommend whether or not the patient is at risk for a more severe reaction, such as systemic hives

- *Treatment with corticoids or immunosuppressive agents:* In some cases, fibrosis may not occur or may be incomplete, with the consequent risk of not achieving occlusion and possible risk of pregnancy. The corticoid acts by inhibiting the inflammatory response to Dacron fibers. After treatment has been completed, it could be suitable for this method
- If a hysterosalpingography check-up needs to be performed, allergy to the contrast agents used in radiology.

Preparation

Interview

Information on the method, complete medical history, gynecological examination, and transvaginal ultrasound if the patient has clinical symptoms or the examination shows that there is disease. Rule out contraindications. Read and sign informed consent.

Day of Insertion

It is important to select the day of insertion taking into account the phase of the cycle. The follicular phase is the ideal period for the procedure. Insertion during the secretion phase may entail several problems: First of all, the endometrium may be hypertrophic. Therefore, the ostia may not be visible and, secondly, the patient may be pregnant. In order to prevent these problems, hormonal contraceptives should be taken one month prior to insertion. This will achieve a hypotrophic endometrium and prevent risk of pregnancy. Moreover, insertion can be performed at any time during the cycle.

Special Situations

- In those patients who have an IUD, it is advisable to remove it one month before the procedure
- In patients who have had a delivery or abortion, there must be an intermediate period of at least 6 weeks before the devices can be inserted.

Pharmacological Preparation

Arjona[11] treats all his patients with 600 mg ibuprofen and 10 mg of diazepam, one hour before the procedure. During the study, 5 to 10 mg of diazepam and 600 mg of ibuprofen were administered to the patients two hours before the procedure.[12] This regimen can be used in patients that have some anxiety because in our experience the majority of patients do not require any type of preparation.

Insertion of Devices

In our experience for most patients, insertion can be done in the consulting room of the gynecologist, as long as he has the infrastructure needed to perform level I diagnostic and therapeutic hysteroscopy. In some specific cases, the procedure must be performed in an outpatient surgery unit with the presence of an anesthetist (e.g. patients with severe cervical stenosis, forced uterine retroflexion, risk of vagal syndrome, significant associated medical condition, and very nervous or uncooperative patients). Nichols[13] in a study with 320 patients demonstrates that there are no differences between the group performed at the outpatient surgery unit and the one performed at the consulting room. They had evaluated the time of the procedure; percentage of successful insertions; complications and adverse effects.

Arjona[11] has published a series of 1630 patients performed at the consulting room without sedation neither paracervical anesthesia, and only a 3.1% of these patients reported pain superior to menstruation.

Insertion Technique

A series of steps must be followed:

Position

The patient should be placed in gynecological position with the thighs well-flexed on the abdomen. This will facilitate insertion of the device in cases in which tube cannulation is difficult due to the anatomy of the inside of the cavity.

Hysteroscopy

Can be performed by speculum and clamp or by vaginoscopy. We prefer the vaginoscopy technique.

Examination

With the Essure™ of the bushing or the infusion pump and with physiological saline, the hysteroscope is inserted inside the cervical canal until it reaches a cavity. Once inside the uterine cavity, the ostia should be visualized by 45° rotation of the hysteroscope to the right and the left. An examination must be performed beforehand in order to evaluate the presence of disease (polyps, myomas, synechiae) or anatomical changes that prevent insertion of the device.

Insertion of Introducer Guide

After it has been verified that the cavity and the ostia are normal, we begin the procedure by placing the introducer guide in the working channel (FIGURE 14.4). This will protect the device when it advances through the working channel.

Orientation of Hysteroscope

Then the device is inserted into the working channel and advanced slowly. Orientation of the hysteroscope must continue until the tubal ostium is centered. Since the distal end of device is curved, this curvature should be adapted to the right or the left, depending on the tube that one seeks to connulate (FIGURE 14.5).

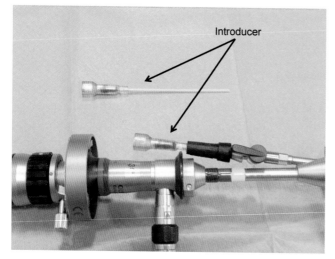

Figure 14.4: Introducer

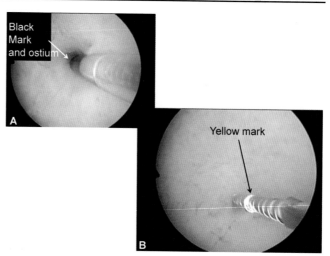

Figures 14.6A and B: (A) Black mark, (B) Yellow mark

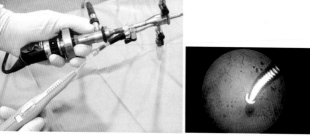

Figure 14.5: Hysteroscopic position for right tubal cannulation

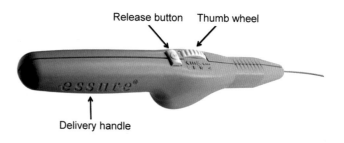

Figure 14.7: Delivery handle

Insertion of Device

Once the tube is in line with the device, then it should be firmly inserted until the black mark is clearly inside the ostium (FIGURE 14.6A).

Unfolding the Device

The next step (FIGURE 14.7) is to move the cog of the handle towards you until it reaches a limit. This ensures that the protective catheter is retracted and the device which is still folded remains inside the tube. The folded device has a yellow mark area in the center. Move the device until this yellow mark area is 1 cm outside of the ostium (FIGURE 14.6B).

Uncoil the Spring

The spring is uncoiled by pressing the button of the applicator handle and rotating the cog towards you

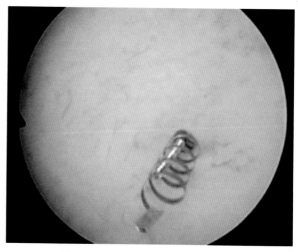

Figure 14.8: Three intracavitary coils

again. From 3 to 10 loops should be visible in the uterine cavity, this is the ideal situation, although between 1 and 14 is also correct (FIGURE 14.8).

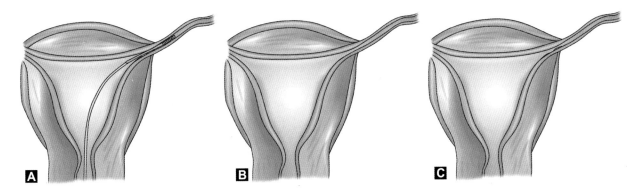

Figures 14.9A to C: (A) Essure insertion, (B) Good situation, (C) Endoluminal fibrosis tree months later

Removal of the Applicator

The next step is to remove the applicator device. This is achieved automatically when we finish rotating the wheel on the handle. Once the device has been released, proceed in the same way with the other tube.

The FIGURES 14.9A to C present a diagram with the complete procedure.

Problems during Procedure

- Stenotic cervix: After paracervical or cervical anesthesia, dilate with Hegar's rods until number 6
- Hypertrophic endometrium that prevents visibility of the ostium: Discontinue the procedure and schedule it for a postmenstrual date or administer oral contraceptives
- Once the procedure is ended, it is important to classify the insertion as satisfactory or unsatisfactory. We considered an insertion as unsatisfactory, when:
  - It has been a difficult insertion
  - It appears an intensive pain during the procedure
  - There are less than 2 visible coils inside the cavity
  - There are more than 14 coils inside the cavity (if there are more than 18 loops it is better to remove the device with a hysteroscopy biopsy forceps). Causes that difficulty or impede the insertion:
  - Spasm of the tube: in this case when we notice a resistance we have to make a continuous pressure until the spasm is solved.
  - Previous obstruction of the tube

- In those failed cases we can try a new insertion after demonstrating with an HSG that both tubes are permeable.
- Patients who are very nervous and have anxiety: In these cases, it is better to interrupt the procedure and try to do it in an outpatient surgery unit, where we can administrate anesthesia for sedation.

Immediate Complications

Although it is infrequent, in some circumstances there may be intense pelvic pain or cramps. This can be resolved by intramuscular or endovenous administration of 50 mg of dexketoprofen. Sometimes, if the pain does not yield, 50-100 mg endovenous of tramadol is needed. The process will be relieved in one or two hours and will not leave any sequelae.

Another possible complication is vaso-vagal syndrome, with onset of nausea, dizziness, bradycardia, and hypotension and, in some cases, syncope. Treatment is intravenous administration of 0.5 to 1 mg of atropine, with immediate resolution of the symptoms.

RECOMMENDATIONS

- Relative rest for 1 to 4 hours, when the procedure has been conducted in the consulting room and there are no complications. If sedation has been required, 6 to 8 hours of rest is recommended.
- Resume normal activity in approximately 24 hours.
- Analgesia is not usually required. If there is pain, 600 mg of ibuprofen every 8 hours is recommended

- Minor uterine bleeding is normal, and may last up to a week
- Begin sexual relations in one week. It is important to remind the patient to use a safe alternative contraceptive during the first three months, and not to wait until the medical check-up.

Three-month Check-up

Simple X-ray of Pelvis

When this protocol was drafted, the three month check-up consisted of performing a simple radiography of the pelvis, with the radiological criteria shown in FIGURE 14.10. Any change in insertion or in the radiographic check-up at 3 months requires performance of a HSG.

Ultrasound

Nowadays in Europe the simple pelvis X-ray is being displaced by the ultrasound.[14-16]

The ultrasound shows us the location of the devices and their relation with the uterus. We considered that the devices are correctly positioned when they cross the intramural portion in a transversal section of the uterus at the fundus level.

If one of them is not correctly inserted or is not visible, we should make an HSG.

Transvaginal ultrasound with contrast (that shows if there is an obstruction[17]) and especially tridimensional[18] ultrasound are likely to be successful in the future. We attached Veugels[14] ultrasound control modified algorithm (FIGURES 14.11A to D).

In FIGURES 14.12A and B, the Figure A demonstrate a correct position of both devices. In Figure B is necessary to make a HSG because the right device is not visible.

Hysterosalpingography

Hysterosalpingography is the gold standard because it is useful to locate the devices and it also informs about the obstruction of both tubes (FIGURE 14.13).

Indications:

- Unsatisfactory insertion (FIGURE 14.14)
- Doubts about ultrasound and/or X-ray

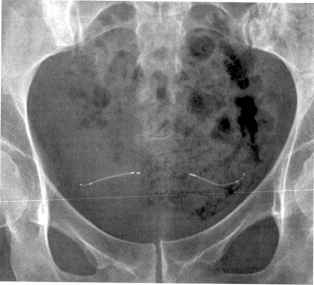

– Symmetrical appearance
– Distance between the ends < 4 cm
– The ends should not cross one another
– Both ends are in the opposite direction
– The devices should not be parallel

Figure 14.10: Correct position of X-ray

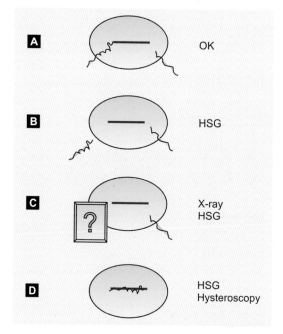

Figures 14.11A to D: Ultrasound control[14]
(Adapted from S Veersema, M Vleugels)

Hysteroscopy

Performed in cases in which ultrasound and/or HSG indicate that a device is nearly completely inside the

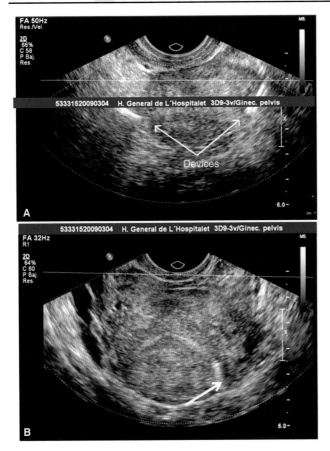

Figures 14.12A and B: Transversal vaginal ultrasound: (A) Devices are in satisfactory position, (B) Only one device is in satisfactory position. A HSG is necessary

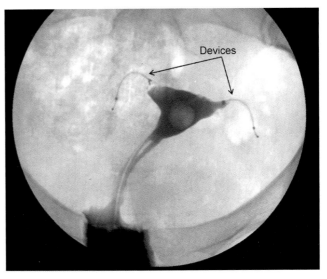

Figure 14.13: Hysterosalpingogram

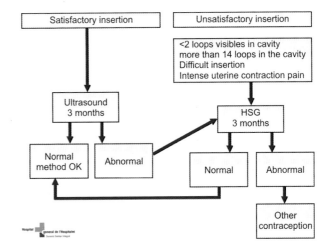

Figure 14.14: Algorithm

uterine cavity. Hysteroscopy is used to verify the number of spiral loops in the cavity. If there are more than 18 loops, it should be removed by hysteroscopy (Conceptus Inc).

The algorithm currently used for ultrasound control in Hospital General Hospitalet is illustrated in FIGURE 14.14.

COMPLICATIONS

Expulsion of Device through the Vagina[7,9,10]

In multicentric studies this complication occurred when there were technical problems, or there were more than 16 intracavitary loops when the device was unfolded. In the personal clinical series presented in this Chapter, there has not been any vaginal expulsion. This can be attributed to technical improvement of the devices and greater experience of the physicians.

Perforation[9,10]

This situation occurred in 3.1% of the phase II cases and 0.9% of the pilot study cases. In clinical patients, occurred in two cases (0.5%) (FIGURE 14.15).

Migration of Device[9-10]

This consists of movement of the device from the inside of the tube to the peritoneal cavity. It can occur in cases in which the device remains in the uterine cavity without any visible loop. In our clinical series, it did not occur in any case.

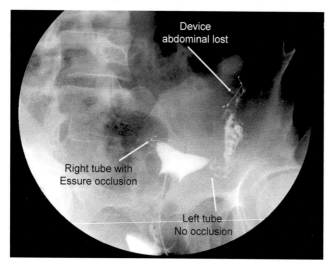

Figure 14.15: HSG with tubal perforation

EXPERIENCE

We present the experience of cases treated in both public and private practice, all carried out by the same team with 462 cases. It is interesting to consider the evolution of the results from the time the studies began up until the present. In the studies,[7,9,10,12] the insertion rate was less than 90%. At this time, the rate is 95 to 99%,[11] even though there are only a few cases. Average insertion time has also varied. At this time, the total duration of the procedure is 9 minutes (TABLE 14.1). There are two factors that have contributed to the change: First of all, the experience of the gynecologist who performs the technique and, secondly, the change in the design of the introducer catheter.

Pivotal and Phase II studies were carried out in the outpatient surgery unit. 42% of the patients needed sedation because of a poor tolerance to the procedure. However, from 2005 upto 2009 a 93.5% (291 patients) of the procedures were carried out in consultation with paracervical anesthesia or without anesthesia. The experience of gynecologist and the improvements in the device has facilitated the procedure that can be performed outpatient. In our experience near to 94% (TABLE 14.2). All patients were questioned about the pain of the procedure using an analogue scale (0 to 10).

Tolerance to the procedure in the group of patients without anesthesia or with paracervical block is really good; 80% marked the pain they had, from 0 to 3 (TABLE 14.3).

Regarding side effects (TABLE 14.4), it can be pointed out that the number of technical problems related to failures in the device mechanism has decreased. As well as the number of vaso-vagal syndrome (2.5%) however are due to the hysteroscopy technique.

Problems have also been detected in the control of three months (1.25%), one of them was a case of perforation, the HSG showed that left tube was

Table 14.1: Experience

	Studies Phase II and Pivotal	Clinical use
Cases	62	400
Positive insertion	55 (88.7%)	386 (96.5%)
Failure insertion	7 (11.3%)	14 (3.5%)
Time	18′	9′

Table 14.2: Use of anesthesia

	291 cases 2005 to 2009
Office Not anesthesia or paracervical block	272 (93.5%)
Ambulatory minor surgery Sedation	19 (6.5%)

Table 14.3: Visual scale to pain

N = 291	N (%)
0 to 3	228 (79.3%)
4 to 6	35 (12%)
7 to 10	28 (9.6%)

Table 14.4: Adverse events

	Studies N: 62	Clinical use N: 400
Relationship to procedure Vagal reflexes	3 (4.8%)	10 (2.5%)
Technical problems	3 (4.8%)	7 (1.8%)
Adverse effects on device control	6 (9.7%)	5 (1.25%)
Tubal perforation	1	2
HSG malposition	0	3
Vaginal expulsion	5	1
– Repeat placement	4 successful	1 (failure)

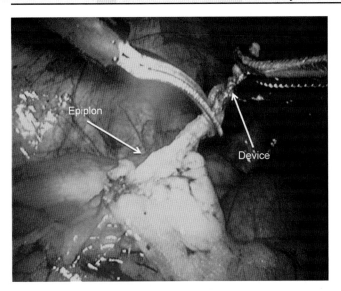

Figure 14.16: Adhesion epiplon to device

permeable and that the device was in the abdominal cavity (FIGURE 14.15). A laparoscopy was performed and the device was found adhered and wrapped by the omentum (FIGURE 14.16).

Extraction was difficult because the omentum was adhered to the PET fibers. Anyway a consensus has been reached not to remove the device when there is a perforation.

In these cases, HSG demonstrated that the devices were not in good location or that tubes were not occluded, so in these cases we cannot rely on the method.

The expulsion rate has also fallen, which we consider is due to the experience of the gynecologists. In our group, there are currently 156 patients with over 5 years of follow-up. We have been using the device as a contraceptive without any pregnancy for over 17757 months (TABLE 14.5).

Table 14.5: Results May, 2009

2009/May	Studies N = 55	Clinical use N = 253 controlled cases	Total
Women months of effectiveness	5406	12351	17757
Women relying Essure for >5 years	55	101	156
First case	9 years		
Number of pregnancies	0	0	0

RESULTS OF MULTICENTRIC STUDIES

A total of 871 patients with demonstrated fertility were selected for this study with the Essure™ method: 269 patients in the phase II study and 602 patients in the pilot study (TABLE 14.6). In 84% (227) of the patients in the phase II study, and in 86% (518) of the patients in the pilot study, satisfactory insertion was achieved in the first attempted tube cannulation. These results improved to 88 and 90%, respectively, if satisfactory second attempts are included (TABLE 14.7). At 6 months, tubal occlusion was 100% in the patients in the phase II study, and 97.7% in the pilot study.

An important objective of the studies was evaluation of the need for anesthesia in order to perform the procedure. According to the protocol, the patient can request anesthesia or sedation depending on the discomfort or pain caused by the procedure. In a total of 43% of the patients in the phase II study and 59% of the patients in the pilot study, no anesthesia was required or only local paracervical anesthesia was practiced.

As regards follow-up, in December 2008 a total of 643 patients had more than 5 years of follow-up. This represents 47.875 months of use as contraceptive without any pregnancy detected to date (TABLE 14.8).

The adverse effects are shown in TABLE 14.9. The most frequent adverse effect is Vaginal Expulsion, as mentioned previously in this Chapter.

Table 14.6: Multicentric studies (Results)

Parameter	Phase II	Pivotal study
Patients enrolled	269	602
Patients attempt	227 (84%)	518 (86%)
Average age	35 (23-45)	32 (21-40)
Gravity	2.6	3.0
Parity	2.2	2.3

Table 14.7: Multicentric placement

	Phase II	Pivotal study
Bilateral placement (1st placement attempt)	197/227 (86%)	446/518 (86%)
Bilateral placement (2nd placement attempt)	200/227 (88%)	464/518 (90%)

Table 14.8: Multicentric results as in December, 2008

Parameter	Phase II	Pivotal study
Bilateral occlusion at 3 months	96.4% n = 187/194	96.1%* n = 416/433
Bilateral occlusion at 6 months	100% n =194/194	97.7% n = 420/433
Women of use > 5 years	194	449
Woman months of effectiveness at 5 years	16.253	31.622
Pregnancies	0	0

* Of the 17 patients not occluded at 3 months, only 4 had undergone repeat HSGs at the time of this data analysis

Table 14.9: Multicentric adverse events

Parameter	Phase II n = 227	Pivotal study n = 518
Expulsion	1 (0.4%)	14 (2.7%)*
Perforation	7 (3.1%)	5 (0.9%)
Undesirable device location	1 (0.4%)	2 (0.4%)
Total	9 (4.0%)	21 (4.5%)

* Of 14 patients experiencing expulsion, 8 had reattempts and successful replacement of the device

Tolerance of women to the Essure™ was ascertained at the 3, 12, 24, 36, 48, 60, 72 and 84 months follow-up, and has been rated as "good to excellent" in 99% of women at all visits, and 95% of them would recommend it as a contraceptive method.

In the follow-up at more than ten years, no significant changes were detected in menstrual patterns, dysmenorrhea, or pelvic pain. (Information on the results of multicentric studies provided by Conceptus).

OTHER INFORMATIONS AND APPLICATIONS

About IUD

In patients who have an IUD, it is advisable prior to the procedure. Nevertheless this is under discussion; Mascaró[19] with 28 cases and Agostini[20] with 6 have demonstrated that it is possible to insert Essure™ devices in patients with IUD. They have not registered any infection case. The advantage of it, is that you can use IUD as a contraceptive method during the following three months after the procedure. More studies have to be done to confirm this tendency.

Essure™ Related Pregnancy Factors

Pregnancies[21-23] in women using Essure™ have been reported; once analyzed them it has been demonstrated that they were not due to a failure in the method.

Conceptus has registered 305 gestations from 1998 up to December 31th 2008, 83% of them were in the USA and 17% outside the USA. During this period 259.746 Essure™ system have been placed.

Patient noncompliance is a large factor in patients that become pregnant; almost 1/3rd of patients who become pregnant (96) did not comply with post-procedure instructions. Following the Essure™ procedure, patients must return for a follow-up confirmation test which will demonstrate proper placement of the devices (and fallopian tube occlusion in the United States); 72 patients who became pregnant did not return for their confirmation test. Additionally, patients must use alternative contraception until they undergo a follow-up confirmation test and are instructed by the physician to discontinue use of alternate contraception and rely on the Essure™ devices for pregnancy prevention; 24 patients who became pregnant did not follow this instruction.

Misinterpreted confirmation test results also contribute to pregnancies in Essure™ users; in this time period, 91 patients became pregnant and their confirmation tests were re-examined and determined to be read improperly. Of these patients, 36 had a perforation, 21 had unsatisfactory placement, 16 had inadequate HSGs, 14 had an expulsion or missing micro-insert, and 4 had a patency that was missed at first review.

The remainder of the contraceptive failure occurred for various reasons. One pregnancy occurred in a clinical trial patient who was wearing a prior device design that was never distributed commercially. Three pregnancies occurred in patients who had an expulsion following their confirmation test. Seventeen pregnancies occurred in patients whose physicians performed the Essure™ procedure off-label, including intentional unilateral placement and not advising their patients to get a

Table 14.10: Essure-related pregnancy factors 1998-2008 (With permission of Conceptus)

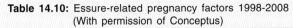
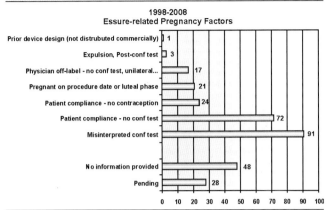

confirmation test. And 21 of them were already pregnant because the insertion took place at the late luteal phase (TABLE 14.10).

Wanted Pregnancy with Essure™

It is not infrequent that women who had decided not to have more children change their mind some years later. Different circumstances can make a woman seek a solution.

Because of the Essure's mechanism of action, that destroys the inside of the tube is not possible, neither to remove the device, except one published case, nor make a restorative surgery. Kerin[24] publishes a pregnancy post Essure™ using IVF. Although we need more studies to confirm it, IVF can be a good method for all women with Essure™ that wish a new gestation.

Essure™ Effects on Pregnancy

Conceptus has followed up pregnancy and delivery of 52 pregnant women wearing Essure™. Of the 52 cases, 3 patients had spontaneous abortion. In the other 49 cases, follow-up was performed on pregnancy, delivery and newborns. No increase in adverse effects (miscarriages, preterm deliveries, premature rupture of membranes, high number of cesarean sections and neonatal pathology) was detected in the mothers or the newborns. Until larger studies are available, the possibility of IVF may be considered in cases of sterilization regret.

Hydrosalpinx and IVF

A different application for Essure™ could be in sterile women with hydrosalpinx before an IVF. According to literature,[25-28] patients with hydrosalpinx have a high number of failures when they undergo an IVF and this number improves after a salpingectomy. The objective of the salpingectomy is to avoid the contact between the liquid from the hydrosalpinx and the embryo transferred.

Essure™ has been used successfully in a patient with hydrosalpinx and serious contraindications for surgery. After inserting an Essure™ in the tube where the hydrosalpinx was, an IVF was practiced and she got a twin gestation with healthy newborns.[29] Mijatovic[30] has published a study with 10 patients with hydrosalpinx, he achieved Essure™ insertion in all cases; 40% of gestations with IVF and 20% of newborns at home.

They are promising results, although more studies have to be done before this one becomes a new indication for Essure™.

Menorrhagia or Hypermenorrhea

Another situation with which we can find is a patient that has Essure™ and her menses are becoming plentiful. Once we have discarded a pathological process this patient could be a candidate for a progesterone IUD, but there are no publications to support IUD with Essure™.

The next option could be endometrial ablation with a monopolar resectoscope but monopolar energy is contraindicated because of risk of burns in the pelvic region (electric current could go to the devices instead of going back to the generator).

There is a bipolar resectoscope that it should not give problems (Conceptus Inc).

Thermachoice (Ethicon) is a method to make an endometrial ablation with an intrauterine balloon filled with hot liquid. Valle[31] practiced in a group of 39 patients an endometrial ablation with thermachoice and sterilization with Essure™ at the same time and there were no complications. Donanadieu[32,33] in a literature review concluded that Essure™ method is compatible with Hydrotermablator (Boston Scientific) which is intrauterine hot liquid and with Novasure (Cytyc Corporation) that consists of use of intrauterine radiofrequency to make an endometrial ablation. However is preferable to wait for new publications with more studies to confirm that there is no problem to use these ablation techniques in the presence of Essure™ devices.

Comparative Economic Study With Laparoscopy Sterilization

Different publications support that Essure™ method is cheaper than laparoscopy.[34,35]

Magnetic Resonance

Use of magnetic resonance in patients with Essure™ devices has been studied. No clinical evidence of complications has been found.[36] Therefore, use can be considered safe.

Finally, when compared with laparoscopic technique, there is only one study designed to compare both methods. The results[37] of the Essure™ method are highly favorable.

Other Rare Adverse Events

In our experience two cases of continuous pelvic pain after placement of Essure™ have been described. In one of the cases in our series, pain began in the right iliac space after satisfactory placement of the device. At three months, the X-ray and ultrasound check-up were normal. Since the pain continued, a diagnostic hysteroscopy and a laparoscopy were performed. Results were normal. A cuneiform resection of the uterine horn, where pain originated was practiced in both patients. In one of the cases, it was documented that the device had dissected the muscular wall of the tube; in the other case, no anatomical cause was found. After surgery the pain was solved.

Connor[38] reviewed the MAUDE database and found 20 reports of post Essure™ pain. Five were caused by a bad position of the devices excluding perforation, in other five cases it was due to a uni- or bilateral perforation. Four of them because of a simultaneous endometrial ablation and for the rest no cause was found.

CONCLUSION AND COMMENTS

Based on the information in the research studies and the clinical information collected to date, the Essure™ method can be considered a significant advancement in the field of permanent contraception. It is a nonsurgical method performed in the hysteroscopy consulting room that hardly ever requires any type of anesthesia. Moreover, this procedure is well-tolerated by women, has few adverse effects, and effective contraception is achieved after waiting just three months. In spite of the fact that it was initially recommended that the procedure be performed in an outpatient surgery center[39] subsequent experience has confirmed that the technique can be performed in an external consulting room.

At the three months check-up, the only procedures probably performed will be a transvaginal ultrasound and, in some cases, a HSG.

No pregnancy has been detected to date in any of the patients with devices properly placed at the three months check-up.

The degree of satisfaction reported in all of the surveys is very high (96%).

Regarding efficacy in pregnancy prevention, Essure™ results were compared with the CREST[40] report. It has been demonstrated that classical tubal sterilizations have a much higher failure rate. Based on this data and statistical calculations, a 99.6% effectiveness rate is forecast.

A disadvantage is that this technique must be performed by hysteroscopy experts. An insertion failure rate of 1-5% has been calculated for expert gynecologists. This figure may increase up to 10-15% in nonexpert hands. For training, use of hysterectomy pieces, as recommended 6 years[12] ago in an article by the authors, is no longer required. One must have experience in hysteroscopy, be familiar with the equipment used, train with models, have a suitable hysteroscope available, and perform the procedure under the guidance of an expert in the first cases.

REFERENCES

1. MacKay AP. Tubal Sterilization in the United States, 1994-1996. Family Planning Perspectives 2001;33:161-6
2. Pantaleoni DC. On endoscopic examination of the cavity of the womb. Med Press Circ 1869;8:26.
3. Hosseinian AH. Hysteroscopic sterilization. In: Siegler AM (Ed): The Fallopian Tube: Basic Studies and Clinical Contributions: New York: Futura 1986; 283.
4. Valle RF, Reed TP. Hysteroscopic Sterilization. In: Diagnostic and operative hysteroscopy. St Louis: Mosby 1999;353-66.
5. Quinones-Guerrero R, Aznar-Ramos R, Duran HA. Tubal electrocauterization under hysteroscopic control. Contraception 1973;7:195-201.
6. Reed TP, Erb RA. Hysteroscopic occlusion with silicone rubber. Obstet Gynecol 1983;61:388-92.
7. Kerin JF, Cooper J, Price T. Van Harendael B, Cayuela E, Cher D, Carignan C. Hysteroscopic sterilization using a micro-insert device: Results of multicentre Phase II study. Human Reprod 2003;18:1223-30.
8. Valle RF, Carignan CS, Wright TC. Tissue response to the Stop microcoil transcervical permanent contraceptive device: Results from prehysterectomy study. Fertil Steril 2001;76:974-80.
9. Kerin JF, Carignan S, Cher D. The safety and effectiveness of a new hysteroscopic method for permanent birth control: Results of the first ESSURE™ pbc clinical study. Aust N Z Obstet Gynaecol 2001;41:364-70.
10. Cooper J, Carignan C, Cher D, Kerin J. For selective tubal occlusion procedure 2000 Investigators Group. Microinsert non incisional hysteroscopic sterilization. Obstet Gynecol 2003;102:59.
11. Arjona JE, Miño M, Cordón P, Povedano B, Pelegrin B, Castelo-Branco C. Satisfaction and tolerance with office hysteroscopic tubal sterilization. Fertil Steril 2008;90:1182-6.
12. Cayuela E, Valle RF, Cos R, Heredia F, Moros S. Programa de adiestramiento y resultados en la inserción histeroscópica de dispositivos para la esterilización tubárica permanente. Prog Obstet Gynecol 2003;46:283-90.
13. Nichols M, Carter JF, Fyltra DL, Childers M. Essure™ system U. post-approval study group. Comparative study of hysteroscopic sterilization performed in-office versus a hospital operating room. J Minin Invasive Gynecol 2006;13:447-50.
14. Veersema S, Vleugels MP, Timmermans A, Brolmann HA. Follow-up of successful bilateral placement of Essure™ microinserts with ultrasound. Fertil Steril 2005;84:1733-6.
15. Weston G, Bowditch J. Office ultrasound should be the first-line investigation for confirmation of correct Essure™ placement. Aust NZJ Obstet Gynecol 2005;45:312-5.
16. Kerin JF, Levy BS. Ultrasound: An effective method for localization of the echogenic Essure™ sterilization micro-insert: Correlation with radiologic evaluations. J Minim Invasive Gynecol 2005;12:50-4.
17. Connor V. Contrast infusion sonography in the post-Essure™ setting. J Minim Invasive Gynecol 2008;15:56-61.
18. Pachy F, Bardou D, Piovesan P, Jeny R. Intérêt de l'echographie 3 D vaginal pour le contrôle du positionnement des dispositifs Essure™. J Gynecol Obstet Biol Reprod Doi 10.1016/j.jgyn.2009.03.014.
19. Mascaro M, Mariño M, Vicens-Vidal M. Feasibility of Essure™ placement in intrauterine device users. J Minim Invasive Gynecol 2008;15:485-90.
20. Agostini A, Crochet P, Petrakian M, Estrade JP, Cravello L, Gamerre M. Hysteroscopic tubal sterilization (Essure™) in women with an intrauterine device. J Minim Invasive Gynecol 2008;15:277-9.
21. Kerin JF. Pregnancies in Women Who Have Undergone the Essure™ Hysteroscopic Sterilization Procedure: A Summary of 37 Cases. J Minim Incas Gynecol 2005;12:S28.
22. Veersema S, Vleugels MPH, Moolenaar LM, Janssen CAH, Brölmann HAM. Unintended pregnancies after Essure™ sterilization in the Netherlands. Fertil Steril 2008 ddoi:10.1016/j.fertnstert.2008.10.005.
23. A Levy B, Levie MD, Childers ME. Summary of reported pregnancies after hysteroscopic sterilization. J Minim Invas Gynecol 2007;14:271-4.
24. Kerin JF, Cattanach S. Successful pregnancy outcome with the use of in vitro fertilization after Essure™ hysteroscopic sterilization. Fertil Steril 2007;87:1212.e1-1212.e4.
25. Strandell A, Lindhard A. Why does hydrosalpinx reduce fertility? The importance of hydrosalpinx fluid. Hum Reprod 2002 17:1141-5.
26. Strandell A, Lindhard A, Waldenstrom U, Thorburn J. Hydrosalpinx and IVF outcome: Cumulative results after salpingectomy in a randomized controlled trial. Hum Reprod 2001;16:2403-10.
27. Camus E, Poncelet C, Goffinet F, Wainer B, Merlet F, Nisand I, Philippe HJ. Pregnancy rates after in vitro fertilization in cases of tubal infertility with and without hydrosalpinx: A meta-analysis of published comparative studies. Hum Reprod 1999;14:1243-9.
28. Johnson NP, Mak W, Sowter MC. Laparoscopic salpingectomy for women with hydrosalpinx enhances the success of IVF: A Cochrane review. Hum Reprod. 2002;17:543-8.
29. Rosenfield R, Stones R, Coates A, Matteri R, Hesla J. Proximal occlusion of hydrosalpinx by hysteroscopic placement of micro-insert before in vitro fertilization–embryo transfer. Fertil Steril 2005;83:1547-50.
30. Mijatovic V, Veersema S, Emanuel MH, Schats R, Hompes PGA. Essure™ hysteroscopic tubal occlusion device for the treatment of hydrosalpinx prior to in vitro fertilization embryo transfer in patients with a contraindication for laparoscopy. Fertil Steril 2009. doi:10.1016/j.fertnstert.2008.11.022.
31. Valle RF, Valdez J, Wright TC, Kenney M. Concomitant Essure™ tubal sterilization and Thermachoice EA: Feasibility and safety. Fertil Steril 2006;86:152-8.
32. Donnadieu AC, Fernandez H; The role of Essure™ sterilization performed simultaneously with endometrial ablation. Curr Opin Obstet Gynecol 2008;20:359-63.
33. Donnadieu AC, Deffieux X, Gervaise A, Faivre E, Frydman R, Fernandez H. Essure™ sterilization associated with endometrial ablation. Int J Gynecol Obstet 2007;97:139-42.
34. Franchini M, Cianferoni L, Lippi G, Calonaci F, Calzolari S, Mazzini M, Florio P. Tubal sterilization by laparoscopy or hysteroscopy: Which is the most cost-effective procedure? Fertil Steril 2009;91:1499-1502.
35. Hopkins MR, Creedon DJ, Wagie AE, Williams AR, Famuyide AO. Retrospective cost analysis comparing Essure™ hysteroscopic sterilization and laparoscopic

bilateral tubal coagulation. J Minim Invasive Gynecol 2007;14:97-102.

36. Shellock FG. New metallic implant used for permanent contraception in women. Evaluation of MR safety. AJR 2002;178:1513-6.

37. Duffy S, Marsh F, Rogerson L, Hudson H, Cooper K, Jack S, Hunter D, Philips G. Female sterilization: A cohort controlled comparative study of Essure™ versus laparoscopic sterilization. BJOG 2005;1512:1522.

38. Connor VF. Essure™: A review six years later. J Minim Invasive Gynecol 2009;16:282-90.

39. Cayuela E, Cos R, Heredia F, Moros S, Torrabadella L. Esterilización tubárica histeroscópica con el método Essure™ en CMA. Cir May Amb 2003;8:42-4.

40. Peterson HB, Xia Z, Hughes JM, Willcoxthe LS, Tylor LR, Trusell J. For the US collaborative review of sterilization working group. The risk of pregnancy after tubal sterilization: Findings from US collaborative review sterilization. Am J Obstet Gynecol 1996;174:1161-70.

15

Complications in Hysteroscopy

Federico Heredia Prim
Enrique Cayuela Font
Ramón Cos Plans

INTRODUCTION

In hysteroscopy, as in all invasive techniques, there is a risk of complications. Over the years the complication rates have been decreasing. This has been demonstrated by improvements in the equipment and the experience of surgeons. In two multicentric interviews of the American Association of Gynecologic Laparoscopists performed by Hulka,[1] the severe complication rate decreased from 1 to 0.2% in 3 years. Jansen et al. performed a survey in 82 Dutch hospitals, and concluded that the complication rate in 11,085 diagnostic hysteroscopies was less (0.13%) than in 2,515 surgical hysteroscopies (0.95%) (TABLE 15.1).[2] These indices can be reduced if a series of precautions are taken before, during, and after the procedure. In this chapter, we will review the different types of complications that can arise in the practice of diagnostic hysteroscopy and surgical hysteroscopy, as well as the preventive measures. Some measures are applicable to both procedures, whereas others are specific. The patient should be informed of the risks, and sign the document that accredits that she is aware of these risks.

DIAGNOSTIC HYSTEROSCOPY

The possible complications associated with diagnostic hysteroscopy have been divided into mechanical, vasovagal reflex, pain, local anesthetics, distension media, and infectious complications.

Mechanical Complications

These are the most frequent. They occur in diagnostic hysteroscopy as well as surgical hysteroscopy.

Cervical Tear

This usually occurs due to excessive traction of the cervix with Pozzi's tenaculum or clamp. Nulliparity, cervical hypoplasia, menopause, and treatment with GnRH analogues are predisposing factors. It occurs most frequently in surgical hysteroscopy when the cervix is dilated with Hegar's rods, or when inserting and removing the hysteroscope through the cervix. Diagnosis is usually easy and immediate. If the cervix does not bleed, treatment is expectant. Otherwise, stitches with reabsorbable material must be applied.[3]

Table 15.1: Complications of hysteroscopy

	AAGL Survey[2]	Nicoloso[8]	Jansen[1]	Spanish Survey[19]
Perforation	1.1%	1.5%	1.3%	1.35%
Bleeding	0.2%	0.11%	0.16%	0.67%
Fluid overload	0.14%	0.11%	0.2%	0.1%

Prevention:
- Handle the hysteroscope carefully.
- Practice a vaginoscopy if possible.
- Dilate the cervical canal with rods by increasing the caliber progressively by 0.5 mm.
- In cases that are expected to be difficult, prepare the cervix with laminaria rods, prostaglandin gel, vaginal misoprostol (200 mcg) or estrogens.

Endocervical or Endometrial Lesions

This occurs during insertion of the hysterometer, dilation with rods, or during insertion of the hysteroscope without actually perforating the uterus. Menopause, cervical stenosis, and retroflexion of the uterus are predisposing factors. Warning signs are difficult insertion, deficient vision or bleeding, and pain. If diagnosis is early, the hysteroscope can be repositioned and proceed with the technique.

Prevention:
- Perform a bimanual examination of the internal genitals in order to determine the position of the uterus before beginning the examination.
- Perform careful dilatation, bypassing only the internal cervical orifice, with prior preparation of the uterus if necessary as described earlier.
- Insert the hysteroscope under direct visual control, bearing in mind the foreoblique viewing angle of the hysteroscope lens. In diagnostic hysteroscopy, this angle is nearly always 30º (FIGURES 15.1 and 15.2).[4]

Uterine Perforation

This occurs during hysterometry, cervical dilatation or hysteroscope insertion (FIGURE 15.3). According to Jansen, the rate is 0.13%.[1] Uterine perforation is particularly important since it may cause a lesion in a major blood vessel or nearby organs such as the bladder, ureters or the intestine.

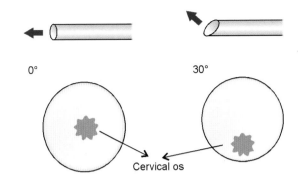

0°   30°

Cervical os

Figure 15.1: If the lens is at 0°, the internal cervical os should be centered on the cervical canal. If the lens is at 30°, the internal cervical os should be visible on the lower part of the canal

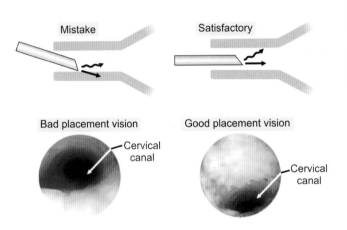

Mistake   Satisfactory

Bad placement vision   Good placement vision

Cervical canal   Cervical canal

Figure 15.2: Insertion of the hysteroscope

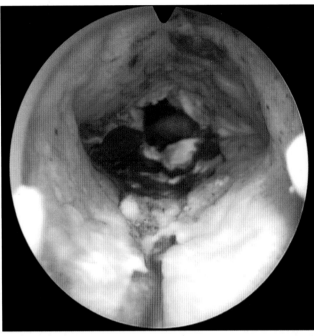

Figure 15.3: Uterine fundal perforation in diagnostic hysteroscopy

There are a series of predisposing physiological factors, such as uterus, in forced anteversion or retroversion, and menopausal uterus. Other predisposing and pathological factors are cervical stenoses after surgery (e.g. conizations), intrauterine synechia, endometrial carcinoma, uterine hypoplasia and/or congenital uterine malformations. Uterine perforation is suspected when the intestine, omentum or bladder are visible through the lens, or when proper distension is not achieved inspite of use of proper distension medium pressure and inflow, and there is high consumption of the medium. The procedure should be concluded immediately. Remove the hysteroscope, and attempt to visualize how and where perforation has occurred. Patient hemodynamic status and uterine bleeding should be evaluated. Perforation is usually of small caliber,

up to a maximum of 5.5 mm. If it has not been caused by a cutting or electrical instrument, there is usually no problem. Medical treatment with a wide spectrum antibiotic is introduced, and the patient is kept under observation for two hours with monitoring of blood pressure, pulse and pain. If there is any doubt regarding a hemoperitoneum, the intra-abdominal organs should be examined by explorative laparotomy or laparoscopy. Diagnostic hysteroscopy can be repeated after 1-2 months with the aid of an ultrasound scan to prevent further perforation.

Prevention:
- If necessary, mature the cervix.
- Gently insert the hysteroscope and always advance towards the interior of the uterus with direct vision.
- If there is not good vision due to the presence of blood and endometrial fragments, do not advance until the continuous flow system provides good image quality.
- Do not perform any maneuver with biopsy forceps or other elements if there is not a good image. At times, when the hysteroscope is inserted in the external cervical orifice, the direction in the endocervix is not visible. To prevent compli-

cations, remove the hysteroscope and use a hysterometer. This not only dilates the cervix, but also provides the direction of the endocervix.

Vasovagal Reflex

This occurs during manipulation of the endocervical canal; presence of pain or anxiety contributes to onset. It presents as weakness, heat, sweating, pallor, nausea and vomiting, bradycardia, and at times, hypotension. In severe cases, there may be a blackout with opisthotonos due to transient cerebral hypoxia. Treatment consists of placing the patient in Trendelenburg position, calming her and monitoring vital signs. Minor symptoms usually subside spontaneously within 30 minutes. If symptoms are severe, administer oxygen, and 0.1 mg/kg of endovenous atropine.[2] In the event of blackout, insert a Mayo tube. Although this situation is very dramatic, recovery is rapid and without sequelae.

In order to prevent onset, avoid sudden manipulation of the cervix when inserting the hysteroscope. In potentially sensitive patients, premedicate the patient with ibuprofen and diazepam type drugs. If the patient has history of previous vagal syndrome, he can be treated with subcutaneous atropine 30 minutes before the examination. Local cervical/paracervical anesthesia can help prevent the syndrome. Nevertheless, this can also be performed in the operating theatre with sedation.

Pain

According to the distension medium,
- *Fluid distension medium:* There may be pain on the level of the hypogastrium during insertion of the hysteroscope, especially when crossing the internal cervical orifice. Distension of the uterus can also cause contractile uterine pain that at times may become very intense.
- *If the distension medium is CO_2:* There may also be oppressive precordial and subscapular pain. This pain is caused by passage of CO_2 through the tubes into the peritoneal cavity that leads to irritation of the subphrenic nerve.

Treatment consists of discontinuing the examination and administering analgesics. If contractile pain is intense, medication should be administered parenterally. Prevention consists of treating the potentially sensitive patients with ibuprofen and diazepam. Use local anesthesia and avoid lengthy examinations that may contribute to uterine contractility.

Local Anesthetics

They may be toxic-allergic and of immediate or late onset, or due to inadvertent passage to the bloodstream that can cause cardiovascular disorders. Therefore, administration of anesthetics of the amide group is recommended, since they cause minimum systemic toxicity, few allergies, and are also easy to manage. This will be dealt with in depth in the chapter on anesthesia in hysteroscopy.

Distension Medium

The distention media used in diagnostic hysteroscopy are physiological saline solution and, in increasingly fewer cases, CO_2.
- CO_2 is a safe medium that is absorbed rapidly and eliminated by ventilation. There is risk of excessive passage to the bloodstream with pressures over 100 mm Hg and/or flows greater than 100 ml/min. This can cause metabolic acidosis associated with an increase in CO_2 partial pressure and decrease in O_2. The risk of gaseous embolization is low; this is nearly always due to use of pressures and flows that are too high. Dyspnea is the most frequent symptom, although there may also be arrhythmia, sudden decrease in O_2 saturation, cyanosis, hypotension, onset of pounding heart beat and tachycardia. Treatment consists of concluding the examination immediately, placing the patient in left lateral recumbent position, hyperbaric oxygen therapy, placement of a PVC catheter to aspirate the gas bubbles in the right heart and, if necessary, cardiopulmonary resuscitation.[2-5]

- Physiological saline solution will only cause problems if there is massive absorption. It can produce massive fluid overload and heart failure in patients with cardiac or renal disease. This is treated by insertion of a PVC catheter, administration of diuretics, oxygen, and if necessary, cardiac stimulants. During a hysteroscopic examination with physiological saline solution as distension medium, it is important that cutting or coagulation electrodes with electrical current not be used due to the risk of causing serious burns.

In order to prevent these complications, appropriate inflow and pressure should be used. This can be achieved by using specific insufflators for hysteroscopy and never using those for laparoscopy. If CO_2 is used, inflow should be 40-60 mL/min, with insufflation pressure of 100 mm Hg (maximum 150). Avoid Trendelenburg position. If fluid media is used, supervise the proper use of free-fall, pressure couplings, or irrigation pumps in order to not surpass 120 mm Hg.[6]

Infectious Complications

These types of complications are usually rare (0.7%)[2] and minor. Moreover, prognosis is good since the uterus has high resistance due to cyclical endometrial shedding.[5] The most frequent complication is endometritis. It is caused by contamination of the hysteroscope or by dragging infected cervical mucus. Risk is slightly greater if a fluid distension medium is used. Clinical symptoms are indicative of endometritis that can progress into salpingitis. It may begin as endometritis and later become salpingitis. Clinical symptoms are those associated with a pelvic infection, with fever and pain in hypogastrium. Treatment is based on rest, antibiotic therapy, and analgesia. In order to prevent complications, use aseptic procedures and sterilize the equipment; disinfect the vagina and cervix before beginning the examination; insert and remove the hysteroscope only when required and, above all, do not practice the examination if there is vaginitis or recent inflammatory pelvic disease. There are no clear indications in the literature as regards antibiotic prophylaxis. Nevertheless, use of antibiotics is recommended in women with cardiac valve disease, as well as patients who are infertile, immuno-suppressed, or have history of inflammatory pelvic disease. The usual regimen is 100 mg of oral doxycycline every 12 hours the day before, after, and on the same day as the examination.

Dissemination of Tumor Cells

In women with endometrial carcinoma, hysteroscopy can disseminate tumor cells towards the peritoneal cavity. The presence of tumor cells in the peritoneal lavage theoretically indicates progression of disease to stage IIIa. Nevertheless, the clinical significance of this finding is not known since dissemination of these cells does not necessarily entail cell implantation. In studies of survival at 5 years, no differences were found.[8]

SURGICAL HYSTEROSCOPY

Complications during surgical hysteroscopy are more frequent than in diagnostic hysteroscopy. TABLE 15.1 shows the statistics provided by Hulka et al. based on a study of 17,298 interventions; Nicoloso et al. with 2,757 cases of surgical hysteroscopy; Jansen et al. with 2,515 cases of surgical hysteroscopy; and the Spanish study prepared by Heredia et al. with 1,776 cases of surgical hysteroscopy. In all of these studies, similar rates were recorded with the exception of bleeding, which was higher in the Spanish study.

Complications that may occur during surgical hysteroscopy can be divided into complications that are mechanical, associated with distension medium, bleeding, electrical, laser-related, infectious, late, or associated with new techniques.

Mechanical Complications

These are exactly the same as in diagnostic hysteroscopy. However, during surgical hysteroscopy a resectoscope with an average thickness over 10 mm is used. Dilatation of the cervix is required, and there is also risk of perforation by the auxiliary instruments (mechanical, electrical, laser, etc.) (FIGURE 15.4). For all of these reasons, lesions may

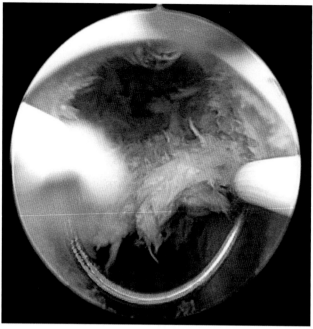

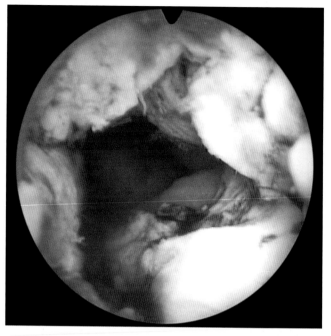

Figure 15.4: Cervical tear in the isthmic upper wall of the uterus

Figure 15.5: Uterine perforation in a surgical hysteroscopy. Abdominal contents are clearly seen

be more frequent and more serious. In some types of surgery, there is greater risk of uterine perforation in serious cases, synechotomy is clearly the procedure with the highest risk, followed by septostomy, type II myomectomies in fundal myomas of the cornual region, endometrial resections in the cornual regions, and tubal cannulation. The presence of complications also varies depending on the technique used. Use of resectoscope loop electrode entails a greater risk of perforation than ball, rolling ball, or laser.[9] If there is uterine perforation during a surgical hysteroscopy, treatment also varies. The procedure to be followed is the same as that described in diagnostic hysteroscopy if perforation was performed with the hysterometer, Hegar's rods, or resectoscope without electrical activation control. If perforation was performed with an electrode or laser, an explorative laparoscopy is indicated in order to evaluate possible damage on the level of the pelvic vessels, urinary system, and small and large intestine (FIGURE 15.5). On occasions perforation may not be noticed. Nevertheless, it should be suspected if two warning signs are present. First of all, there is a loss of uterine distension and, secondly, there is a high level of consumption of the distension medium within a short period of time.

In order to prevent mechanical lesions during surgical hysteroscopy, follow the same advice as in diagnosis. Moreover, vessels that obstruct vision should be coagulated, and procedures with electrical energy should not be performed if the distal end of the working component used is not visible (resection loop, rolling ball, laser, etc.). Although we are not completely in agreement, in cases with high-risk of perforation, some authors practice a simultaneous laparoscopy.[2,4,5]

Complications Associated with Distension Medium

The mission of the distension medium is to expand the uterine cavity, and cleanse the cavity of blood and tissue remains to ensure optimal vision. The ideal fluid is transparent; isosmotic, to prevent aqueous intoxication; non-conducive, to prevent dispersion of the electrical current; non-metabolizable, so that it will be eliminated rapidly by circulation; non-hemolytic; nontoxic; sterile and inexpensive. Presently the media used most frequently are glycine,

Cytal (mannitol-sorbitol), dextrose and physiological saline, all of which have low viscosity. There are also fluids with high viscosity, such as Hyskon, that are hardly ever used. This topic is further explained from the anesthesiologist point of view in Chapter 18.

Glycine

A nonessential amino acid solution with 1.5% water, limited miscibility with blood and mucus, ion-free, hypotonic (200 mOsm/L), metabolizes in the liver, and is excreted by the kidney after conversion into glyoxylic acid and ammonia. It can cause three types of complications: Those related to aqueous intoxication, glycine toxicity, and byproducts.

Aqueous intoxication: Present in 0.2-6% of the cases.[1] This involves rapid intravascular absorption of a non-electrolytic fluid through the exposed venous sinuses, causing dilutional hyponatremia, acute fluid overload, high blood pressure, and reflex bradycardia. This is very similar to the so-called Transurethral Resection of the Prostate (TURP) syndrome. Pathophysiology and treatment are nearly the same. It can present intraoperatively or postoperatively. The pathophysiology of this complication in women begins with passage of glycine to the bloodstream through the vascular apertures in the interior of the uterine muscle and its subsequent passage from the peritoneal cavity through the tubes. The amount of fluid absorbed is directly dependent on the number of vascular apertures, duration of the intervention, and the lavage flow pressure one is working at. Ideally, pressure should not be greater than average patient blood pressure. Intravasation of glycine produces hypervolemia with the consequent hemodilution. Therefore, it leads to decreased osmolarity and electrolyte concentrations, particularly of sodium, and hematocrit. After approximately 85 minutes the glycine moves to the intracellular space and causes hypo-osmolar hyponatremia (FIGURE 15.6). The low osmolarity intravascular free water moves towards the interstitial and intracellular space (high osmolarity) in order to achieve a balance.[6,10] This can cause pulmonary edema and cerebral edema. It leads to

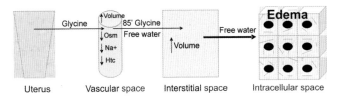

Figure 15.6: Pathophysiology of fluid overload

increased intracranial pressure, decreased blood flow, and causes hypoxia on this level. The increase in intracranial pressure is shown by high blood pressure and bradycardia. A 5% increase in cerebral volume can cause herniation, and a 10% increase is incompatible with life. Hyponatremia alone can be toxic for the skeletal and cardiac muscle, and alter membrane potentials and nerve impulses. The increase in antidiuretic hormone produced by the glycine and surgical stress, associated with the increase in renin and aldosterone, can also contribute to this overload.[6] Aqueous intoxication should be suspected if neurological symptoms such as nausea, cephalea, blurred vision, agitation, or confusion, that can develop into convulsive symptoms, are present during the course of or after completion of surgery. It is important that the type of anesthesia allow the patient to remain awake, so that the surgeon can be warned of initial symptoms. There may be cardiovascular signs such as those described above: High blood pressure, increased central venous pressure, bradycardia or irregular ECG (arrhythmia, widening of QRS complex, ST-elevation or T-wave inversion). Finally, respiratory signs and symptoms such as dyspnea, cyanosis and hypoxemia may also present. The clinical course will depend on the level of natremia and the speed of onset of this condition. Significant symptoms develop when natremia descends below 120-125 mEq/L. If it is under 120 mEq/L, the patient presents confusional state and restlessness. If it is under 115 mEq/L, he may report nausea, cephalea, drowsiness, or present negative inotropic cardiac effects and minor hypotension. Natremia under 110 mEq/L causes arrhythmias (tachycardia or ventricular fibrillation), severe hypotension, convulsions, coma and death (TABLE 15.2).

The velocity of onset is also important since acute hyponatremia is usually highly symptomatic. Unlike

Table 15.2: Symptoms of hyponatremia

Natremia	Symptoms
135-145	Normal
120-135	Restlessness
115-120	Confusion, restlessness
110-115	Nausea, headache, sleepiness, cardiac irregularities, minor hypotension
< 110	Tachycardia, arrhythmia, fibrillation, severe hypotension, convulsions, coma and death

Table 15.3: Treatment of hyponatremia

Natremia	Treatment
135-145	No
135-130	Control
120-130	Supplemental oxygen Ventilatory support if pulmonary edema 0.9% saline solution Furosemide 40-60 mg EV
110-120	3% hypertonic saline solution Furosemide 1 mg/kg/4-6 hour Sedatives if convulsive

hyponatremia with slow progression, it causes serious and irreversible neurological damage. If aqueous intoxication is diagnosed, discontinue the intervention immediately, introduce oxygen therapy, and perform strict hemodynamic control and urgent analyses of blood count and ionogram.[11]

Treatment of aqueous intoxication depends on the amount of fluid absorbed and the degree of dilutional hyponatremia.[10] The fluid absorbed can be controlled easily if there is an irrigation pump with distension medium equipped with collection container.

If there has been aqueous intoxication but natremia is normal, only vital signs and diuresis need to be monitored. If, on the other hand, natremia is low but higher than 120 mEq/L, treatment will consist of administration of 0.9% saline solution to maintain intravascular volume and force diuresis with 40-60 mg of endovenous furosemide. If natremia is under 120 mEq/L, treatment will be performed with 3% hypertonic saline solution and furosemide 1 mg/kg weight/4-6 h.[5] If the patient has convulsions, intravenous administration of midazolam (2-4 mg), diazepam (3-5 mg), or thiopental (50-100 mg) is recommended (TABLE 15.3).

It should be taken into account that excessively rapid correction of natremia leads to the pathological process of central pontine myelinosis or osmotic demyelination syndrome. The course of the condition includes severe neurological deterioration with symptoms of paresis, akinetic mutism, pseudobulbar paralysis with dysarthria and dysphagia, behavioral changes, uncoordinated movement, and convulsions that can lead to irreversible neurological sequela and death. Onset of this syndrome is most frequent after 2 days of hyponatremia less than or equivalent to 105 mEq/L. It occurs invariably if correction has been

greater than 12 mEq/L/day (0.5 mEq/L/hour). This is the reason why there are guidelines for treatment of hyponatremia.[11]

Asymptomatic hyponatremia should be treated by correcting the cause, if possible, and restricting water allowance if the fluid balance shows evidence of excess water. Serum calcemia, kaliemia and natremia should be monitored. Endovenous administration of 10-20 mg furosemide should be considered.

Regardless of whether it is acute or chronic, symptomatic hyponatremia is an authentic urgency. Plasma sodium should be elevated by administering sodium at a rate of 0.5-1 mEq/L/hour.

If sodium is administered, and in any type of hyponatremia, plasma sodium should not be elevated over 12-15 mEq/day, nor more than 25 mEq/L in the first 48 hours of treatment, and it should not be over 120 mEq/L in the first 24 hours. Normal levels of plasma sodium (i.e. 135-140 mEq/L) should not be surpassed under any circumstances.

Glycine toxicity: It can cause decreased visual acuity and transient blindness. This is due to a direct inhibitory effect of the glycine on neurotransmission in the retina. The patient presents blindness with highly dilated pupils, absence of photomotor reflex and adaptation, conserving the blinking reflex. He will return to normality within 24 hours without residual symptoms.

Convulsions can also be caused. The glycine increases the effects of N-methyl-D-aspartate (NMDA), an excitatory neurotransmitter. The magnesium acts as a negative control on the NMDA receptor. Dilutional hypomagnesemia increases susceptibility to convulsions.

Toxicity of glycine byproducts: The liver and kidneys metabolize the glycine in glyoxylic acid, which is eliminated in urine in the form of oxalate. This leads to hyperoxaluria that is nephrotoxic, and ammonia that can produce hyperammonemic encephalopathy, cortical edema, nausea and vomiting.[9]

To prevent the complications associated with distention media, the following should be performed.[2,4]

- Continuous fluid balance: Discontinue intervention with losses between 1000-1500 cc
- Monitor blood pressure, pulse oximetry and ECG
- Control intrauterine pressure: Not greater than 150 mm Hg. An infusion pump with fluid balance should be used, with flows of 300-400 mL/min and pressure of 80-120 mm. Work with intrauterine pressure similar to average blood pressure is recommended.[20] Practice of surgical hysteroscopy with resectoscope without strict control of distension fluid inflow and outflow can not be justified at present. Therefore, there is significant risk of aqueous intoxication in uterine distension performed with pressure couplings
- Prevent long interventions: Actual surgery time should not be greater than 60 minutes. If necessary, perform the intervention in two visits
- Proper intraoperative patient hydration: Intraoperative hydration reduces uterine venous pressure and contributes to increased absorption
- Proper surgical technique and experience
- Use locoregional anesthesia since it allows to detect early symptoms of hyponatremia such as nausea, vomiting and mental confusion
- Discontinue intervention if there is uterine perforation
- Suitable previous pharmacological preparation with GnRH analogues (2-3 months) in large or type II myomectomies. Administration facilitates reduced endometrial thickness, myoma size and vascularization.[21] This leads to reduced surgical time, bleeding, absorption of distension medium, and increases patient hemoglobin in the event of preoperative anemia
- Special attention should be given to patients with heart disease or chronic obstructive lung disease.

Physiological Saline

Used with the Versapoint™ and bipolar resectoscope. Use of these instruments with physiological saline is not necessarily associated with onset of aqueous intoxication syndrome. Although the distension medium is physiological saline, massive inflow of saline can cause serious hydroelectric problems with pulmonary edema. The same controls should be used.

Cytal

This is a solution with 0.54% mannitol and al 2.7% sorbitol. Mannitol is a diuretic and sorbitol is eliminated rapidly from plasma. This reduces the likelihood of vascular overload. When aqueous intoxication occurs, there is hyperglycemia and hemolysis, in addition to the conventional symptoms.

Dextrose (2.5-4%)

Not used often since it causes significant hyperglycemia.

Dextran 70 (32%) or Hyskon

Presently in disuse. The consistency is highly viscous. Therefore, it has a caramelizing effect and hinders instrument cleaning. It is hyperosmolar. It can cause anaphylactic reaction, respiratory distress syndrome, pulmonary edema and coagulation irregularities.[2,4]

Physiological Saline

Only used if the working material uses bipolar electrical energy or laser, in order to prevent electrical accidents. Intravascular passage of excess physiological saline during surgery can also cause severe disorders such as pulmonary edema.

A side effect of all distention media is hypothermia. This occurs particularly in elderly women when significant volumes are handled during a lengthy surgical procedure. It predisposes the patient to present arrhythmias, decreases myocardial contractility and interferes in coagulation. Therefore, it is recommendable to heat the irrigation fluids.[9]

Bleeding

Infrequent. The prevalence of bleeding depends on the type of energy used. In endometrial ablation with rolling ball and loop, incidence is 2.57%; with loop alone 3.57%; with laser 1.17%; and with ball alone 0.97% (FIGURE 15.7).[8] It is caused by lesion to the vessels of the disease to be resected (myomas, polyps, adherences), lesion of intramyometrial veins (endometrial resection, myomectomy) and/or continuous bleeding due to lesion of the submucosal capillary network. There may also be dilutional thrombocytopenia associated with excessive bleeding.[10] A distinction is made between intra-operative bleeding and postoperative bleeding. In the first case, treatment is to increase intrauterine pressure of the distension medium. It should be taken into account that this will lead to increased intravasation and/or selective coagulation of bleeding vessels by electrical ball/loop or laser. If there is postoperative bleeding, spontaneous hemostasis usually occurs when the uterus contracts. Treatment consists of performing uterine compression by Foley catheter or a specific uterine balloon (FIGURE 15.8) inserted in the cervix. A total of 30 cc of physiological saline is instilled. After 6 hours the balloon is deflated. Without removing the catheter, bleeding is verified with the patient in semi-Fowler position. If there is limited blood loss, the catheter is removed completely. If bleeding continues, the balloon is inflated again and kept in place for 24 hours. After this time, it is very rare for bleeding to continue.[2-4]

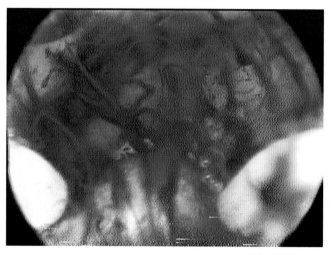

Figure 15.7: Hemorrhage during a loop endometrial resection

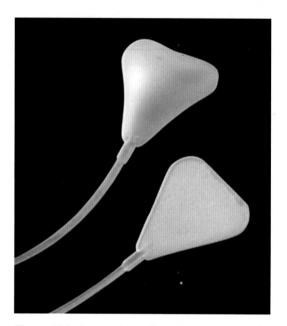

Figure 15.8: Intrauterine balloon *(Courtesy: Cook™)*

Electrical Complications

These complications are caused by transmural thermal diffusion of electrical energy with rolling ball, loop or ball in endometrial ablations; cutaneous electrical lesions due to improper plate placement; use of electrical equipment in poor condition or monopolar electrical current with a distension medium with ions (physiological saline or Ringer's solution). In order to prevent these, electrical equipment should be checked prior to the intervention. Verify that it is in good condition; inspect the electrical connections, particularly the insulation; ensure proper application of the plate whenever monopolar current is used; and place it as close as possible to the surgical lesion. Use suitable current power (100 W cutting and 80 W coagulation) and distention media with ions whenever monopolar electrical current is used.[2-4]

Laser-related Complications

Coaxial fibres should be avoided, particularly those with sapphire tip since they require continuous cooling with gas or fluid, and can cause excess absorption, or even embolism.[3,5] Laser can cause thermal lesions to nearby organs such as the intestine or major vessels. Moreover, laser can cause distance lesions from the perforation site since, after having passed through the myometrium, it can vaporize the next surface that it finds in its path.

Infectious Complications

Described during diagnostic hysteroscopy (Chapter 3).

Complications Associated with New Techniques

Intrauterine instillation of heated saline solution: A study by Perlitz[12] with 14 patients did not show evidence of complications. No complications were recorded by Das Dores,[13] Weisberg,[14] Richart[15] or Bustos-López[16] either, after practicing endometrial ablation with this technique for treatment of metrorrhagia. They are prospective, observational studies with a small number of patients.

Late Complications

Hematometra

Occurs in 1-2% of endometrial resections. This condition, which is secondary to obstruction of the internal cervical orifice or intrauterine adherences, causes chronic, cyclic pain in the hypogastrium. Treatment consists of drainage by hysteroscope or guided by ultrasonography. In order to prevent this, the isthmus region of the uterus should be respected in the resections, excluding the internal orifice of the cervix.[2,17]

Synechia

Intrauterine adherences can appear after surgical hysteroscopy, especially after myomectomy in which two myomas are located on opposite walls of the uterus. In this case, it is better to perform the myomectomy in several surgical interventions in order to prevent adherences.

Postablation-tubal Sterilization Syndrome

Focal development of a hematometra on the cornual level secondary to endometrial remains on the uterine horns after an ablation. The patient reports unilateral or bilateral cyclic pain that begins after two months. In some cases, there is genital bleeding. Treatment is bilateral salpingectomy and/or hysterectomy.[17]

Uterine Breakage

There is risk of uterine breakage during pregnancy or childbirth after specific procedures: Septoplasty, adhesiolysis, and myomectomy. The primary etiological factor is uterine perforation (scissors, loop electrode-scalpel or laser) and surgical lesion of the myometrium.

Placental Accretion

A total of 26% placenta accretes have been described in postablation pregnancies.[18]

Hysteroscopic complications are rare, but they may be serious. Knowledge of these complications, as well as the instruments and techniques, in conjunction with the experience acquired, are essential to reduce incidence and severity.

REFERENCES

1. Jansen FW, Vredevoogd CB, van Ulzen K, Hermans J, Trimbos JB, Trimbos-Kemper TC. Complications of Hysteroscopy: A Prospective, Multicenter Study. Obstet Gynecol 2000;96(2):266-70.
2. Hulka JF, Peterson HB, Phillips JM, Surrey MW. Operative hysteroscopy. American Association of Gynecologic Laparoscopists 1991 membership survey. J Reprod Med 1993; 38:572-3.
3. Valle RF. Possible complications of hysteroscopy. In Taylor & Francis (Ed): Manual of clinical hysteroscopy. London 2005;39-45.
4. Vilos GA. Hysteroscopic surgery: indications, contra-indications and complications In: A practical manual of hysteroscopy and endometrial ablation techniques. Pasic RP, Levine RL (Eds): Taylor & Francis. London 2004;237-57.
5. Baggish MS. Complications of Hysteroscopic Surgery. In: Baggish MS, Barbot J, Valle RF (Eds): Diagnostic and operative hysteroscopy. Mosby Inc. St Louis.1999:367-79.
6. Cayuela E. Instrumentación en histeroscopia. Medios de distensión. In: Comino R, Balagueró L, del Pozo J (Eds):

Cirugía endoscópica en Ginecología. Prous Science SA, Barcelona 1998;261-73.

7. Obermair A, Geramou M, Gucer F, Denison U, Graf AH, Kapshammer E, Medl M, Rosen A, Wierrani F, Neunteufel W, Frech I, Preyer O, Speiser P, Kainz C. Impact of hysteroscopy on disease-free survival in clinically stage I endometrial cancer patients. Int J Gynecol Cancer 2000;10:275-9.

8. Nicoloso E, Cravello L, d'Ercole C, Boubli L, Blanc B. Les complications de hystéroscopie: Enquete nationale prospective a propos de 2757 hystéroscopies. Rev Fr Gynecol Obstet 1997;92:91-8.

9. Overton C., Hargreaves J, Maresh A. A national survey of the complication of endometrial destruction for menstrual disorders. The Mistletoe study. Br J Obstet Gynecol 1997;104:1351-59.

10. Giannakikou I, Vlahos N. Síndrome de intoxicación acuosa en cirugía ginecológica. In: Obstetricia y Ginecología de Postgrado. Revista Quincenal de Obstetricia y Ginecología Clínica 2005;2(5).

11. Mosquera JM. Trastornos del metabolismo del sodio. In: Gil J, Díaz-Alersi, Coma MJ, Gil D (Eds): Principios de Urgencias, Emergencias y Cuidados Críticos. http://tratado.uninet.edu/c050202.html

12. Perlitz Y, Rahav D, Ben-Ami M. Endometrial ablation using hysteroscopic instillation of hot saline solution into the uterus. Eur J Obstet Gynecol Reprod Biol 2001;99 (1):90-2.

13. Das Dores GB, Richart RM, Nicolau SM. Evaluation of Hydro ThermAblator for endometrial destruction in patients with menorrhagia. J Am Assoc Gynecol Laparosc. 1999; 6(3):275-8.

14. Weisberg M, Goldrath MH, Berman J, Greensteinn A. Hysteroscopic endometrial ablation using heated saline for the treatment of menorrhagia. J Am Assoc Gynecol Laparosc 2000;7(3):311-6.

15. Richart RM, das Dores GB, Nicolau SM, Focchi GR. Histologic studies of the effects of circulating hot saline on the uterus before hysterectomy. J Am Assoc Gynecol Laparosc 1999;6(3):269-73.

16. Bustos-Lopez HH, Baggish M ,Valle RF, Vadillo-Ortega J. Assessment of the safety of intrauterine instillation of heated saline for endometrial ablation. Fertil Steril. 1998;69(1):155-60.

17. Shveiky A. Complications of hysteroscopic surgery. Beyond the learning curve. JMIG 2007;14:530-1.

18. Hare AA, Olah KS. Pregnancy following endometrial ablation: a review article J Obstet Gynaecol 2005;25(2):108-14.

19. Heredia F, Cos R, Cayuela E. Encuesta española sobre histeroscopia. Presented in the II° Congreso Español de Endoscopia Ginecológica. Madrid 2000.

20. Garry R, Hasham F, Kokri MS. The effect of pressure on fluid absorption during endometrial ablation. J Gynecol Surg 1992;8:1-10.

21. Lemay A, Maneux R. GnRH agonist in the management of uterine leiomyoma. Inf Reprod Med Clin North Am 1996;7:33-5.

16

Transcervical Embryoscopy

Tirso Pérez-Medina
Jennifer Rayward

INTRODUCTION

Transcervical embryoscopy (TE) is an endoscopic technique consisting in the introduction of an optical lens through the cervical canal in order to visualize the gestational sac and the embryonic structures between the 5th and 12th weeks of pregnancy.

One out of every 6 clinical pregnancies ends in spontaneous miscarriage and 2 out of every 3 spontaneous miscarriages are attributed to chromosomal abnormalities.[1] Generally speaking, the samples obtained by curettage don't contain any embryonic tissue and if they do, the samples are so severely damaged[2] that morphological study is extremely limited.

Embryonic development is a precisely programmed choreographic event made up of developmental steps that demand the collaboration of many genes to regulate growth and morphogenesis. In early missed abortion specimens, the cytogenetic analysis is an important component in evaluating human malformations when trying to elucidate etiological factors. The detection of aneuploidy or polyploidy provides a causal explanation for the developmental defect and it has been found that the risk of recurrence in these couples is not substantially increased.[3] These factors are not usually considered to be etiologically related to the early pregnancy loss and the trend is not to look for chromosomal disorders. This prevents the diagnosis of genetic causes.

TE in missed abortion is a technique for the direct visualization of the deceased embryo inside the uterus, and allows the endoscopist to perform directed biopsies. The samples from TE are not damaged like the ones obtained by instrumental or spontaneous evacuation, making evaluation more precise.

DEVELOPMENT OF THE TECHNIQUE

In 1945, Westin[4] published a study entitled "Hysteroscopy in early gestation". He introduced transcervically McCarthy's panendoscope into the uterus and directly observed the embryo in 3 patients scheduled for pregnancy termination. The fetuses measured 21, 19 and 10 cm. In 1966, Agüero et al[5] published "Hysteroscopy in pregnant patients, a new diagnostic tool". They used transcervically three 20, 24 and 28 Fr. diameter hysteroscopes in a patient population of 118 women from 8 to 40 weeks of gestational age, to observe the aspect of the ovular membranes, the presentation, the cervical canal and the uterine walls. They also observed prolonged gestations, ruptured membranes, third semester hemorrhages, Rh incompatibility, fetal death and hydatidiform moles. In 1972, Valenti[6] used the term "endoamnioscopy" to refer to the technique used in his series of 6 patients scheduled for pregnancy termination with a gestational age between 14 and 18 weeks. An 18 Fr. cystoscope was used, inserting the endoscope via transmyometrial laparotomy, facilitating the direct visualization of the fetus. In 1978, Gallinat[7] published a study entitled "A preliminary report about transcervical EC", in a first try to standardize the technique.

The widespread use of the transvaginal sonography (TVUS) in gynecology made these techniques fall into disuse due to their excessive invasiveness and the high rate of fetal loss. In the 90's, when endoscopic instruments were developed with smaller diameters and improved optic features, new interest in embryoscopy and fetoscopy flourished due to minimizing the aggression and giving way to the possibility of performing minor surgical interventions.

Some authors like Cullen in 1990,[8] Ghirardini in 1991[9] and Reece in 1993[10] began to call the technique "embryoscopy". They inserted 2 to 4 mm diameter endoscopes transcervically into patients scheduled for pregnancy termination between weeks 5 and 13. These authors were able to visualize the embryo in 96, 75 and 100% respectively of the procedures, with a dramatically reduced complication rate. Only Cullen reported an immediate fetal death. In 1991, Cullen[11] performed transcervical endoscopy for verification of congenital anomalies in the second trimester of pregnancy.

Dumez[12] in 1992 performed TE by means of a 1.7 mm endoscope in a series of 39 patients with pregnancies between 8 and 13 weeks with high risk for dominant autosomic genetic diseases including facial and limb alterations. He succeeded in 97% of the cases when embryo was clearly visualized. Subsequent miscarriage occurred in 12.8%.

In 1993, Quintero et al,[13] performing transabdominal embryoscopy, documented a 25% failure rate in visualizing the embryo in a series of patients scheduled for pregnancy termination between 9 and 18 weeks. They used 18 and 19 G needles. One patient experienced uterine wall bleeding. In pregnancies below the 11th week the success rate dropped 10% lower because in some cases the needle punctured the amniotic cavity. This can be explained because after the 10th week, the chorionic cavity is almost virtual. They also report a transabdominal diagnosis of Meckel syndrome when finding polydactyly and occipital encephalocele in an eleven weeks pregnancy.

Later on, Yin[14] performed transcervical endoscopy by means of a flexible hysteroscope with apparent good results.

MATERIAL AND METHODS

The first sign that TE may be performed is the observation in routine TVUS of a missed abortion. Sonography also later helps correlate the findings with the TE results. By comparing the LMP and the CRL it allows a precise estimate of the gestational age in which embryonic growth stopped.

The main indication for TE is a missed abortion diagnosed by TVUS under 10 embryonic weeks or 12 weeks of amenorrhea and fulfilling at least one of the following criteria defined by Filly:[15]
- Clear visualization of an amniotic sac with no embryonic structures (blighted ovum)
- Absence of heart beat in a 5 mm embryo
- Absence of vitellin vesicle in a 13 mm diameter gestational sac
- Absence of embryo in a 18 mm diameter gestational sac.

Technique

The TE is performed in an operating theater under general or regional anesthesia. If regional anesthesia is the choice, the patient must not be able to see the screen for obvious reasons.

By means of vaginoscopy, without need for cervical tenaculum or cervical dilation, a 5.5 mm continuous-flow diagnostic hysteroscope with a 5 Fr. working channel is atraumatically guided through the cervical canal with normal saline as distension medium, with flow manually regulated with the key of the hysteroscopic sheath. A physiological pressure is obtained by gravity when two 3 liter interconnected saline bags situated 1 meter above the patient to obtain a pressure of about 70 mm Hg until the internal cervical os is passed and uterine cavity is reached.

The examination of the uterine cavity begins by observing its regularity, paying special attention to the presence of intrauterine malformations or morphologic alterations such endometrial polyps, submucous myomas, or uterine septa. Subsequently the endometrial decidualization and its vascularization are studied. Then the location, size, number and characteristics of the gestational sac(s) are observed.

For biopsy, the decidua just opposite to the implantation site, where the membranous or capsular decidua is thin and avascular, is chosen. The decidua is carefully penetrated with a biopsy grasper or microscissors and the hysteroscope is slowly introduced. The chorion is gently dissected with the tip of the hysteroscope, reaching the chorionic membrane. The membrane is then penetrated in the same way, entering the extracoelomic space or chorionic cavity.

Before 10th week of pregnancy, a spherical space in the chorionic cavity where the amniotic sac anchors will appear. It is joined by a delicate stalk with the vitellin vesicle. Next, a hole is drilled through the amniotic membrane to be in direct contact with the embryo. The whole embryo is visualized, changing its position by means of the endoscopic ancillary graspers or with jets of saline when opening the entrance via saline in the sheath. This is an important moment and much care must be taken with the instruments not to damage the delicate embryo. Once the visualization of the embryo is completed, directed biopsies can be performed.

FINDINGS

Endocervical Canal

When inserting the optical lens through the external cervical os, a glandular epithelium with decidualization characteristics is observed. Dense, opaque mucus is visualized that progressively clears as saline solution flows. The cervical os will be totally or partially occluded, but sometimes the os is free of decidua (FIGURE 16.1).

Uterine Cavity

Upon entering the cavity, the first thing visualized is the projection of the gestational sac towards the cavity. As pregnancy progresses, the sac invades the uterine walls and then it is distinguished by the differences between the capsular and the parietal decidua. The parietal decidua is highly vascularized with irregular angiogenetic-type patterns with lacunar vascular spaces. Despite the deceased embryo, the surrounding tissues can still exhibit normal vascularization. Other times depending on the degree of vascular stasis and anoxia the tissue may appear anywhere from white to a darker color on a dark brown background instead of a live physiological red.

Gestation Sac

The membrane that covers the gestation sac is the capsular or membranous decidua and differs considerably with the parietal decidua. At 5 weeks there are hardly any differences between the capsular and the parietal decidua except for their localization on the sac but these differences evolve with pregnancy. At first they are homogeneously the same width but as the sac grows, it advances and ends up being a thin layer that covers it, until it embeds in the parietal decidua. This capsular decidua doesn't present venous lakes and its vascularization is scarce. Its evolution will be less obvious.

Chorionic Membrane and *Chorion Laeve*

Immediately under the capsular deciduas, the chorionic decidua is distributed evenly around the sphere of the chorionic sac in the first week of

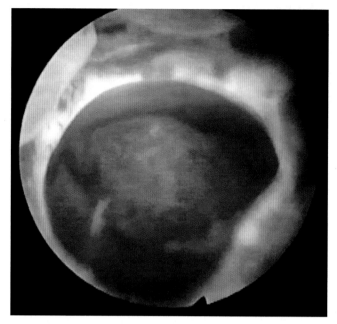

Figure 16.1: The internal cervical os with the opened decidua parietalis in a view from the canal

amenorrhea. As the base of implantation spreads, the *Chorion frondosum* or future placenta will be formed.

Upon examination, the first membrane is the *Chorion laeve* that will gradually disappear. The thinnest part is in this anatomical portion, before the chorionic membrane, that defines the chorionic sac containing the extracoelomic space or chorionic cavity. The *Chorion laeve* is digitiform, with different extents of ramifications depending on gestational age (FIGURE 16.2). The time of embryonic death will be decisive in the degree of hydrophic degeneration reached. Macroscopic diagnosis of hydatidiform mole may be contemplated. The chorionic membrane is semitransparent and different chorial vessels may be individualized.

Extracoelomic Space and Chronic Cavity

Upon entering in the spherical chorionic cavity, its space is delimited by the chorionic membrane that due to its transparency allows the visualization of a whitish tubular network on a reddish background. The extracoelomic space is translucent with trabecular structure (FIGURE 16.3). The earlier the gestation, the more fibrous and trabecular is the intrachorionic material. Inside this spherical cavity, in the

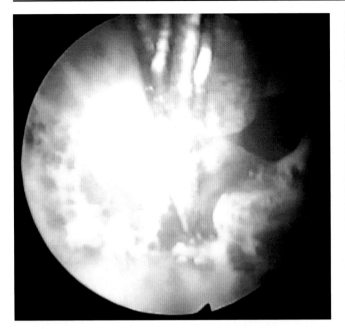

Figure 16.2: Endoscopic scissors opening the *chorion laeve*

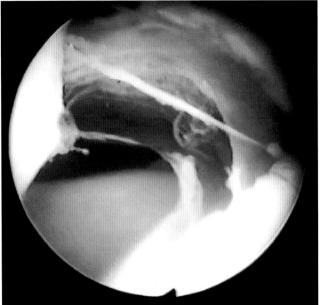

Figure 16.4: Endoscopic scissors opening the amniotic sac

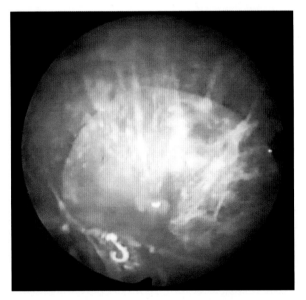

Figure 16.3: Extracoelomic space.
Note the dense, trabecular aspect

extracoelomic space, two suspended globular off-centre formations differing in size with transparent membranes and joined by a delicate cord are seen that corresponds to the amniotic sac joined to the secondary vitellin vesicle and its stalk.

Amniotic Sac and Vitellin Vesicle

The embryo is located inside the amniotic sac (FIGURE 16.4), along with the chorionic membrane,

in which the omphalomesenteric conduit and the allantoids are located in the first stages of the development although later on, the umbilical cord will be the only structure observed. The amnion grows with gestational age until it contacts with the chorion in the 10 week. The amniotic membrane is totally transparent which allows visualization of the embryo, so, in the embryoscopy where no intervention is needed opening is not required.

The earlier the gestation, the closer the vitellin vesicle will be to the embryo and the amniotic sac and its conduct will be shorter and wider. As the gestation evolves, the vitellin vesicle with a granulated membrane disappears and gives way to the secondary vitellin vesicle in the 3rd week (FIGURE 16.5). Later, when the amnion fuses with the corion, it completely obliterates the extracoelomic space. The vitellin vesicle will be displaced peripherally and eventually it will become very small and difficult to visualize.

EMBRYO

The embryonic period extends from 5th week, i.e. from the date of the last menstrual period (or 3 weeks after ovulation), until 12 weeks from the date of the last menstrual period (or 10 weeks after ovulation).

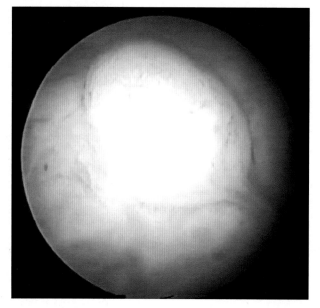

Figure 16.5: Solitary secondary vitellin vesicle in the 3rd week

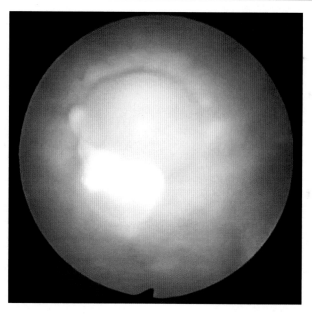

Figure 16.6: Three weeks embryo measuring 2 mm

At 10 weeks, the embryo will measure 6 cm. At this point in time the fetal period begins.

The embryonic development classification, dated in weeks, starting from the date of ovulation is the one described by Carnegie[16] and proposed and adapted by O'Rahilly and Muller[17] in 1987. In Obstetrics, gestational age is counted from the last menstrual period, so a 3rd week embryo in the Carnegie classification is equivalent to a 5th week embryo in "obstetric language."

According to Carnegie classification, the following description by weeks is what is observed:

2nd Week

Between days 7 and 13, an intense decidualization is observed. A whitish, polypoid proliferative endometrium is visualized. The same image is observed in other situations like when there is progesterone activity. In this early stage, the hysteroscopic diagnosis of pregnancy is very difficult. Even in the first days of blastocyst implantation, no difference in the endometrium can be observed.

3rd Week

Towards the end of 2nd week and during 3rd week, i.e. between days 14 and 21, the embryo undergoes gastrulation during which the bilaminar disk formed by the ventral region or hypoblast, and the dorsal region or epiblast becomes a trilaminar disk where mesenchymal cells migrate located between both regions. These three layers are denominated ectoderm, endoderm and the new layer, mesoderm. These three layers form the primitive pit. The embryo changes daily. It begins to fold, thus beginning the so-called notochordal process. The heart and the corporal cavities originate from the notochordal canal and the neural fold, as well as the intraembryonic celoma. The amnion contains the embryo and the secondary vitellin vesicle begins to disappear. The length of the embryo is 2 mm at this time (FIGURE 16.6).

4th Week

In the course of 4th week (between day 22 and 28), the embryo's body shape changes dramatically.

At days 22 and 23, the embryo is almost straight and some pairs of somites produce bumps on the surface. The neural canal is formed between the opposite somites, but both neuropores are still open.

At days 24 and 25, one or two pharyngeal or branchial arches are visible: The first arch is also called the mandibular arch and the second, the hyoid arch. Now the embryo, the head, and tail are bending towards each other and the heart begins to pump blood.

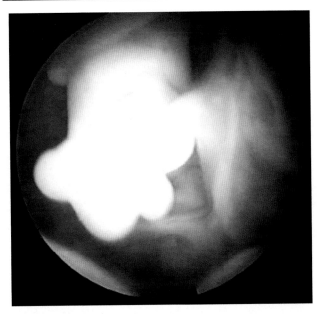

Figure 16.7: The upper and lower limb buds in the 4th week

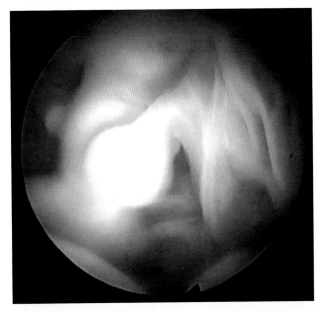

Figure 16.8: The tail is clearly visible between the lower limb buds

On days 26 and 27, a third branchial arch appears and rostral neuropore closes. The anterior brain produces an important prominence of the head and the embryo has folded to its characteristic C-shape. A long curved tail is evident. The buds of the upper limbs are small swellings on the ventrolateral walls of the body (FIGURE 16.7). The otic placodes are also visualized. This is the first evidence of the internal ears. On both sides of the head, ectodermic elevations are seen, the pit of the future lens of the eyes, called lens placode of the crystalline.

Towards, the end of 4th week (day 28), the fourth pair of branchial arches and the buds of the lower limbs are formed. At the end of week 4 the tail is less evident and the caudal neuropore closes. The embryo now measures 3.5 mm.

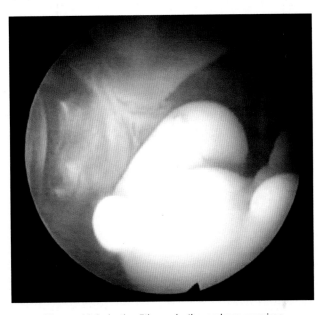

Figure 16.9: In the 5th week, the embryo acquires a human aspect

5th Week

Between days 29 to 35 the changes in body shape are small in comparison with those that took place during 4th week. There is rapid growth of the head. This growth implies development of the brain and of the facial prominences that contact with the heart prominence. The buds of the upper limbs are palette-like while the buds of the lower limbs are finlike. The tail is clearly visible (FIGURE 16.8). The embryo measures between 4 and 8 mm (FIGURE 16.9).

6th Week

Between days 36 to 42, the upper limbs show accelerated differentiation as elbows and hands are developing. Digital rays, primordium of the fingers begin to develop into buds of the hands or the hand plates. Embryos in 6th week show spontaneous movements, a kind of shaking of the trunk and the

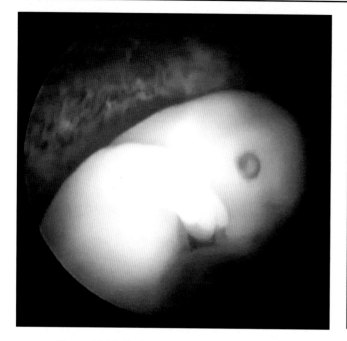

Figure 16.10: Retinal pigment is easily recognized from the 6th week

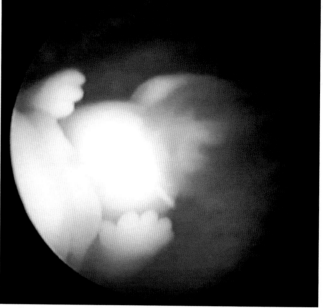

Figure 16.11: Physiological umbilical hernia in the 7th week

limbs. The lower limbs develop after the upper limbs, forming the foot plates. Between the first two branchial arches several small swellings called auricular hillocks develop around the branchial arch. This arch will form the external acoustic meatus (external auditory conduit) and the auricular hillocks fuse to their surrounding structures to form the external auditory pavilion and the ear. Retinal pigment has formed making the eyes visible (FIGURE 16.10). The head is much bigger than the trunk and leans more over the great cardiac prominence that marks the neck that begins to differentiate. The tail is long and thick. At this time the embryo measures between 8 and 13 mm.

7th Week

In 7th week (Days 43 to 49), the embryo now has the aspect of a fetus. The trunk straightens. The head is still disproportionate, the face is almost formed with a still flat nose, the former lids are perceptible and the heart is less prominent. Herniated intestines in the extraembryonic celoma form the so-called physiological hernia where the umbilical cord enters the abdomen (FIGURE 16.11). The genitalia are still

undetermined. The tail is still visible, but is thick and short and will disappear by end of this week of development. The hands show the fingers beginning to differentiate. The limbs change dramatically during this week. Furrows appear among the digital rays in the buds of the hands representing a clear indication of the future fingers. Towards the end of 7th week, the ossification of the upper limb bones has begun and the CRL is now 18 mm.

8th Week

In the early part of the last week of the embryonic period (Days 50 to 56), the upper limbs are longer and bent at the elbows. The fingers are well defined (FIGURE 16.12). They are membranous. Now, obvious furrows are seen among the digital rays of the toes in a fan shape. Towards the end of the eighth week the limbs are differentiated and the fingers lengthen and completely separate. The tail can no longer be seen.

During this week, for the first time, intentional movements of the limbs appear. During the eighth week lower limbs bone ossification begins in the femur. The vascular plexus of scalp forms a band near

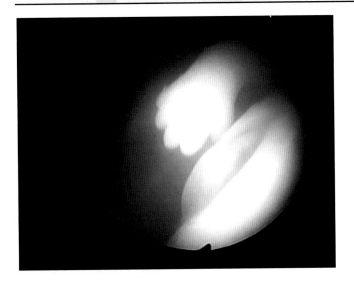

Figure 16.12: In the 8th week, the fingers are independent

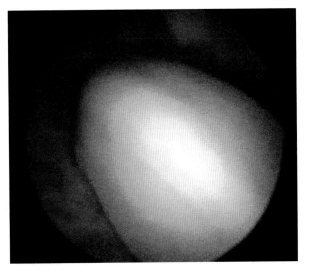

Figure 16.13: The spinal cord in a 9th weeks embryos

the vertex of the head. The hands and the feet turn inward. The embryo measures between 20 and 30 mm.

9th Week

At 9th week (Days 57 to 64), except for the external genitalia (in their final differentiation stage) the embryo is totally formed. The head is still disproportionately large and makes up almost half of the embryo. The neck region is well defined and the lids are more obvious, now in the preocclusion phase. The spinal cord is closed (FIGURE 16.13). The external ears begin to acquire their final shape, but their implantation in the head is still low. At the end of this week, the Crown-rump length reaches the 50 mm.

10th Week

During the tenth week (Days 64 to 70) the embryo grows to a CRL of 60 mm. Towards the end of the 10th week, the embryo has evident human characteristics. The intestine is now inside the fetal abdomen. The genitalia are totally defined (FIGURE 16.14). Toward the end of the tenth week the eyelids fuse by epithelial coalition. From this point on in time, the fetal period begins.

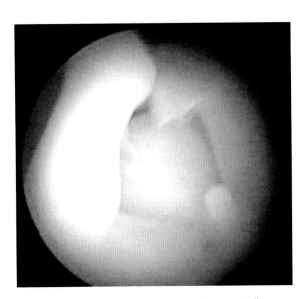

Figure 16.14: The external genitalia are totally defined since the 10th week

INDICATIONS FOR TRANSCERVICAL EMBRYOSCOPY

Morphological alterations are very difficult to observe and diagnose in the embryos between the fourth and the sixth week unless they are very evident, like if a sac is anembryonic or not.[18]

Philipp and Kalousek[19] described and documented a series of embryonic neural tube defects in 10 selected cases, concluding that embryoscopy is able to accurately diagnose development defects in cases of early pregnancy loss.

The embryo's morphology changes quickly. This process is very dynamic and, when correctly understood, allows to conclude that in some cases, when studying a detained pregnancy, some changes are observed in those embryos in which the only alteration seems to correspond to a delay of the development of just some corporal segments with regard to other segments of the same embryo or even compared with the development of other structures of the sac that have continued its development in spite of having a dead embryo, as is stated by Ferro,[20] pioneer of embryoscopy in Spain.

It is from 7th week on when a diagnosis of a craniofacial, branchial arches, vertebrae or limb defects can be observed. These alterations can be clearly demonstrated when dating the embryo or if all segments have developed synchronously.[21] There are other morphological alterations with a well-described presentation like myelomeningocele, anencephaly, encephalocele, leporine lip, palatine fissure, polydactyly, the cord cysts and the evident pathologies beginning at week 7-8.[22]

There is no doubt of the value of TE in twin or multiple gestations in which the technique allows to obtain independent samples of each of the embryos and membranes.[23]

An interesting field with research and diagnostic applications is legal pregnancy termination. A report by Greco et al[24] on endoscopic examination of the fetus in early gestation, suggests this procedure. In the near future, this technique could become the preferred examination to accurately solve diagnostic doubts. At present, the sonographic diagnosis of embryonic anomalies in early gestations, especially those below week 10 is not possible.

TE in cases of missed abortion could thus reveal morphological abnormalities undetectable by TVUS,[25] increasing the diagnoses spectrum and posterior evaluation of the pregnancy loss. This technique could establish a favorably characterized cohort of abortion specimens with seemingly normal chromosomes as a starting point for extensive detailed genetic studies. Such studies are needed to reach a better understanding of the embryopathogenesis and, consequently early pregnancy loss.

It is still debatable if TE and cytogenetic studies should be offered to every woman with missed abortion. These examinations provide etiologic data, but it is an invasive procedure and extra costs are required in addressing a condition with a low recurrence risk rate. However, a detailed embryoscopic examination of the deceased embryo could prove to be useful in couples suffering recurrent abortion. In these cases, chromosomic analysis is generally recommended.[26] TE could be indicated prior to the D&C in these patients to carry out chromosomic analysis in order to achieve a better understanding and diagnosis of the aetiology of this entity. It is important to remember that independent samples of the embryo and villosities must be performed since, as stated in many studies, chromosomic discrepancies between fetus and placenta may exist.[27] These biopsies will be able to be studied in morphological, cytogenetic and immuno-histochemical research. Another potential application for the TE is the chorionic villous sampling under direct visual control. Some authors explore this possibility suggesting that the number of abortions equals that produced in the classical ultrasonographic CVS, but the number of inconclusive diagnosis or placental mosaicisms is reduced.[28]

TE may be used to collect umbilical cord blood for confirmation of genetic diseases. It may also allow the potential of isolating fetal mesenchymal stem cell in first trimester.[29]

CONCLUSION

TE is a fascinating endoscopic technique that has broadened our understanding of the first days of human life. The data obtained from this procedure, along with other examinations will help us better understand, now and in the future, which pathology is important for our patients' reproductive future. TE opens up a little known inner world that can also enrich our scientific knowledge with minimal consequences for the patient.

REFERENCES

1. Tariverdian G, Paul M. Genetische Diagnostik in Geburtshilfe und Gynaekologie. Ein Leitfaden für Klinik und Praxis. Springer-Verlag, Heidelberg, 1999;191-4.
2. Kalousek DK. Anatomical and chromosomal abnormalities in specimens of early spontaneous abortions: Seven years experience. Birth Defects 1987;23:153-68.
3. Warburton D, Kline J, Stein Z, Hutzler M, Chin A, Hassold T. Does the Karyotype of a spontaneous abortion predict the karyotype of a subsequent abortion? Evidence from 273 women with two cariotipod spontaneous abortions. Am J Hum Genet 1987;41:465-83.
4. Westin B. Hysteroscopy in early pregnancy. Lancet 1954;267:872.
5. Agüero O, Aure M, López R. Hysteroscopy in pregnant patients: A new diagnostic tool. Am J Obstet Gynecol 1966;94:925-8.
6. Valenti C. Endoamnioscopy and fetal biopsy. Am J Obstet Gynecol 1972;141:561-4.
7. Gallinat A, Lueken RP, Lindemann HJ. A preliminary report about transcervical EC. Endoscopy 1978;10:47-50.
8. Cullen MT, Reece EA, Whetham J, Hobbins JC. EC: Description and utility of a new technique. Am J Obstet Gynecol 1990;162:82-6.
9. Ghirardini G. EC: old technique new for the 1990s? Am J Obstet Gynecol 1991;164:1361-2.
10. Reece EA, Whetham J, Rotmensch S, Wiznitzer A. Gaining access to the embryonic-fetal circulation via first-trimester endoscopy: A step into the future. Obstet Gynecol 1993;82:876-9.
11. Cullen MT, Whetham J, Viscarello RR, Reece EA, Sanchez-Ramos L, Hobbins JC. Transcervical endoscopic verification of congenital anomalies in the second trimester of pregnancy. Am J Obstet Gynecol 1991;165:95-7.
12. Dumez Y, Mandelbort L, Dommergues M. Embryoscopy in continuing pregnancies. In: Evian (Ed): Proceedings of the annual meeting of the international fetal medicine society. France 1992.
13. Quintero RA, Romero R, Mahoney MJ, Abuhamad A, Vecchio M, Holden J, Hobbins JC. Embryoscopic demonstration of hemorrhagic lesions on the human embryo after placental trauma. Am J Obstet Gynecol 1993;168:756-9.
14. Yin CS, Liu JY, Yu MH. Transcervical flexible endoscopy for first trimester embryonic/fetal evaluation. Int J Gynaecol Obstet 1996;54:149-53.
15. Filly RA. Appropriate use of ultrasound in early pregnancy. Radiology 1988;166:274-5.
16. Carnegie JA, McCully ME, Robertson HA. The early development of the sheep trophoblast and the involvement of cell death. Am J Anat 1985;174:471-88.
17. O'Rahilly R, Müller F. Developmental stages in human embryos. Washington DC Carnegie Instn Publ 1987.
18. Philipp T, Kalousek DK. Neural tube defects in missed abortions: Embryoscopic and cytogenetic findings. Am J Med Genet 2002;107:52-7.
19. Philipp T, Kalousek DK. Amnion rupture sequence in a first trimester missed abortion. Prenat Diagn 2001;21:835-8.
20. Ferro J, Martinez MC, Lara C, Pellicer A, Remohi J, Serra V. Improved accuracy of hysteroembryoscopic biopsies for karyotyping early missed abortions. Fertil Steril 2003;80:1260-4.
21. Yin CS, Chen WH, Wei RY, Chan CC. Transcervical embryoscopic diagnosis of conjoined twins in a ten-week missed abortion. Prenat Diagn 1998;18:626-8.
22. Philipp T, Kalousek DK. Generalized abnormal embryonic development in missed abortion: Embryoscopic and cytogenetic findings. Am J Med Genet 2002;111:43-7.
23. Philipp T, Philipp K, Reiner A, Beer F, Kalousek DK. Embryoscopic and cytogenetic analysis of 233 missed abortions: Factors involved in the pathogenesis of developmental defects of early failed pregnancies. Hum Reprod 2003;8:1724-32.
24. Greco P, Vimercati A, Bettochi S, Loverro G, Selvati L. Endoscopic examination of the fetus in early pregnancy. J Perinat Med 2000;20:190-3.
25. Blaas HG. The examination of the embryo and early fetus: How and by whom? Ultrasound Obstet Gynecol 1999;14:153-8.
26. Wolf GC, Horger EO. Indication for examination of spontaneous abortion specimens: A reassessment. Am J Obstet Gynecol 1995;5:1364-7.
27. Petracchi F, Colaci DS, Igarzabal L, Gadow E. Cytogenetic analysis of first trimester pregnancy loss. Int J Obstet Gynecol 2009;68:243-4.
28. Nordenskjold F, Gustavii B. Direct-vision chorionic villi biopsy for prenatal diagnosis in the first trimester. J Reprod Med 1984;29:572-4.
29. Chan BC, Hui PW, Leung WC, Leung KY, Pun TC, Lee CP. Application of transcervical hysterofetoscopy and cord blood collection at first trimester termination of pregnancy for fetal anomalies. Prenat Diagn 2008;28:939-42.

17

Hysteroscopic Treatment of Intrauterine Adhesions

Rafael F Valle

Intrauterine adhesions are scars that result from trauma to a recently pregnant uterus. In over 90% of the cases, they are caused by curettage. Usually the trauma has occurred because of excessive bleeding requiring curettage 1-4 weeks after delivery of a term or preterm pregnancy, or an abortion. During this vulnerable phase of the endometrium any trauma may denude or remove the basalis endometrium causing the uterine walls to coapt each other and form a permanent bridge, distorting the symmetry of the uterine cavity.[1-3] In rare circumstances, conditions such as abdominal metroplasty or abdominal myomectomies may cause intrauterine adhesions, but these adhesions are usually due to misplaced sutures rather than the true coaptation of denuded areas of myometrium that occurs following postpartum or postabortal curettage. The type and consistency of these adhesions varies; some are focal, some extensive, some mild and filmy, and some thickened and dense, with extensive fibromuscular or connective tissue components. The extent and type of uterine cavity occlusion correlates well with the extent of trauma during the vulnerable phase of the endometrium following a recent pregnancy. Fibrosis usually follows the longevity and duration of these adhesions, the adhesions become thickened and dense and formed by connective tissue.

Intrauterine adhesions frequently result in menstrual abnormalities, such as hypomenorrhea or even amenorrhea, depending upon the extent of uterine cavity occlusion. Patients with long-standing intrauterine adhesions may also develop dysmenorrhea. Over 75% of women with moderate and severe adhesions will have either amenorrhea or hypomenorrhea.[4]

DIAGNOSIS

The most important clue to the diagnosis of intrauterine adhesions is a history of trauma to the endometrial cavity, particularly following a delivery or an abortion. Secondary to that it is a history of amenorrhea or hypomenorrhea. Because intrauterine adhesions are not related to hormonal events, an intact hypothalamic-pituitary-ovarian-axis should result in a biphasic basal body temperature curve, suggesting

ovulation; failure to withdraw from a progesterone challenge test in a patient with amenorrhea will strengthen the diagnosis. Uterine sounding has been used to assess obstruction of the internal cervical os, but this test should be abandoned, because of the increased danger of uterine perforation as well as inaccuracy of diagnosis. The most useful screening test for intrauterine adhesions is a hysterosalpingogram. It provides evaluation of the internal cervical os and uterine cavity; delineation of the adhesions, and information about the condition of the rest of the uterine cavity, if adhesions do not completely occlude this area. Hysterosalpingography is useful in determining the extent of uterine cavity occlusion, but it cannot provide an appraisal of the consistency and type of intrauterine adhesions. For this reason, hysteroscopy becomes a useful adjunct to hysterosalpingography by confirming the extent and type of intrauterine adhesions.

METHODS OF TREATMENT

Treatment of intrauterine adhesions is surgical, consisting of removing these adhesions by division. In the past, blind methods of division were used with curettes, probes or dilators, or hysterotomy-assisted division of these adhesions under direct vision. These techniques have failed to produce acceptable results and have been largely abandoned. Introduction of modern hysteroscopy has permitted transcervical division of the adhesions under visual guidance; hysteroscopic methods have used mechanical means, such as hysteroscopic semi-rigid scissors, the resectoscope, fiberoptic lasers, and of late, bipolar vaporizing electrodes.

Because intrauterine adhesions in general are avascular they can be divided and not removed, results have been similar to that of division of a uterine septum. The adhesions are divided centrally, allowing the uterine cavity to expand upon division of the adhesions. This is performed utilizing flexible, semi-rigid, and occasionally rigid or optical scissors. The most commonly used method is with the semi-rigid hysteroscopic scissors because of the increased facility in manipulating the scissors and by selectively dividing these adhesions that retract upon cutting.

Occasionally, thick connective tissue adhesions are present and form very thick stumps, and they benefit not only from division but also from removal. This is particularly true at the lateral uterine walls and the uterotubal cones. To achieve these goals a sharp punch biopsy forceps sometimes becomes most useful to divide and remove these types of adhesions. If electrosurgical methods are used, it is preferable to use thin, sharp electrodes through the operating channel of the hysteroscope than the resectoscope. The resectoscope which in general is 9 mm in diameter becomes a cumbersome tool in these contracted and shrunken uterine cavities, particularly if extensive adhesions are encountered and the electrical energy may unnecessarily damage the already denuded and damaged peripheral endometrium that will be the reservoir for subsequent re-epithelialization. While this peripheral scattering may be reduced with the utilization of fiberoptic lasers, also, this phenomenon should be taken into consideration when lasers are elected as a tool for dividing the adhesions, to use those fiber lasers of the sculpted or sharpened type, to avoid peripheral scattering. Similar precautions should be taken when using vaporizing electrodes (FIGURES 17.1 to 17.6).

The advantages of using hysteroscopic scissors for the division of intrauterine adhesions are those of mechanical methods. Mechanical tools provide excellent landmarks when dividing these adhesions,

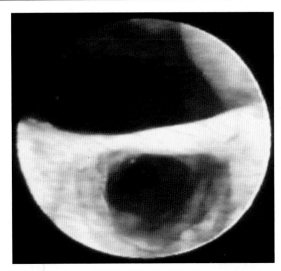

Figure 17.2: Lower segment fibrous adhesions distorting the uterine cavity's symmetry

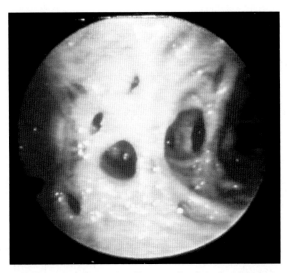

Figure 17.3: Extensive fibrous adhesions involving a large portion of the uterine cavity

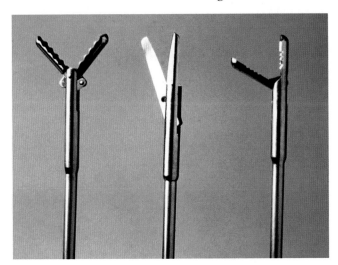

Figure 17.1: Semi-rigid 7-f hysteroscopic instruments (left to right: Grasping forceps, sharp and pointed scissors, cup biopsy forceps)

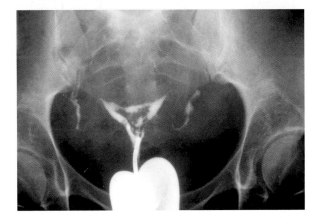

Figure 17.4: Hysterosalpingogram shows extensive central intrauterine adhesions

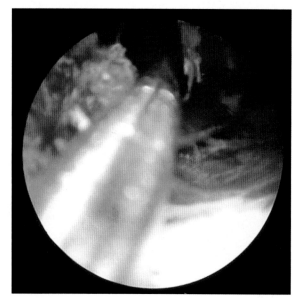

Figure 17.5: Hysteroscopic division of the adhesions from the internal cervical os

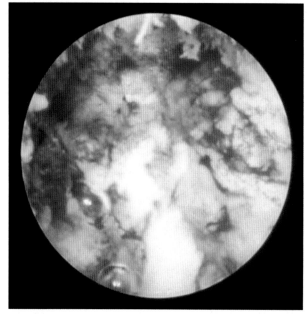

Figure 17.6: Following lysis of adhesions, the uterine cavity achieves symmetry

endometrium can be found when extensive intrauterine adhesions are present. The disadvantages are that it may be sometimes difficult to manipulate semi-rigid instrumentation, particularly to the lateral walls of the uterine cavity (FIGURES 17.7 to 17.12). Scissors do not provide the sharpness of mechanism to cut these adhesions, as the scissors do not close uniformly at their distal tip and need to be readjusted and sharpened frequently.[5,6]

The treatment of severe intrauterine adhesions remains a challenge and several methods have been suggested in an attempt to improve the therapeutic

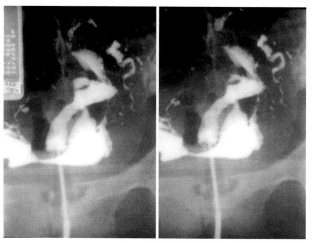

Figure 17.7: A semi-lunar shaped adhesion at the right cornu is seen on hysterosalpingogram.

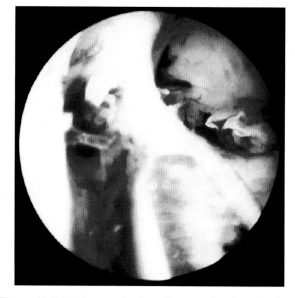

Figure 17.8: Hysteroscopic view of same adhesion with tip of scissors reaching the adhesion.

particularly when approaching the juxtaposed myometrium. Bleeding may be observed at the myometrial junction and this warns the hysteroscopist to stop the dissection, so as to avoid perforation. No scattering of energy is produced to damage the small areas of healthy endometrium which are the reservoir for future re-epithelialization. This is an important consideration, because no extensive healthy

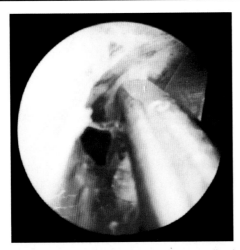

Figure 17.9: Hysteroscopic lysis of the adhesion

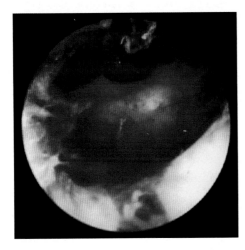

Figure 17.10: Following hysteroscopic treatment, the uterine cavity's symmetry has been re-established

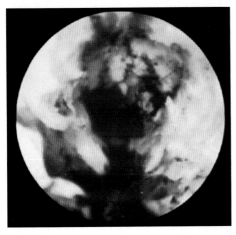

Figure 17.11: After initial hysteroscopic lysis of severe and extensive intrauterine adhesions some remaining stumps of the divided adhesions can be seen

results, such as concomitant fluoroscopy or sonography, transfundal uterine injection of dyes, coaxial injection of radiopaque materials, vital dyes to distinguish fibrous adhesions from residual endometrium, endometrial electrosurgical scoring, blind lateral sounding of the uterine cavity between myometrium and adhesions for conversion to a "septum" division, and hysterotomy for transfundal dissection of the adhesions. However, all these procedures have been attempted in few patients and their efficacy and safety has not been consistently and definitely confirmed.[7-15]

POSTOPERATIVE ADJUNCTIVE THERAPY

The principle of therapy is to remove the adhesions surgically. Because most of these patients have a sclerotic or destroyed endometrium, they need other adjunctive therapy to promote re-epithelialization and also a temporary mechanical separation of the uterine walls to prevent reformation of adhesions. These adjuncts are intrauterine splints, prophylactic antibiotics, and estrogens and progesterone to promote re-epithelialization.

Prophylactic antibiotics are given preoperatively, with cephalosporins or doxycycline and when a uterine splint is left in the uterine cavity for a week, and then the prophylaxis should extend for one week to avoid possible infection. While there are different splints that can be used for this purpose, in the form of IUDs or balloons, a pediatric number 8 Foley catheter with a trimmed tip and inflated with 3-3.5 ml of sterile saline becomes most useful. Once in place it is wrapped with sterile gauze and attached to the side of the patient and she is taught how to take care of this catheter to avoid cross contamination. At the conclusion of seven days of wearing, she removes the catheter by cutting the distal portion allowing the fluid to escape. Natural conjugated estrogens in the form of Premarin 2.5 mg twice a day for 30-40 days are used to stimulate endometrial re-epithelialization and progesterone 10 mg during the last ten days is added to allow withdrawal bleeding. Upon completion of the hormonal therapy, and once withdrawal bleeding has ceased, a hysterosalpingogram is performed to observe the results of the operation and decide upon further therapy or initiation of attempts for conception. Those patients with initial filmy, focal adhesions may not require hysterosalpingography but an in-office hysteroscopy to assess uterine cavity symmetry.

Results of Therapy

The results of hysteroscopic treatment of intrauterine adhesions have correlated well with the extent of uterine cavity occlusion and the type of adhesions present. Normal menstruation is restored in over 90% of the patients. Therapeutic outcome correlates well with the type of adhesions and extent of uterine cavity occlusion. Of 187 patients treated hysteroscopically by Valle and Sciarra, removal of mild, filmy adhesions in 43 cases gave the best results, with 35(81%) term pregnancies; in 97 moderate cases of fibromuscular adhesions, 64(66%) term pregnancies occurred, and in 47 severe cases of connective tissue adhesions, 65 (32%) term pregnancies occurred. Overall restoration of menses occurred in 90% of the patients, and the overall term pregnancy rate was 79.7%. These results demonstrate a much better reproductive outcome than was previously obtained with blind methods of therapy[3] (TABLE 17.1).

DIAGNOSIS AND CLASSIFICATION

Reproductive outcome seems to correlate well with the type of adhesions present and the extent of uterine cavity occlusion. It is useful to have a way of classifying these adhesions as filmy and composed of endometrial tissue, moderate or fibromuscular, and severe or composed of connective tissue. The degree of uterine cavity occlusion also is important. Attempts to classify intrauterine adhesions by hysterosalpingography alone give a good appraisal of the extent of uterine cavity occlusion, but it is impossible to determine by hysterosalpingography alone the type of adhesions that are present. When using hysteroscopy alone, it is difficult to assess the extent of uterine cavity occlusion by visualization, because the access of the hysteroscopist is from the cervix to the fundus, and not perpendicular to the uterine body, as hysterography is, outlining in the

Table 17.1: Reproductive performance after treatment of intrauterine adhesions (1298 patients from 15 reports)*

	Number of patients (%)
• Normal menses	1060 (87.5)
• Pregnancy	718 (72.3)
• Term pregnancy	603 (87.2)

*Valle RF. Intrauterine Adhesions: A Review. December, 2000.

uterine cavity from a different axis. For this reason, the combination of hysterosalpingography and hysteroscopy has been used most commonly to assess not only the extent of uterine cavity occlusion, but also the type of adhesions found by hysteroscopy at the time of treatment. Valle and Sciarra utilized a three stage classification of the extent and severity of intrauterine adhesions (mild, moderate, and severe), based on the degree of involvement shown on hysterosalpingography, and the extent and type of adhesions found on hysteroscopy. Three stages of intrauterine adhesions are defined:

Mild Adhesions

Filmy adhesions composed of basalis endometrial tissue producing partial or complete uterine cavity occlusion (FIGURE 17.12B).

Moderate Adhesions

Fibromuscular, characteristically thick, still covered with endometrium that may bleed upon division, which partially or totally occlude the uterine cavity (FIGURE 17.12C).

Severe Adhesions

Composed of connective tissue only, lacking any endometrial lining and not likely to bleed upon division. These adhesions may partially or totally occlude the uterine cavity[3] (Figure 17.12D).

Recently the American Fertility Society (now the American Society for Reproductive Medicine) has proposed a classification of intrauterine adhesions based on the findings of hysterosalpingography and hysteroscopy, and their correlation with menstrual patterns. The classification in four stages is based on assigned points for each stage. Using a uniform

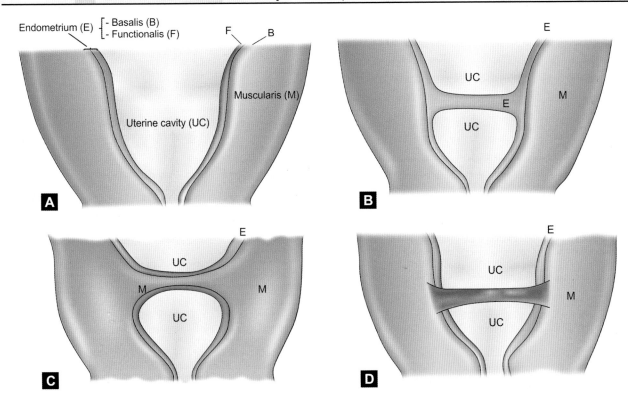

Figures 17.12A to D: Diagrammatic representations of normal endometrial layers and types of intrauterine adhesions: (A) Normal endometrium; (B) Endometrial adhesion, filmy; (C) Fibromuscular adhesion, dense; (D) Connective tissue adhesion, thick and lacking endometrium

classification for intrauterine adhesions greatly enhances our ability to report, evaluate and compare results of different treatments of intrauterine adhesions, particularly when utilizing these variables following the hysteroscopic approach.[16]

The treatment of intrauterine adhesions can be accomplished by four different techniques: Scissors, resectoscope, fiber optic lasers, and bipolar vaporizing electrodes. All have advantages and disadvantages that must be used with knowledge of each particular technology and its drawbacks. Each technique should be tailored not only to the anatomy and etiology of each process, but also to the experience and knowledge of the operator. The operator should select the appropriate method and technique for each patient. The results of therapy should be a successful pregnancy for those patients with impaired reproduction, keeping in mind the safety of the patient with the least morbidity possible, absence of complications and the overall effectiveness and diminution of unnecessary cost. Versatility plays a significant role in the selection of therapeutic alternatives, the surgeon has to intelligently select the best method for each individual patient.

CONCLUSION

Intrauterine adhesions may impair reproductive function. Prevention and early diagnosis remain important factors in the avoidance and successful treatment of the adhesions when they occur. Because these adhesions or scars usually form following trauma to the uterine cavity, particularly curettage following a delivery or an abortion, when these procedures are required to explore or empty the uterine cavity, utmost care must be exercised to do that gently and, if needed, using suction devices rather than metal curettes to diminish undue trauma to the endometrial lining. Patients who develop menstrual abnormalities following trauma to a recently pregnant uterus need to be evaluated promptly to rule out intrauterine adhesions and, if present, a plan of therapy established.

The hysteroscopic treatment of intrauterine adhesions should be considered the standard treatment for this condition and selection of the specific method of hysteroscopic treatment must be done according to individual experience, and extent and type of intrauterine adhesions present.

REFERENCES

1. Asherman JG. Traumatic intrauterine adhesions. J Obstet Gynaecol Br Emp 1950;57:892-6.
2. Klein SM, Garcia CR. Asherman's syndrome: A critique and current review. Fertil Steril 1973;24:722-35.
3. Valle RF, Sciarra JJ. Intrauterine adhesions: Hysteroscopic diagnosis classification, treatment and reproductive outcome. Am J Obstet Gynecol 1988;158:1459-70.
4. Schenker JG, Margalioth EJ. Intrauterine adhesions: An updated appraisal. Fertil Steril 1982;37:593-610.
5. Valle RF. Lysis of Intrauterine Adhesions (Asherman's Syndrome). In: Sutton C, Diamond M (Eds): Endoscopic Surgery for Gynaecologists. WB Saunders Company Ltd., London, Philadelphia, Toronto, Sydney, Tokyo. 1993;338-44.
6. Valle RF. Intrauterine Adhesions (Asherman's Syndrome). In: Marty R, Blanc B, deMontgolfier R (Eds): Office and Operative Hysteroscopy. Springer-Verlag, France, Paris, Berlin, Heidelberg: New York, 2002;229-42.
7. Thomson AJM, Abbott JA, Kingston A, Lenart M, Vancaillie TG. Fluoroscopically guided synechiolysis for patients with Asherman's syndrome: Menstrual and fertility outcomes. Fertil Steril 2007;87:405-10.
8. McComb PF, Wagner BL. Simplified therapy for Asherman's syndrome. Fertil Steril 1997;68:1047-50.
9. Protopapas A, Shusham A, Magos A. Myometrial scoring: A new technique for management of severe Asherman's syndrome. Fertil Steril 1998;69:860-4.
10. Reddy S, Rock JA Surgical management of complete obliteration of the endometrial cavity. Fertil Steril 1997;67:172-4.
11. Fernandez H, Al-Najjar A, Chauveaud-Lambling A, Frydman R, Gervaise A. Fertility after treatment of Asherman's syndrome stage 3 and 4. J Minim Invasive Gynecol 2006; 13:398-402.
12. Abbott J, Thomson A, Vancaillie TG. Spray gel following surgery for Asherman's syndrome may improve pregnancy outcome. J Obstet Gynaecol 2004;24:710-1.
13. Robinson JK, Colimon LM, Isaacson KB. Postoperative adhesiolysis therapy for intrauterine adhesions (Asherman's syndrome). Fertil Steril 2008;90:409-14.
14. Yu D, Li TC, Xia E, Huang Y, Liu Y, Peng X. Factors affecting reproductive outcome of hysteroscopic adhesiolysis for Asherman's syndrome. Fertil Steril 2008; 89:715-22.
15. Yu D, Wong YM, Cheong Y, Xia E, Li TC. Asherman's syndrome-one century later. Fertil Steril 2008;89:755-79.
16. The American Fertility Society: Classifications of adnexal adhesions, distal tubal occlusion, tubal occlusion secondary to tubal ligation, tubal pregnancies, Mullerian anomalies and intrauterine adhesions. Fertil Steril 1988; 49:944-55.

18

Anesthesia in Hysteroscopy

Teresa Tijero
Marta De Vicente

INTRODUCTION

Hysteroscopy is a widely used technique in diagnosis and treatment of diverse gynecological conditions. Technical advances in hysteroscopes and the use of the appropriate distension media have allowed an increase in number and variety of indications. Almost all the diagnostic hysteroscopies are performed in office, without the presence of an anesthesiologist, whereas most of the operative hysteroscopies are performed in an ambulatory setting, provided that selection criteria for ambulatory surgery and anesthesia are met.

When anesthesia is required, different anesthetic techniques adapt to the range of interventions and to patient preferences,[1] from local anesthesia supplemented or not with sedation[2] to regional or general anesthesia.[3]

Hysteroscopy is a relatively safe procedure, but the possibility of complications is always present (more in the operative hysteroscopy than in the diagnostic one). It is the anesthesiologist's duty the early recognition of complications and prompt intervention in order to prevent adverse sequelae.

INDICATIONS FOR ANESTHESIA IN HYSTEROSCOPY

A great number of diagnostic hysteroscopies and some operative ones can be performed without the need of anesthesia.[4] In the remaining interventions, some kind of anesthesia may be required due to factors related to the surgery or to the patient.

Related to Surgery

Operative hysteroscopy can be divided into three groups according to complexity (TABLE 18.1). Minor and intermediate surgery is generally office-based, with local anesthesia, mild sedation or without anesthesia, provided a correct patient selection and an experienced gynecologist. Major hysteroscopies are programmed in a day-surgery facility, under loco-regional or general anesthesia. The anesthetic technique depends on several factors: Type and duration of surgery, chosen surgical technique and instrumental, and surgeon's experience.[5]

Table 18.1: Classification of operative hysteroscopy according to complexity

Minor	Intermediate	Major
Guided biopsies	Tubal sterilization	Myomectomies
Small polypectomies	Tubal ostia canulization	Large polypectomies
Intrauterine dispositive extraction		Endometrial ablation / resection
Simple adhesiolysis		Resection of uterine septa Severe adhesiolysis

Type and Duration of Surgery

Hysteroscopic myomectomy and resection of uterine septum are associated with a greater risk of complications, especially excessive fluid absorption, whereas hysteroscopic polypectomy and endometrial ablation are less risky.[6] Regional anesthesia may be more appropriate in the former, because it allows early detection of signs and symptoms of dilutional hyponatremia and fluid overload. However, in a study comparing epidural versus general anesthesia there was significant less glycine absorption in the general anesthesia group.[3] General anesthesia may be preferable in short interventions to allow for a faster recovery, essential in day-case settings.

Surgical Technique and Instrumental

Although mechanical instruments are still used, more popular techniques consist of resection or ablation of intrauterine tissue with either electrodiathermy or laser, using a hysteroscope in conjunction with a distension fluid to permit clear visibility within the uterus. The use of laser is less practical due to the need to follow strict safety rules and regular maintenance. Electrosurgical devices can use monopolar or bipolar coagulation. The last one permits the use of electrolyte-containing distension media, and can be employed in patients with pacemakers.

The size of the hysteroscope is related to the degree of discomfort and can determine the type of anesthesia. Hysteroscopes with diameters of 5.5 mm or less permit manipulation within the uterine cavity with less cervical dilation, which is a recognized risk factor for procedure-associated pain, total resection failure, and complications such as cervical lacerations. Smaller instruments (e.g. a pediatric cystoscope) have been employed to improve patient compliance.[7] Regional or general anesthesia are necessary when using larger sizes that involve cervical dilation, because pain in hysteroscopy occurs with cervical os dilation and uterine cavity distension.[8]

Surgeon's Experience

Hysteroscopies done by general gynecologists have lower rates of surgical complications than those performed by other surgeons.[6] Therefore, surgeon's skills can influence the choice of anesthetic technique in favor of regional or general anesthesia that provide better operative conditions and are safer in case of complications.

Related to Patient

Pain and anxiety are influential factors in patient acceptability of outpatient hysteroscopy. History of vaginism, discomfort in previous hysteroscopies, nulliparity, or young age are factors that can determine the need of anesthesia, due to the high levels of anxiety as well as the existence of cervical stenosis in many of these patients.

Therefore, some women are likely to opt to undergo the procedure under general anesthesia. Other patients choose locoregional anesthesia, sedation or both, out of fear of general anesthesia or because they wish to watch the intervention on the video screen.

HYSTEROSCOPY SETTING

Outpatient or Ambulatory Setting

One possible definition of the term "ambulatory surgery" is the process by which surgical procedures that need simple postoperative care are carried out, under any type of anesthesia, without hospital admission.

Operative hysteroscopy belongs to the groups I and II of Davis' classification, and therefore fulfils the requirements to be included in ambulatory surgery programs (TABLE 18.2).[5] Still, there is great variability in the choice of treatment system

Table 18.2: Davis' classification of surgical procedures according to intensity

Type	Definition
I	Office-based procedure. No specific postoperative care
II	Surgical setting. Specific postoperative care
III	Surgical setting. Hospital postoperative care
IV	Surgical setting. Specialized postoperative care (e.g. intensive care)

(inpatient, outpatient, office-based) according to a national survey of gynecologists in UK.[9]

It is mandatory to have a preoperative assessment of patients scheduled for hysteroscopy in a surgical setting in order to decide their inclusion as outpatients. The aim is to minimize and control surgical and anesthetic risks, thus reducing the number of unplanned hospital admissions. A correct patient selection takes into account personal factors such as age, weight and ASA grade of anesthetic risk (TABLE 18.3) but, above all, a full comprehension and acceptance of the process, and a willingness to cooperate. There are also some social criteria to be met: An accompanying adult for the first postoperative for 24 hours, a private means of transport, adequate living conditions, hospital distance less than 1 hour, telephone.

The following groups of patients are generally excluded from ambulatory surgery: ASA groups IV and V, morbid obesity, coagulopathies, risk of malignant hyperthermia, hemoglobinopathies, drug

Table 18.3: Preoperative physical status classification of patients according to the American Society of Anesthesiologists

Class	Definition
I	A normal healthy patient
II	A patient with mild systemic disease and no functional limitations
III	A patient with moderate to severe systemic disease that result in some functional limitation
IV	A patient with severe systemic disease that is a constant threat to life and functionally incapacitating
V	A moribund patient who is not expected to survive 24 hours with or without surgery
VI	A brain-dead patient whose organs are being harvested
E	If the procedure is an emergency, the physical status is followed by "E"

addictions, active infections, severe psychiatric or psychomotor disorders, and extremes of age.[10]

Office Setting

Diagnostic hysteroscopy is routinely performed in office, without anesthesia in most cases. Office-based operative hysteroscopy is feasible in selected patients, with a success rate of up to 80-90% of cases. Factors related to an improved rate of resection are multiparity, absence of intense pelvic pain, and small polyp size. Anesthetic paracervical block does not consistently increase the rate of resection,[11] although success rate may be higher when some form of analgesia (nonsteroidal anti-inflammatory drugs) or anesthesia (locoregional techniques) is employed, since pain, together with cervical stenosis and poor view have been implied as reasons for failure.[12]

ANESTHETIC TECHNIQUES

The ideal anesthesia for operative and diagnostic hysteroscopy should provide good surgical conditions without discomfort to the patient, and should seek to minimize complications by allowing early detection of fluid overload and hyponatremia.

Diagnostic or minor operative hysteroscopy can be carried out using various forms of anesthesia, ranging from no anesthesia,[4] topical and local anesthesia infiltration and paracervical block. These techniques do not require the presence of an anesthesiologist unless associated to intravenous sedation. Regional or general anesthesia are required for those who cannot tolerate the procedure otherwise, and in most operative hysteroscopies. In all cases, it is recommended that remote and near premeditation be given, the night before and 1 hour before the procedure, with a short half-life benzodiazepine (e.g. midazolam).

Patient monitoring for all operative hysteroscopies, and for those diagnostic ones in which any form of anesthesia is administered, includes electrocardiography (ECG), arterial oxygen saturation ($Sat O_2$), and non-invasive blood pressure (NIBP). Oceanography (end-tidal carbon dioxide concentration) is necessary in general anesthesia, and whenever CO_2 is used as a distending medium. In high-risk patients (cardiopulmonary or renal disease), control of central venous pressure (CVP) may be necessary for the early diagnosis and treatment of fluid overload.

Locoregional Anesthesia

It is the temporary loss of painful stimuli from a part of the body by effect of local anesthetic blockade (TABLE 18.4) on nerve endings. Local anesthetics can be applied over mucous membranes (topical anesthesia), by a subcutaneous injection (infiltrative anesthesia), over a bundle of nerves conforming a plexus or a ganglion (paracervical block) or administered within the spinal canal, into the subarachnoid space (spinal anesthesia) or into the epidural space (epidural anesthesia).[13]

Neuroanatomy of the Uterus and Cervix

The uterus and cervix are supplied by nociceptive afferents that pass to the spinal cord by accompanying sympathetic nerves in the inferior, middle and superior hypogastric plexus. They pass through the lumbar and lower thoracic sympathetic chain and enter the spinal cord through the posterior nerve roots of T10-L1. Frankenhäuser's ganglia contain all the visceral sensory nerves originating from the uterus, cervix and upper vagina. Parasympathetic innervation is not thought to be important in the mediation of uterine and cervical pain. The pudendal nerve (S2-4) supplies the vagina and the perineum.[14]

Table 18.4: Maximum recommended doses of more commonly used local anesthetics

	Lidocaíne	Prilocaíne	Mepivacaíne	Bupivacaíne	Ropivacaíne	Levobupivacaíne
Maximum safe dose (mg/kg)	4	6	5	2	2-2.3	2
Maximum safe dose with vasoconstrictor (mg/kg)	7	10	7	2.5	2-2.3	2-2.5
Toxic threshold (mg/ml)	5-6	7-9	5-6	1.6	–	–
Seizure-provoking dose (mg/kg)	14.2	18.1	18.8	4.4	4.9	5

Topical Anesthesia

This technique is performed over cervix and uterine cavity and it has been reported to reduce pain and attenuate vasovagal reactions. Different topical anesthetics have been used: Lidocaine gel and spray, benzocaine 20% gel, mepivacaine and tetracaine solution, cocaine spray, etc. but the best-studied is EMLA (an eutectic mixture of lidocaine 2.5% and prilocaine 2.5%), which is well tolerated and provides good pain relief for procedures involving the surface tissues, and also diminishes the discomfort of local anesthetic injection.[15]

Paracervical and Intracervical Block and Infiltrative Anesthesia

Paracervical block is the most frequently used anesthetic technique by surgeons in diagnostic or operative hysteroscopy, associated or not to intracervical and intrauterine infiltration (FIGURE 18.1).

Before the cervix is dilated, local anesthetic is injected with a 18-20 Gauge spinal needle, submucosally (2-3 mm deep) in the vagina at the level of uterosacral ligaments (paracervical) (FIGURES 18.2 and 18.3) or on either side of the cervix at the 3 and 9 o'clock positions (intracervical) (FIGURES 18.4 and 18.5). Optionally, more local anesthetic may be injected into the substance of the cervix and in 10-15 points into the myometrium to a depth of 1 cm around the uterine fundus and cornua, because these are the least

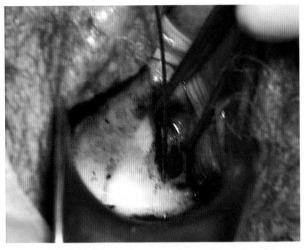

Figure 18.2: Left side paracervical injection. Note the white area reflecting the submucosal location of the local anesthetic

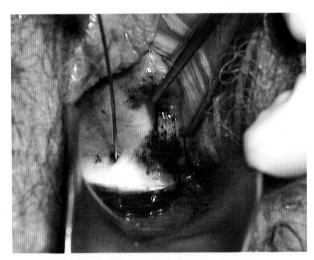

Figure 18.3: Right side paracervical injection

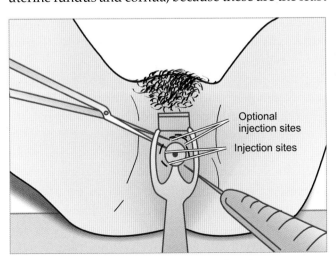

Figure 18.1: Local anesthetic injection sites for paracervical block

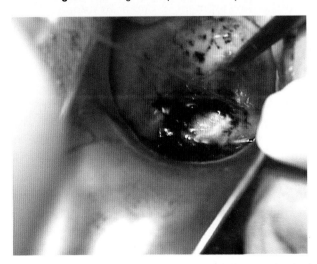

Figure 18.4: Left side intracervical injection. At least a depth of 2 cm is needed to achieve a correct analgesia

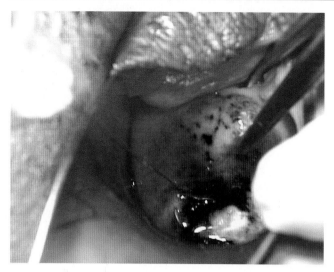

Figure 18.5: Right side intracervical injection

anesthetized areas by the cervical block. The uterus and cervix are rich in blood vessels and aspiration should always be performed to prevent intravascular injection.[16] The most commonly used local anesthetic is 1% lignocaine with 1:200000 epinephrine (30 to 40 ml).

Regional Anesthesia

The use of spinal anesthesia in day case surgery has grown in detriment of epidural anesthesia in part due to the combinations of short-acting local anesthetics and opioids and nonopioids which provide early postoperative ambulation and discharge, as well as to the development of small atraumatic needles (pencil-point) that have contributed to significantly reduce the incidence of postspinal headache and its severity, which would make it feasible to be treated without need of admission.[14]

For short procedures such as diagnostic hysteroscopy, hyperbaric lidocaine historically has been popular, but reports of cauda equina syndrome and transient radicular irritation symptoms related to lidocaine have contraindicated its use. Mepivacaine can provide a short acting alternative, while bupivacaine offers a longer-lasting one. Transient radicular irritation symptoms are rare with these drugs.

Advantages of regional anesthesia over general anesthesia are: A better recovery in the immediate postoperative period (lower incidence of post-operative nausea and vomiting, shivering, cognitive dysfunction and somnolence), early detection of signs and symptoms of dilutional hyponatremia and fluid overload, less surgical stress, and more residual analgesia in the immediate postoperative period.

However, regional anesthesia has some disadvantages such as the possibility of urinary retention and hypotension due to the sympathetic block, postdural puncture headache, slow block recovery (a drawback in outpatient surgery), and a very low incidence of prolonged neurological damage. Also, it is important to take into account that regional anesthesia does not abolish the obturator reflex (external rotation and leg adduction, secondary to obturator nerve stimulation by electrocautery current passing through the lateral uterine wall). That reflex is only reliably blocked by using muscle relaxants during general anesthesia.

Absolute contraindications for regional anesthesia are: Patient refusal, local anesthetic allergy (very rare in the amide group) and local infection in the injection site or signs of bacteriemia. Some relative contraindications are coagulopathy, psychiatric disorders (due to lack of cooperation with the technique), aortic stenosis and lumbar spine alterations.[17]

Sedation

The term "monitored anesthesia care" refers to monitoring the patient during a procedure performed with local anesthesia administered by the surgeon, supplemented or not with intravenous sedation by the anesthesiologist.

The objective of supplemental medication is to induce sedation and anxiolysis during the surgical procedure, and to provide additional analgesia for the minor discomforts that occur even with a successful local anesthetic block. Thus, patient's satisfaction with local anesthetic techniques can be greatly increased.[18]

Sedative drugs for hysteroscopy should have a short onset and duration of action and few side effects. A favorable cost-effectiveness ratio is also desirable. Benzodiazepines such as midazolam, the hypnotic propofol, and opioids such as fentanyl and alfentanyl can be used. Inhalation analgesia is also possible, with agents such as nitrous oxide[2] or sevoflurane. Medication can be administered by intravenous bolus or by a continuous pump infusion, controlled by the anesthesiologist or by the patient.[19] When carbon dioxide is used as a distension medium the use of nitrous oxide is not recommended due to its high solubility in blood, which might worsen the clinical consequences of an air embolism by increasing the size of the gas bubble.

General Anesthesia

The basic components of general anesthesia are hypnosis, amnesia, analgesia and, when necessary, muscle relaxation. Generally, these effects are provided by several combined drugs, inhaled or intravenously administered.

Monitoring is helpful in the early diagnosis of complications such as uterine perforation or air embolism, as well as essential in the control of a general anesthetic technique. Apart from the routine monitoring (done previously), measuring depth of anesthesia is now possible with the bispectral index (BIS), a numeric value derived from bispectral analysis of the electroencephalogram. It has potential clinical and economic applications, such as avoidance of intraoperative awareness, reduction of recovery times by better drug titration, and cost reductions by accurate drug titration and by improving out-patient units performances through earlier patient discharge.

Medication

In short ambulatory hysteroscopies, general anesthesia using short-acting agents may be indicated as an alternative to regional anesthesia, which has longer discharge times. The ideal general anesthetic in ambulatory surgery should provide a rapid onset, adequate intraoperative amnesia and analgesia, optimal surgical conditions, a predictable effect in intensity and duration, a fast recovery with none or few adverse effects, and a good cost-effectiveness ratio.

Anesthetic induction can be intravenous with propofol, or inhalational with sevoflurane. The use of intravenous induction is more extended, and preferred by adults. Anesthesia can be maintained with oxygen/air or oxygen/nitrous oxide, and an inhalational agent (sevoflurane, desflurane) or a propofol infusion, but total intravenous anesthesia (TIVA) with oxygen/air and a propofol infusion may be preferable because it is a technique associated to less postoperative nausea and vomiting (PONV).

An opioid is added to provide analgesia. Although fentanyl remains the most frequently used opioid, the role of remifentanyil in hysteroscopy has been investigated. Remifentanil has unique pharmaco-kinetic characteristics with potential applications in outpatient anesthesia. Its properties are minimally altered by extremes of age or renal or hepatic dys-function, and its context-sensitive halftime (the time required for the drug's plasma concentration to decrease by 50% after stopping its infusion) is very short, which permits a rapid recovery from anesthesia.[20] That advantage can turn into an inconvenience if the treatment of postoperative pain is not anticipated, but hysteroscopy is a relatively painless procedure, and a NSAID administration before emergency can provide adequate postoperative analgesia. High costs of drug and continuous infu-sion systems offset the potential advantages of remifentanil and, when compared to fentanyl, the cost-effectiveness ratio was similar in both groups.[21]

A concern about general anesthesia is post-operative cognitive dysfunction (POCD) in the elderly. It is evident after major surgery, but it has also been reported 24 hours after minor surgery such as hysteroscopy, without significant difference between anesthetic drugs (propofol or sevoflurane).[22]

Airway Control

Airway management includes spontaneous or mechanical ventilation (maintaining a ventilatory peak pressure inferior to 20-25 cm H_2O) through a standard or a Proseal Laryngeal Mask (LMA) (FIGURE 18.6), or through an endotracheal tube when the LMA is not indicated.

The laryngeal mask is an airway device initially developed by Brain in 1981. In clinical anesthesia, it

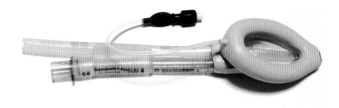

Figure 18.6: The Proseal laryngeal mask

plays an intermediate role between the facemask and the endotracheal tube, since it provides a safer airway than the former, but no real protection as with the latter. Its use is limited by cases of reduction of thoracopulmonary compliance and full stomach, since it does not protect against regurgitation and aspiration.[23] To minimize the risk of regurgitation, Brain developed a modified laryngeal mask (the Proseal LMA) that includes a second lumen through which a gastric tube can be inserted, and additional design features that provide a better seal around the glottis.

In hysteroscopy, the laryngeal mask may be indicated in short surgeries where steep Trendelenburg position is not used. In the remaining cases, a Proseal LMA or an end tracheal tube are preferred.

ANESTHETIC MANAGEMENT OF COMPLICATIONS

Complications of operative hysteroscopies are relatively rare events, which occur more frequently with operative than with diagnostic hysteroscopy. Frequency varies among series: From 2.7 to 13.6%.[7,24] Adequate training of surgical techniques and of treatment of potential complications, as well as good communication between specialists is required for safe management of these procedures. Thus, all staff members should be familiar with the equipment, careful when positioning the patient and vigilant during the procedure. An accurate calculation of irrigation fluid deficit and close monitoring of the patient are essential (the surgical management is revised in Chapter 17).

Related to Distension Media

The ideal distension medium should be nontoxic, isotonic, nonhemolytic, not metabolized, rapidly eliminated, and permit good visibility. Saline and Ringer's lactate fulfil these requirements but, being electrolyte-containing fluids, disperse the electric current and are not suitable for most electro-diathermy devices. In diagnostic hysteroscopy, carbon dioxide and normal saline are currently used, whereas in operative hysteroscopy the most widely used fluid is glycine 1.5% (a low viscosity electrolyte-free medium). All fluids used in hysteroscopic procedures can be associated with complications (TABLE 18.5).

Gas Embolism

It is a rare complication, but of catastrophic consequences. It can be caused by carbon dioxide or ambient air trapped in the tubing used for surgery. Prevention measures could be, purging of all tubing prior to surgery, avoidance of steep Trendelenburg position, using a low pressure insufflator and covering the cervix when instruments are removed. Gas embolism should be suspected if there is a decrease in end-tidal CO_2, hypoxia, tachycardia, tachypnea, and hypotension. Later, bradycardia and electromechanical dissociation or asystole may appear. Precordial Doppler may help in the diagnosis, but it is not routinely used because of its high false-positive rate.

Table 18.5: Complications related to distension media

Complications	Distension media
CO_2 embolism	Carbon dioxide
Anaphylaxis, pulmonary edema, coagulopathy, renal failure	32% dextran—70 (Hyskon®)
Fluid overload	32% dextran—70, glycine 1.5%, sorbitol 5%, mannitol 5%, normal saline, Ringer's lactate
Hyponatremia	glycine 1.5%, sorbitol 5%, mannitol 5%
Hipo-osmolality	glycine 1.5%
Hyperammonemia, hyperglycinemia	glycine 1.5%
Hyperglycemia	sorbitol 5%

If suspected, the following measures should be carried out: Administer 100% oxygen and discontinue nitrous oxide if it is in use, stop the procedure and flood the operative site with saline, occlude the vagina, turn the patient to the left lateral position and try to aspirate air through a central venous catheter, if available, and initiate cardiovascular resuscitation measures as needed.

Absorption of Distension Media

Absorption of large volumes of any distension medium can provoke fluid overload, but only electrolyte-free fluids cause hyponatremic hypervolemia and, when glycine is involved, hypo-osmolality can also appear due to its hypotonicity. Other possible complications of glycine use are hyperglycinemia (direct toxicity) and hyperammoniemia (indirect toxicity, through liver degradation). In an attempt to minimize these complications, bipolar operative hysteroscopes have been developed. They allow to surgeon to use low-viscosity electrolyte-containing fluids whose excessive absorption is less dangerous and easier to treat.

To prevent fluid overload, it is essential to have an accurate estimation of fluid deficit (it is recommended to end the surgery when a 1000 ml deficit is reached), as well as controlling the irrigation pressure preferably by pressure-controlled pumps. A correct preparation of the endometrium with gonadotropin release hormone (GnRH) agonist therapy and an atraumatic surgical technique that reduces vascular damage can diminish intraoperative uterine fluid absorption. Monitoring serum electrolytes is recommended in case of prolonged surgery, a fluid deficit superior to 500 ml and when indicated by clinical signs, but fluid overload can also happen in short surgeries.

The clinical picture caused by hyponatremic hypervolemia and irrigation media toxicity had already been described by urologists and anesthetists as transurethral resection of the prostate (TURP) syndrome. It occurred when electrolyte-free fluids (glycine 1.5%, sorbitol 5%, and mannitol 5%) were used.

Most of the clinical signs and symptoms of TURP syndrome are manifestations of fluid overload (congestive cardiac failure) and hyponatremia (neuro-logical symptoms). They can appear either in the intraoperative or in the postoperative period, and are more obvious in the conscious patient: Nausea and vomiting, dyspnea, headache, chest pain, confusion and seizures. Suspicion arises in both conscious and unconscious patients if the following appear: Hypertension, hypothermia, dilated pupils and a decrease in oxygen saturation. Eventually, cerebral edema and cardiovascular collapse may occur if appropriate treatment is not initiated. Symptoms of hyponatremic encephalopathy appear when serum sodium concentration decreases below 120 mEq/l. Severe hypo-osmolality can lead to hemolysis, hemoglobinuria and anemia. Hyperglycinemia higher than 1000 mg/l has been reported to cause transient blindness. Hyperammonaemia higher than 155 µmol/l may produce cerebral dysfunction, visual disturbances and muscle weakness. Sorbitol metabolism can lead to hyperglycemia, which can be marked in diabetic patients. Absorption of mannitol can exacerbate fluid overload.

Treatment of TURP syndrome depends on early detection and should be based on the severity of the symptoms. In all cases of fluid overload, monitoring should include arterial and central venous pressure, urine output, and frequent serum electrolytes and osmolality counts as well as a full blood count if hemolysis is suspected. Treatment aims at eliminating absorbed fluid and avoiding hypoxemia and hypoperfusion. To achieve this, we employ diuretics (furosemide), oxygen therapy, vasodilators and morphine. Mild hyponatremia can be treated with fluid restriction and diuretics, but severe hyponatremia may require therapy with hypertonic saline 3-5%, at a rate not faster than 100 ml/h to avoid an abrupt decrease in cerebral blood volume that could cause intracranial hemorrhage and central pontine mye-linolysis. Seizures can be treated with midazolam (2-4 mg), diazepam (3-5 mg) or thiopental (50-100 mg). In severe cases of fluid overload or when neurological symptoms are present, endotracheal intubation and management in an intensive care unit are advisable.[25]

Dextran Syndrome

It is a clinical picture produced by excessive Hyskon® absorption. Symptoms can be varied: Hypotension, noncardiogenic pulmonary edema, anemia, coagulopathy not explained by hemodilution and acute renal failure due to vacuolization of tubular cells. The following risk factors have been described: long surgeries, infusion of great amounts of dextran and large areas of traumatized endometrium. On rare occasions (1:1500 to 1:300000) and due to its antigenicity, Hyskon® can produce anaphylactic reactions without need of prior exposure to dextran. Treatment involves maintenance of oxygenation, controlled ventilation and promotion of dieresis.[26]

Related to Surgical Instrumentation

The main complications are uterine perforation and bleeding, and may be entry-related, or secondary to surgical instrumentation.

Uterine Perforation

Uterine perforation can be provoked when the hysteroscope is not introduced under direct vision or by surgical instruments during the procedure. It can be detected by direct vision, or indirectly by a sudden fall in distension pressure and a loss of visibility due to a rapid absorption of fluid through the wall defect. Also, a brusque patient movement (during general anesthesia without muscle relaxants) or changes in the monitor (bradycardia) may be seen. The use of any energy source must be stopped, and damage to surrounding organ and vessels must be excluded by laparoscopy or laparotomy if needed. In any case, the patient will be admitted overnight for adequate vigilance and treatment.

Prevention measures are: Entering the uterine cavity under direct vision, avoiding cervical dilation when not necessary by employing small-diameter instruments, and taking extreme care in patients with higher risk of perforation (nulliparity, menopause, GnRH agonist use, retroverted uterus and previous cone biopsy).[28]

The use of muscle relaxants during hysteroscopy under general anesthesia may generate controversy. On one side, its use may mask the patient response to the perforation and subsequent peritoneum stimulus. On the other, if depth of anesthesia is not adequate, a patient movement secondary to a surgical stimulus can be the cause of the perforation (e.g. obturator reflex).

Hemorrhage

Intraoperative bleeding may be due to entry-related cervical lacerations or due to the rupture of blood vessels during the surgical procedure. Hemodilution by the distension medium contributes to mask detection of the problem. Even clinical signs such as hypotension and tachycardia can be offset by the hypertension and bradycardia secondary to the distending fluid. However, the distension pressure probably tends to occlude the open vessels and diminish the intraoperative hemorrhage. Therefore, bleeding can be more troubling in the postoperative period, and this fact is especially hazardous since hysteroscopy is an outpatient procedure. If the patient is not absolutely fit for discharge, no matter how feeble the suspicion may be, we recommend hospital admission for observation.

Vaginal bleeding can be stopped by keeping inflated the balloon of a urinary catheter with 30-50 ml of normal saline during 24 hours. Other measures are intracervical oxytocin injection or packing. If unsuccessful, bilateral uterine artery embolization or eventually an emergency hysterectomy must be performed.[26] Intraperitoneal bleeding can happen if there has been a uterine perforation, and suspicion arises when there is postoperative abdominal pain, tachycardia and hypotension. Abdominal cavity inspection is mandatory to repair the damage and stop the hemorrhage. At the same time, anesthetic management comprises adequate fluid therapy and other supporting measures.

Related to Patient Positioning

A correct lithotomy position is necessary to avoid complications such as peripheral neuropathy. The peroneal nerve can be injured if compressed between the leg stand and the lateral aspect of the upper fibula, and the internal saphenous nerve can be compressed against the tibia. A forced leg flexion against the hip can result in injury of the crural and the obturator nerves and an excessive external rotation of the hip may result in distension of the sciatic nerve. Finally, a bilateral compartment syndrome of multifactorial etiology (long surgery, predisposed patients) is also possible.[27]

Special care should be taken to prevent this complication, which is in most cases iatrogenic. If it appears, a thorough neurological examination is mandatory to determine the extent of the deficit. An electromyogram may be necessary to establish the degree of damage to the nerve and the prognosis. When there is a concomitant regional anesthesia, a correct differential diagnosis is essential to avoid that the damage be erroneously attributed to the anesthetic technique.

REFERENCES

1. Lotfallah H, Farag K, Hassan I, Watson R. One-stop hysteroscopy clinic for postmenopausal bleeding. J Reprod Med 2005;50(2):101-7.
2. Tawfeek S, Hayes T, Sharp N. Three-year experience in outpatient microwave endometrial ablation. Obstet Gynaecol Surv 2005;60(4):234-5.
3. Goldenberg M, Cohen SB, Etchin A, Mashiach S, Seidman DS. A randomized prospective comparative study of general versus epidural anaesthesia for transcervical hysteroscopic endometrial resection. Am J Obstet Gynaecol 2001;184(3):273-6.
4. Bettocchi S, Ceci O, Nappi L, Di Venere R, Masciopinto V, Pansini V et al. Operative office hysteroscopy without anaesthesia: Analysis of 4863 cases performed with mechanical instruments. J Am Assoc Gynaecol Laparosc 2004;11(1):59-61.
5. García Triguero A. Cirugía Mayor Ambulatoria en Ginecología. In: Porrero JL (Ed): Cirugía Mayor Ambulatoria Manual Práctico. Madrid (Ed): Doyma 1999;299-308.
6. Propst. AM, Liberman RF, Harlow BL, Ginsburg ES. Complications of hysteroscopic surgery: Predicting patients at risk. Obstet Gynaecol 2000;96(4):517-20.
7. Pansky M, Feingold M, Bahar R, Neeman O, Asiag O, Herman A, Sagiv R. Improved patient compliance using pediatric cystoscope during office hysteroscopy. J Am Assoc Gynaecol Laparosc 2004;11(2):262-4.
8. Guida M, Pellicano M, Zullo F, Acunzo G, Lavitola G, Palomba S et al. Outpatient operative hysteroscopy with bipolar electrode: A prospective multicentre randomized study between local anaesthesia and conscious sedation. Hum Reprod 2003;18(4):840-3.
9. Clark TJ, Khan KS, Gupta JK. Current practice for the treatment of benign intrauterine polyps: A national questionnaire survey of consultant gynaecologists in UK. Eur J Obstet Gynaecol Reprod Biol 2002;103(1):65-7.
10. Aguilera L, Martínez A. Estudio preoperatorio de los pacientes y criterio de selección. In: Carrasco MS (Ed):
11. Garuti G, Cellani F, Colonnelli M, Grossi F, Luerti M. Outpatient hysteroscopic polypectomy in 237 patients: Feasibility of one-stop "see-and-treat" procedure. J Am Assoc Gynaecol Laparosc 2004;11(4):500-4.
12. Readman E, Maher PJ. Pain relief and outpatient hysteroscopy: A literature review. J Am Assoc Gynaecol Laparosc 2004;11(3):315-9.
13. Sala-Blanch X, De Andrés J. Conceptos y material general para la realización de técnicas regionales. In: De Andrés J y Sala-Blanch X, editors. Manual de bolsillo de anaesthesia regional (1st edn). Barcelona: Caduceo Multimedia 2004;10-13.
14. Mushambi Mc, Williamson K. Anaesthetic considerations for hysteroscopic surgery. Best Pract Res Clin Anaesthesiol 2002;16(1):35-51.
15. Zilbert A. Topical anaesthesia for minor gynaecological procedures: A review. Obstet Gynaecol Surv 2002;57(3):171-8.
16. Elliott CJR, Page VP. Anaesthesia for endometrial resection. In: Lewis BV, Magos AL (Eds): Endometrial ablation. Churchill Livingstone, London 1993;55-66.
17. Tetzlaff JE. Spinal, epidural and caudal blocks. In: Morgan GE, Mikhail MS (Eds): Clinical Anaesthesiology (2nd edn). Stamford, CT: Appleton & Lange 1996;211-44.
18. Philip BK. Local anaesthesia and sedation techniques. In White PF (Ed): Outpatient anaesthesia (1st edn). New York: Churchill Livingstone1990;262-91.
19. Lok IH, Chan M, Tam WH, Leung PL, Yuen PM. Patient-controlled sedation for outpatient thermal balloon endometrial ablation. J Am Assoc Gynaecol Laparosc 2002;9(4):436-41.
20. Beers R, Camporesi E. Remifentanil update: Clinical science and utility. CNS Drugs 2004;18(15):1085-104.
21. Beers RA, Calimlim JR, Uddoh E, Esposito BF, Camporesi EM. A comparison of the cost-effectiveness of remifentanyl versus fentanyl as an adjuvant to general anaesthesia for outpatient gynecologic surgery. Anaesth Analg 2000; 91(6):1420-5.
22. Rohan D, Buggy DJ, Crowley S, Ling FK, Gallagher H, Regan C et al. Increased incidence of postoperative cognitive dysfunction 24 hr after minor surgery in the elderly. Can J Anaesth 2005;52(2):137-42.
23. Stone DJ, Gal TJ. Control de la vía aérea. In: Miller RD (Ed): Anaestesia (4th edn). Madrid: Harcourt Brace 1998;1371-1402.
24. Pasini A, Belloni C. Day-surgery operative hysteroscopy with locoregional anaesthesia. Minerva Gynecol 2001; 53(1):13-20.
25. Morgan JE, Mikhail MS. Anaestesia for genitourinary surgery. In Morgan JE, Mikhail MS (Ed): Clinical Anaesthesiology (2nd edn). Stamford, CT: Appleton & Lange 1996;601-10.
26. Murdoch JAC, Gan TJ. Anaesthesia for hysteroscopy. Anaesthesiol Clin North America 2001;19(1):125-40.
27. Bradley LD. Complications in hysteroscopy: Prevention, treatment and legal risk. Curr Opin Obstet Gynaecol 2002;14(4):409-15.
28. Ullrich W, Biermann E, Kienzle F, Krier C. Lesiones posturales en anaesthesia y cirugía (1ª parte). Anästh Intensivmed (Spanish edition) 1999;1:8-22.

Anaesthesia para la cirugía ambulatoria I. Barcelona, Edika Med 1998;71-80.

INDEX